RELAXIN

ADVANCES IN EXPERIMENTAL MEDICINE AND BIOLOGY

Recent Volumes in this Series

RELAXIN

Edited by

Ralph R. Anderson
University of Missouri-Columbia
Columbia, Missouri

SPRINGER SCIENCE+BUSINESS MEDIA, LLC

Library of Congress Cataloging in Publication Data

Midwest Conference on Endocrinology and Metabolism (15th : 1979 : University of Missouri-Columbia) Relaxin.

(Advances in experimental medicine and biology ; v. 143)
"Proceedings of the 15th Midwest Conference on Endocrinology and Metabolism, held October 11-12, 1979, at the University of Missouri, Columbia, Missouri" — T.p. verso.
Bibliography: p.
Includes index.
1. Relaxin — Congresses. I. Anderson, Ralph Robert, 1932- . II. Title. III. Series.
QP572.R46M5   1979   599.01'6   81-19962
ISBN 978-1-4613-3370-8   ISBN 978-1-4613-3368-5 (eBook)   AACR2
DOI 10.1007/978-1-4613-3368-5

Proceedings of the Fifteenth Midwest Conference on Endocrinology and Metabolism, held October 11-12, 1979, at the University of Missouri, Columbia, Missouri, and sponsored by:

National Science Foundation

University of Missouri-Columbia
  Graduate School and Office of Research
  School of Medicine
  University Assembly Lectures
  Division of Biological Sciences
  College of Veterinary Medicine
    Department of Anatomy-Physiology
    Department of Veterinary Medicine and Surgery
    Department of Pathology
    Veterinary Medicine Diagnostic Laboratory
  Department of Medicine
  Department of Obstetrics and Gynecology
  Department of Physiology
  Sinclair Comparative Medical Research Farm
  College of Agriculture

Harry S. Truman Memorial Veterans Administration Hospital

Merck and Co., Inc.

© 1982 Springer Science+Business Media New York
Originally published by Plenum Press, New York in 1982
Softcover reprint of the hardcover 1st edition 1982

CONFERENCE CHAIRMAN

Ralph R. Anderson, Ph.D., Professor of Dairy Science, University of
Missouri-Columbia

PLANNING COMMITTEE

Robert P. Breitenbach, Professor of Biological Sciences, University
of Missouri-Columbia.

John D. David, Ph.D., Associate Professor of Biological Sciences
University of Missouri-Columbia.

C. William Foley, Ph.D., Professor of Veterinary Anatomy and Physiology,
University of Missouri-Columbia.

Leonard R. Forte, Ph.D., Associate Professor of Pharmacology, University of Missouri-Columbia.

John M. Franz, Ph.D., Associate Professor of Biochemistry, University
of Missouri-Columbia.

James Green, Ph.D., Professor of Anatomy, University of Missouri-
Columbia

Murray Heimberg, M.D., Ph.D., Professor, Chairman of Pharmacology,
University of Missouri-Columbia.

David M. Klachko, M.D., Professor of Medicine, University of
Missouri-Columbia.

Harold Werner, M.D., Assistant Professor of Medicine, University
of Missouri-Columbia.

Walter T. Wilkening, Ph.D., Director of Conferences and Short Courses,
University of Missouri-Columbia.

Warren L. Zahler, Ph.D., Associate Professor of Biochemistry,
University of Missouri-Columbia.

SPEAKERS

Lloyd L. Anderson, Ph.D., Professor, Department of Animal Science,
Iowa State University, Ames, Iowa.

Sylvia A. Braddon, Ph.D., Research Chemist, Southeast Fisheries
Center, Charleston Laboratory, Charleston, South Carolina.

Gillian D. Bryant-Greenwood, Ph.D., Associate Professor, Department
of Anatomy and Reproductive Biology, University of Hawaii,
Honolulu, Hawaii.

Hugh D. Niall, Ph.D., Lecturer, Howard Florey Institute of Experi-
    mental Physiology and Medicine, University of Melbourne,
    Parkville, Victoria, Australia.
Christian Schwabe, Ph.D., Associate Professor, Department of
    Physiology and Biophysics, University of Illinois, Urbana,
    Illinois.
Bernard G. Steinetz, Ph.D., Manager, Endocrinology and Metabolism
    Section, Pharmaceutical Division, CIBA-GEIGY Corporation,
    Ardsley, New York.

MINI-PAPER PRESENTERS

Ralph A. Bradshaw, Ph.D., Professor, Department of Biological
    Chemistry, Washington University, St. Louis, Missouri.
S. H. Cheah, Ph.D., Research Associate, Department of Physiology
    and Biophysics, University of Illinois, Urbana, Illinois.
Michael J. Fields, Ph.D., Assistant Professor, Department of Animal
    Science, University of Florida, Gainsville, Florida.
Edward H. Frieden, Ph.D., Professor, Department of Chemistry,
    Kent State University, Kent, Ohio.
M. Gast, M.D., Assistant Professor, Department of Pharmacology,
    Washington University, St. Louis, Missouri.
Fred Greenwood, Ph.D., Professor, Department of Biochemistry and
    Biophysics, University of Hawaii, Honolulu, Hawaii.
Simon C. M. Kwok, Ph.D., Research Associate, Department of Bio-
    chemistry, University of Chicago, Chicago, Illinois.
Barbara M. Sanborn, Ph.D., Associate Professor, Department of
    Reproductive Medicine and Biology, University of Texas, Medical
    School at Houston, Texas.
Lila C. Wright, M.S., Research Assistant, Department of Dairy
    Science, University of Missouri-Columbia, Columbia, Missouri.

MODERATORS

Ralph R. Anderson, Ph.D., Professor, Department of Dairy Science,
    University of Missouri-Columbia.
Irving Boime, Ph.D., Associate Professor, Department of Pharmacology,
    School of Medicine, Washington University, St. Louis, Missouri.
Ralph R. Bradshaw, Ph.D., Professor, Department of Biochemistry,
    School of Medicine, Washington University, St. Louis, Missouri.
John J. Jeffrey, Ph.D., Associate Professor, Departments of Bio-
    chemistry and Medicine, Washington University, St. Louis,
    Missouri.

DISCUSSANTS

Adams, Walter, Kent State University, Kent, Ohio.
Bylander, John, Kent State University, Kent, Ohio.
Diehl, John, Clemson University, Clemson, South Carolina.
Kendall, June, University of Texas Medical School, Houston, Texas.
Mercado-Simmen, Rosalia, University of Hawaii, Honolulu, Hawaii.
Rawitch, Allen, University of Kansas, Lawrence, Kansas.
Soloff, Melvin, Medical College of Ohio, Toledo, Ohio.
Uchima, Francis-Dean, University of Hawaii, Honolulu, Hawaii.
Wixom, Robert, University of Missouri-Columbia.

PREFACE

The Fifteenth Midwest Conference on Endocrinology and Metabolism, held at the University of Missouri-Columbia on October 11 and 12th, 1979, hosted the most prominent active researchers in the world on the subject of the hormone relaxin. Each speaker presented an in-depth coverage of his chosen topic and area of expertise. Some of the data presented in this book are findings which have not been published in a scientific journal. The topic of this conference is especially timely in light of the fact that this is a first conference devoted specifically to the hormone relaxin. Progress on this hormone has been exceedingly rapid in recent years and many significant breakthroughs are documented in these pages. Lively discussions following each presentation attest to the enthusiastic research effort being pursued at the present time concerning relaxin.

Traditionally the Midwest Conferences on Endocrinology and Metabolism have emphasized breadth as well as depth of coverage. The present Conference has covered the many active areas of research in relaxin, including morphological aspects of the hormone's origin, chemical purification and chemical structure, bioassays, radioimmuno-assays, receptors, mechanism of biochemical action and physiological responses to the hormone. Advances in relaxin were slow since its discovery by Dr. Frederick Hisaw, Sr. in 1926 until the availability of homogenous preparations some seven years ago. In the suceeding seven years, activity in the subject has accelerated remarkably. Because of the noteworthy advances in recent years, the topic of the present conference was especially timely. In recognition of the original contribution by Dr. Hisaw in his discovery of relaxin, we dedicate this volume in his honor.

The Editor is most appreciative of the excellent manuscripts which the speakers provided for the Proceedings. The Moderators and staff of Conferences and Short Courses for the abilities in organizing and presenting this Conference. The Planning Committee is grateful for financial support from various sources, especially the National Science Foundation.

Ralph R. Anderson

CONTENTS

RELAXIN LOCALIZATION IN PORCINE AND BOVINE OVARIES

BY ASSAY AND MORPHOLOGIC TECHNIQUES

L. L. Anderson

Department of Animal Science

Iowa State University, Ames, IA 50011[1]

INTRODUCTION

Relaxin is a polypeptide hormone produced primarily by the ovaries during pregnancy in several mammalian species. Investigations beginning more than 50 years ago on isolation of hormones from the corpus luteum eventually showed that the lipid-soluble fraction yields progesterone and estrogens, whereas the water-soluble fraction contains relaxin. A brief report by Hisaw in 1926 describes induced relaxation of the pubic ligament of virgin guinea pigs within 6 to 8 hours after the subcutaneous injection of blood serum from pregnant rabbits. Hisaw (1925) previously had documented the relaxation of the pubic bones during late pregnancy in the guinea pig by expansion of the connective tissue at the symphysis, allowing separation of the pubic bones. During the early postpartum period, the ligaments shortened, and the pubic symphysis again appeared similar to that found in unmated guinea pigs. In the spring-breeding pocket gopher, he noted that the pubic symphysis was lost, usually before pregnancy occurs, and that the interpubic ligament response was controlled by the ovary. Fevold *et al.* (1930) developed extraction and purification methods for this hormone and proposed the name relaxin. Several investigators questioned the existence of relaxin since pelvic relaxation could be produced in ovariectomized guinea pigs by estrogen alone or by combinations of estrogen and progesterone. Hisaw *et al.* (1944) demonstrated that relaxin possessed neither chemical or physiological properties in common with those steroids; water-soluble extracts of

---
[1]This work was partly supported by NIH Grant No. 5 S05RR 07034-09. Purified porcine relaxin (CM-B) was generously provided by Dr. B. G. Steinetz, Research Department, Pharmaceuticals Division, CIBA--GEIGY Corp. Ardsley, NY and purified porcine relaxin (NIH-R-P1) from NIH, Bethesda, MD. Journal Paper J-9691 of the Iowa Agriculture and Home Economics Experiment Station, Ames, IA Projects 2092 and 2273.

porcine corpora lutea produced relaxation of pubic ligaments within
6 hours, whereas ovarian steroids required 96 hours for a maximal
response.

In addition to relaxation of the interpubic ligaments, relaxin
affects the uterus, both the myometrium and endometrium as well as
the cervix, and the mammary glands. The hormone inhibits uterine
motility, induces cervical dialation, and alters milk secretion.
Although these tissue responses are well documented and provide useful
criteria for assessing biological actions, the physiological roles
of endogenously produced relaxin are not clearly defined. Relaxin
has been detected in ovarian tissue or blood serum in at least 15
mammalian species, as well as in the placenta of the cat and rabbit
(for references refer to Schwabe *et al.*, 1978). These species
include the opossum, dog, cat, rat, mouse, hamster, guinea pig, rabbit,
pig, cow, horse, whale, rhesus monkey, baboon, and human. The
testes of armadillos, domestic roosters, and boars also contain relaxin
(Schwabe *et al.*, 1978; Dubois and Dacheux, 1978).

For a considerable period of time, progress on elucidation of the
physiological actions of relaxin was limited by available quantitative
measures and the relative purity of relaxin preparations. A perspective on biochemical and physiological aspects of relaxin is collated
in reviews by Hisaw and Zarrow (1950), Frieden and Hisaw (1953) and
Steinetz *et al.*, (1959). The recent resurgence of interest in the
physiology of relaxin has been enhanced mainly by determination of
the sequence of the amino acid chains of porcine relaxin and the
development of sensitive radioimmunoassay procedures for the hormone.
An excellent account of the chemical composition and structure of
relaxin as well as biological effects of the hormone is presented
in a review by Schwabe *et al.* (1978). Porcine relaxin consists of
2 peptide chains (5600 daltons) and has structural features
indicating partial homology to insulin (Sherwood and O'Bryne, 1974;
Schwabe *et al.*, 1976, 1977; Schwabe and McDonald, 1977; James *et al.*,
1977; and Schwabe *et al.*, 1978).

The following discussion reviews evidence on the localization
of relaxin primarily in the porcine and bovine ovary, but with
reference to findings in a few other domestic and laboratory species.
Presentation of cytological and fine structural features of the ovary
will be followed by the determination of relaxin concentrations in
ovarian tissue and evidence for the localization of relaxin within
the cell.

GENERAL ASPECTS OF PROTEIN AND STEROID SYNTHESIS BY ENDOCRINE CELLS

The respective roles and sequence of participation by cell
organelles in endocrine and exocrine secretory processes will be
considered briefly. This will provide an orientation primarily to

the later discussion on the functional cytology of granulosa lutein cells. The reader is referred to excellent reviews by Fawcett *et al.* (1969), Christensen and Gillim (1969), Enders (1973), and Palade (1975), and to Jamieson and Palade (1971a; 1971b) for some detailed accounts of these intracellular processes.

Information encoded in DNA of the nuclear chromatin is transported to the cytoplasm in the form of messenger RNA, which presumably leaves the nucleus via pores in the nuclear membrane. In the cytoplasm, various numbers of ribosomes become associated with molecules of messenger RNA to form linear arrays of interconnected particles 150 Å, and these are recognized as polysomes. There is a series of subsequent steps in the secretory process that typify endocrine and exocrine cells. These include synthesis, segregation, intracellular transport, concentration, intracellular storage, and discharge. Proteins for export are synthesized on polysomes attached to the membrane of granular (rough) endoplasmic reticulum, and these polysomes are maintained in a regular pattern of rather constant geometry. There exist two subclasses of attached polysomes one synthesizing proteins for export and the other involved in production of endoplasmic reticulum membrane (Palade, 1975). The newly synthesized secretory proteins are segregated in the cisternal space of granular endoplasmic reticulum. The growing polypeptide chain is extruded through the microsomal membrane into the cisternal space of the granular endoplasmic reticulum. This segregation process is the result of vectorial transport of the synthesized polypeptide from the large ribosomal subunit through the endoplasmic reticulum membrane to the cisternal space (Figure 1). Segregation of the protein into these cisternae seems to be an irreversible process.

From the cisternae of the granular endoplasmic reticulum, the secretory products are transported to the Golgi apparatus. The secretory proteins move from the granular endoplasic reticulum to

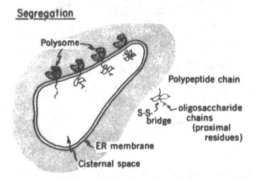

Figure 1. *Diagram of the segregation of newly synthesized secretory protein in cisternal space of granular endoplasmic reticulum. From Palade (1975).*

transitional elements, then to small peripheral vesicles on the cis
side of the Golgi apparatus, and finally to condensing vacuoles
(Figure 2). The secretory proteins reach the condensing vacuoles in
a dilute solution that is progressively concentrated into mature
secretory granules. Concentration is accomplished in trans Golgi
condensing vacuoles of the Golgi stack. From the Golgi apparatus, the
secretory product is transferred from the highly permeable membrane
of the endoplasmic reticulum to a low permeability lipid-containing
membrane where the protein is afforded protection from intracellular
dispersion. The secretory proteins are stored temporarily within
the cell as secretion granules. Their outer membrane is derived from
the Golgi apparatus, and their content is the product of attached
polysomes. Secretion granules discharge their contents into the intracellular space by a fusion of granule and cytoplasmic membranes.
There results a continuity between the granule membrane with the
cytoplasmic membrane. Membranes of secretion granules fuse only with
the cytoplasmic membrane and not to other membrane-bound granules or
cellular organelles. Exocytosis is energy dependent and has a
requirement for calcium ion. Thus, exocytosis results in discharge
of a secretory product and relocation of granule and cystoplasmic
membranes. Endocrine cells producing peptide or protein hormones
follow this sequence but can discharge their secretory products
within the membrane-bounded granule anywhere along the inner surface
of the cytoplasmic membrane. Some cells produce primarily lysosomes,

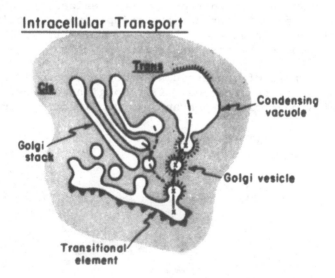

Figure 2.   Diagram of intracellular transport with pathway of
             secretory proteins leading from the rough endoplasmic
             reticulum to transitional elements, then to small
             peripheral vesicles on the cis side of the Golgi apparatus,
             and finally to condensing vacuoles. From Palade (1975).

and these acid phosphatase-reactive granules are also synthesized and secreted in the same manner. Furthermore, some cells are capable of producing a mixture of protein granules and lysosome-containing granules presumably within the same organization of endoplasmic reticulum. The lysosomal hydrolases provide a mechanism for degrading excess secretory protein within the cytoplasm as well as maintaining a suitable balance of secretory granules.

The intracellular synthetic pathway for endocrine glands secreting protein and polypeptide hormones is qualitatively similar, but there are quantitative differences in the degree of development of cell organelles concerned especially with the endoplasmic reticulum (Fawcett *et al.*, 1969). There are large differences in the volumes of protein produced and temporarily stored by different endocrine glands.

In steroid-secreting endocrine glands, the cell organelles associated with protein synthesis are relatively inconspicuous. Ultrastructural features that characterize steroid-secreting cells include a) an extensive agranular (smooth) endoplasmic reticulum, b) a prominent Golgi apparatus, c) mitochondria of variable size and often unusual internal structure, d) numerous lysosomes, and e) conspicuous lipid droplets (Belt and Pease, 1956; Fawcett *et al.*, 1969; Enders, 1973). The agranular endoplasmic reticulum often appears in direct communication with Golgi cisternae.

Granulosa lutein cells are of special interest because of their ability to secrete both steroid and protein hormones. Although there is increasing evidence for the existence of two cell sizes of granulosa lutein cells persisting throughout the estrous cycle and pregnancy in different mammalian species, there is no indication that certain lutein cells secrete primarily steroids while others secrete mainly proteins. These granulosa lutein cells possess typical ultrastructural features for steroid synthesis (e.g., an abundance of agranular endoplasmic reticulum), but they also contain features required for protein synthesis (e.g., granular endoplasmic reticulum, secretory granules). The evidence for localization of steroid synthetic pathways is based primarily upon presence of steroid dependent enzymes within certain organelles of the lutein cell. The structural features involved in secretion of progesterone by lutein cells remains undefined a) since lutein cells presumably do not accumulate steroids and b) since cellular membranes are readily permeable to steroids. Progesterone secretion by granulosa lutein cells, however, was thought to involve hormone diffusion through the cytoplasmic membrane since the steroid is released from functional cells on a continuous basis (refer to Christensen and Gillim, 1969; Enders, 1973). Recent morphologic evidence suggests that progesterone secretion by lutein cells may involve specific intracellular trans- port mechanisms associated with the secretion of protein granules from the cell.

The primary focus of this discussion relates to synthesis, localization, and secretion of relaxin by the mammalian ovary. A secondary consideration is that of progesterone secretion by lutein cells, particularly as related to the secretion of these two hormones, relaxin and progesterone, presumably by the same cell.

FINE STRUCTURE OF THE OVARY AND RELAXIN IN PIGS AND CATTLE

Pig

The corpus luteum of the pig is the primary source of relaxin and progesterone. A brief descriptive account of ovarian changes during the estrous cycle, during pregnancy, and after hysterectomy precedes a consideration of fine-structural changes throughout these reproductive stages.

Estrous Cycle

The length of the estrous cycle is about 21 days. The pig is polyestrous throughout the year; only pregnancy, hysterectomy, or endocrine dysfunction interrupts this cyclicity. The estrous cycle may be categorized into a follicular phase (proestrus and estrus) and a luteal phase (diestrus). During the pro-estrous phase, about 10 to 20 ovarian follicles approach prevolutory size. These maturing follicles produce estrogenic hormones, which induce sexual behavior patterns typical of a gilt or sow in estrus.

After release of the ovum, there is rapid proliferation of granulosa cells lining the inner wall of the ruptured follicle. These granulosa cells become luteinized to form the corpus luteum. Initially, the corpus is considered a corpus hemorrhagicum because of the blood-filled central cavity, but within 6 to 8 days, the corpus lutuem rapidly developes into a solid mass of luteal cells with an overall diameter of 8 to 11 mm and weighs 350 to 450 mg. The luteal phase of the estrous cycle lasts about 16 days. This period is characterized by the transition of the corpus hemmorhagicum into a fully developed corpus luteum that maintains its cellular integrity and hormone-secreting capabilities to <u>day 16</u> and then rapidly regresses to a nonsecreting corpus albicans. Peripheral blood plasma concentrations of estrogen and progesterone are indicated throughout the estrous cycle in this species (Figure 3). Progesterone levels are low at estrus (<u>day 0</u>), begin to increase abruptly after <u>day 2</u> to peak values by <u>days 8-12,</u> and then decline precipitously thereafter to day 18. These steroid profiles in the peripheral blood correspond to patterns of progesterone secretion in ovarian venous blood throughout the cycle (Masuda *et al.*, 1967). These progesterone levels also follow a pattern similar to morphological development and decline of the corpus luteum. Estrogen concentrations in peripheral plasma begin to increase coincident with the

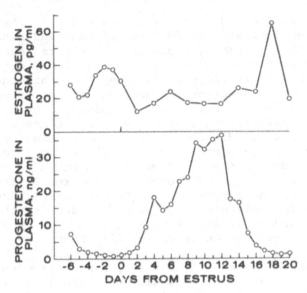

Figure 3. *Peripheral blood plasma concentrations of estrogen and*
progesterone throughout the estrous cycle in the pig.
Adapted from Guthrie et al. (1972) and Parvizi et al.
(1976).

decline and disappearance of progesterone. Peak values occur 2
days preceding estrus and reflect rapid growth and maturation of
graafian follicles during the last proestrous phase. Soon after
estrus, estrogen decreases markedly and remains low during the luteal
phase of the cycle.

Since the classical work of Corner (1919) on the origin of the
corpus luteum of the sow, considerable information has been obtained
concerning the structure and function of this gland, yet many of
the factors responsible for its devlopment, maintenance, and regression
remain obscure. Bjersing (1967), Goodman *et al.* (1968) and Cavazos
et al. (1969) have presented descriptions of the fine structure of
the porcine corpus luteum. In the following description of the fine-
structural alterations of the corpus luteum of the pig during the
estrous cycle, the events are separated into phases of luteinization
(day 1), secretion (days 4, 8 and 12), and regression (days 14, 16
and 18) by recovering corpora lutea at laparotomy for electron microscopy (Cavazos *et al.*, 1969).

During luteinization (day 1), granulosa cells at the periphery
of the ruptured follicle are cuboidal to columnar and separated by
irregular extracellular spaces, presumably of the residual antrum,
which contain a fine flocculent fluff, probably representing precipitated liquor folliculi (Figure 4). Deeper within the corpus
luteum, the cells are hypertrophied, and the nucleus is eccentrically
located. In the peripheral cells, the cytoplasm contains long cisternae of granular endoplasmic reticulum (rough endoplasmic reticulum)
and many free polysomes. Mitochondria are represented by circular
(about 2.0 μm), elliptical, and elongate (1.5-2.0 μm) profiles. The
Golgi complex consists of flattened membranous saccules with
associated small vesicules. Although theca interna in the pig
contributes cells to the corpus luteum (Corner, 1919), these lutein
cells in this species maintain their separate identity throughout the
life span of the corpus luteum. By day 4, in the early part of the
secretory phase, luteinization is essentially complete.

During secretion (days 4 through 12), the cells have hypertrophied and contain masses of agranular endoplasmic reticulum
(smooth endoplasmic reticulum). Polysomes are restricted to sub-

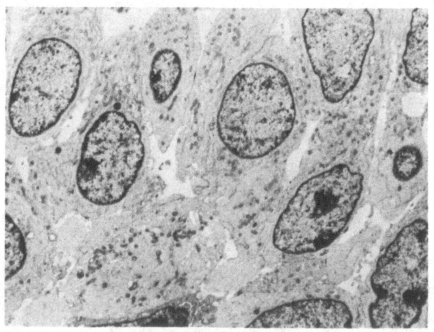

Figure 4.   Adjacent cells of membrana granulosa from day 1 of porcine
             estrous cycle at a site near the basement membrane show
             little evidence of luteinization. The irregular extra-
             cellular spaces are the remnant of the follicular antrum
             and probably still contain liquor folliculi. Mitochondria
             are numerous. From Cavazos et al. (1969).

plasmalemmal and perinuclear locations. Mitochondria exhibit profiles
that are usually circular or short ovals, and the intermal matrix is
moderately dense. Small coated vesicles are abundant in association
with the Golgi complex, whereas the large coated vesicles are numerous
in relation to the plasmalemma. Luteal tissue progesterone concentrations are maximal between <u>days</u> 8 and <u>12</u> of the cycle.

During regression (<u>days</u> <u>14</u> through <u>18</u>), there is an increase in
cellular droplet lipid, cytoplasmic disorganization, and vacuolation
of agranular endoplasmic reticulum (Figures 5 and 6). The tubules
of agranular endoplasmic reticulum appear dilated and frequently are
present in early stages of regression as swirling arrays and later
appear as isolated vesicles. As the concentration of progesterone
declines in the terminal phase of the cycle, there is an increase
in number of lysosomes, a marked vacuolation of the agranular endoplasmic reticulum, and invasion of connective tissue. These events
result in formation of the corpus albicans. Once lysosomal activity
is initiated, particularly at <u>days</u> <u>16</u> and <u>18</u>, the process is
irreversible.

During the estrous cycle there are structural indications of
functional activity in the tissue. For example, the cells are packed

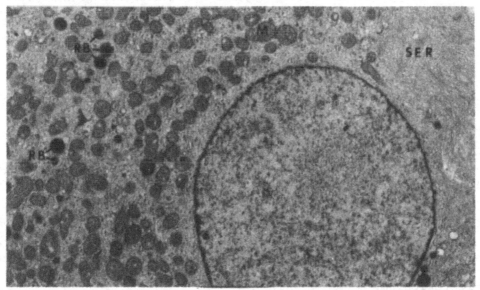

*Figure 5.   A portion of porcine granulosa lutein cell at day 16 of
the cycle. Numerous residual bodies (RB) are encountered
in the cytoplasm. Note the organization of smooth endoplasmic reticulum (SER) in tubular form and the concentration of mitochondria (M). X 9,360. From Anderson et al.
(1969).*

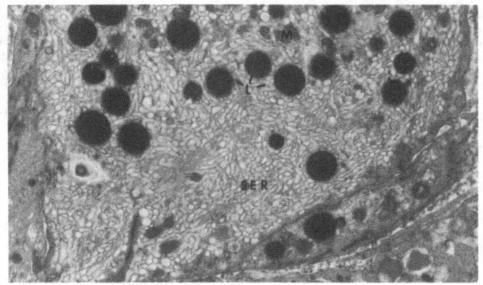

*Figure 6.   The smooth endoplasmic reticulum (SER) is becoming dilated,
            but in this lutein cell, remains tubular in form.
            Numerous lipid droplets (L) are dispersed in the cytoplasm.
            M, mitochondrion.   X 10,350.   From Anderson et al. (1969).*

with agranular endoplasmic reticulum; there are large numbers of
mitochondria, with abundant tubular cristae creating a richly membranous internum.   The fine-structural aspects of agranular endoplasmic reticulum and their implications in the biosynthesis of
steroid hormone are similar in Leydig cells and adrenal cortex as
well as in the corpus luteum (Fawcett *et al.*, 1969).   The coated
vesicles found in luteal cells during the cycle are of particular
interest because they are implicated in protein synthesis and uptake
and in a transport mechanism from the cell.   In the granulosa lutein
cell, this is suggested by the continuity of the coated vesicles
with Golgi saccules and their abundance in the region of the Golgi
complex, but directional movement of the coated vesicles into or
out of the cell could not be ascertained.   As the lutein cell develops,
the abundant cisternae of granular endoplasmic reticulum are replaced
by a more extensively pervading system of tubules of agranular endoplasmic reticulum.

Pregnancy

After mating or artificial insemination, the ovulated eggs are
fertilized within a few hours by spermatozoa migrating to anterior

regions of the oviducts. The porcine embryos enter the uterus approximately 90 hours after fertilization. At days 4 to 12 of pregnancy, embryos migrate within the uterine lumen, rapidly develop into blastocysts, which then form extremely elongated (e.g., > 60 cm) filamentous membranes. Intra-uterine spacing is essentially complete by day 13, which results in an even distribution of the conceptuses throughout both uterine horns (Anderson, 1978). Each of these embryos is arranged end-to-end with no overlap of the extended filamentous membranes. Implantation occurs between days 14 and 18, and the conceptuses develop rapidly. The first 30 days after breeding represent a period of fertilization, embryo migration and spacing, implantation, and placentation, as well as a time when the greatest embryonic loss occurs.

Pregnancy lasts about 115 days in the pig. Unlike corpora lutea in cyclic sows, those corpora lutea that develop soon after mating reach their greatest weight within a few days and then continue cellular integrity and hormone secretion to near term. Within a few hours of delivery, the corpora lutea lose their vascularity, regress rapidly, and continue to decline as corpora albicantia during the lactational phase. Corpora lutea are essential for the maintenance of pregnancy to term because they are the primary source of progesterone; ovariectomy any time during gestation in this species results in abrupt abortion within 36 hours (du Mesnil du Buisson and Dauzier, 1957; Belt *et al.*, 1971; Kertiles and Anderson, 1979).

The porcine corpus luteum develops to its greatest weight by day 8 and is sustained to late pregnancy (Figure 7). After day 114, there is a precipitous decline in luteal weight soon after delivery. Progesterone concentrations in peripheral blood increase to peak values by day 12 and gradually decrease to levels of 20 to 25 ng/ml to day 104. Near the onset of parturition, progesterone concentrations in the blood steadily decline, and they reach basal levels of 1 to 2 ng/ml during lactation (Anderson *et al.*, 1979; Hard and Anderson, 1979; Figure 8).

In enzymically disassociated granulosa lutein cells recovered at days 30, 60 and 90 of pregancy, there appear two luteal cell populations of 30–50 μm diameters and 15–20 μm diameter (Lemon and Loir, 1977). The larger cells produce approximately 5 times more progesterone under *in vitro* conditions. Both sizes of cells respond to porcine luteinizing hormone by an increase in progesterone release, but the steroid responses decrease in magnitude in corpora lutea obtained in later stages of pregnancy. Thecal lutein cells and granulosa lutein cells are present in porcine corpora lutea at all stages of the estrous cycle and pregnancy (Cavazos *et al.*, 1969; Belt *et al.*, 1970). Although the origin of the two sizes of cells is unresolved, the appearance and localization of the cells suggest that the larger ones originate from granulosa and the smaller cells from theca interna (Lemon and Loir, 1977).

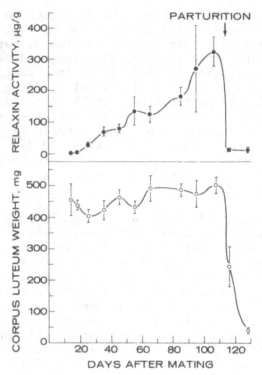

Figure 7.   Relaxin activity in NIH units and corpus luteum weight
            during pregnancy and lactation in the pig.   Parturition
            occurs about day 115.   Mean and SE.   From Anderson et al.
            (1973b).

Plasma concentrations of unconjugated estrone and estradiol-17β
in peripheral blood are measurable by day 80 and rapidly increase to
peak values just preceding parturition (Robertson and King, 1974).
Two peaks of estrone sulfate occur at day 30 and day 112.   All three
plasma estrogens drop at onset of parturition.   These estrogens,
measured in peripheral blood, are produced primarily by the feto-
placental unit rather than the ovaries.   Although blood levels of
estrogens are greater during late pregnancy, they do not induce
behavioral estrus because of the overriding effects of ovarian
progesterone, which suppress the central nervous system and inhibit
uterine myometrial activity.

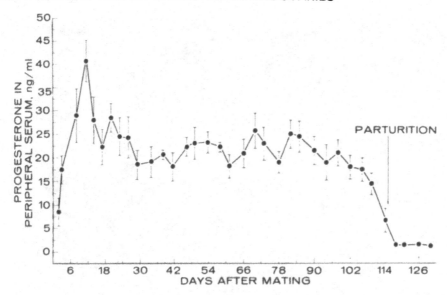

Figure 8. Progesterone concentrations (ng/ml, mean ± SE) in peripheral blood serum during pregnancy and lactation in the pig. From Anderson et al. (1979) and Hard and Anderson (1979).

After Hysterectomy

Corpora lutea in hysterectomized pigs develop and are maintained for periods equivalent to or exceeding those during pregnancy (Anderson *et al.*, 1963, 1969; Anderson, 1973). In 15 gilts hysterectomized between days 8 to 12 of the estrous cycle and the corpora lutea marked with silk sutures, luteal tissue was recoverd by laparotomy for electron microscopy on days 18, 40, 60 and 100 (Belt *et al.*, 1970). The corpora lutea were maintained in a manner similar to those found in pregnant gilts. Progesterone levels in corpora lutea of pregnant or hysterectomized gilts are similar at comparable stages.

Fine Structure of Porcine Granulosa Lutein Cell During Pregnancy and After Hysterectomy

The histological features of the corpus luteum of pregnancy in the pig have been described by Corner (1915, 1919). The fine structure of porcine corpora lutea was examined after recovery of ovarian tissue at laparotomy for electron microscopy on days 18, 28,

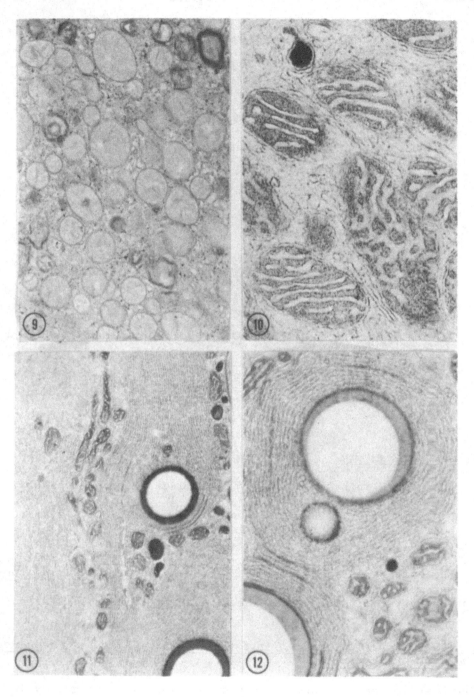

Figure 9.   *A portion of granulosa lutein cell at day 18 in hysterec-*
            tomized pig depicts abundance of mitochondria.   X 16,000
            From Belt et al. (1970).

Figure 10. *Granulosa lutein cell from porcine corpus luteum of 60-*
            day hysterectomy reveals a dense population of mitochondria.
            The mitochondria is rather dense and devoid of mitochondrial
            granules.   X 42,500.   From Belt et al. (1971).

Figure 11. *Granulosa lutein cell from corpus luteum of 40-day hyster-*
            ectomy.   Fenestrated cisternae of agranular (smooth) endo-
            plasmic reticulum and concentrically arranged around
            lipid droplets.   X 22,500.   From Belt et al. (1970).

Figure 12. *Arrays of agranular endoplasmic reticulum surrounding*
            lipid droplets in granulosa lutein cell of 40-day hyster-
            ectomy.   X 27,600.   From Belt et al. (1970).

40, 60, and 106 of pregnancy and after hysterectomy at days 18, 40, 60 and 100 (Belt *et al.*, 1970). Progesterone concentrations in luteal tissue from these animals were correlated with fine-structural changes in the lutein cells at these stages during pregnancy and after hysterectomy.

The granulosa lutein cells have a similar fine structure whether they are from corpora lutea of pregnancy or from those after hysterectomy, and there are few structural differences considered as significant at any of the stages examined. Thus, the following description applies to granulosa cells from gilts (nulliparous pigs) at several stages during pregnancy and after hysterectomy.

Granulosa lutein cells in porcine ovaries either during pregnancy or after hysterectomy are large, frequently 40-50 µm, and generally ovoid or polyhedral. The cytoplasm is abundant, whereas the relatively small nucleus is irregularly spherical, often deeply indented on one side, and without unusual internal features. Mitochondria are abundant within the cytoplasm. Their profiles are mostly circular or oval, and the mitochondrial matrix is quite dense (Figure 9). Mitochondrial granules are rare. The membranous internum displays profiles interpretable as a mixture of plate-like and tubular cristae (Figure 10).

The cytoplasm is filled with agranular endoplasmic reticulum that appears as a system of anastomotic fine membraneous tubules, which prevade the entire cytosome (Figure 11). Arrays of fenestrated cisternae are found more frequently in later stages of pregnancy or after hysterectomy. Massive cisternae whorls often are present about lipid vacuoles (Figure 12). Fenestrated cisternae of agranular endoplasmic reticulum often appear in parallel array and near the cytoplasmic membrane. The agranular endoplasmic reticulum appear in two compartments, an area almost devoid of other organelles or inclusions and one rich in these cellular components.

Cisternae of glandular (rough) endoplasmic reticulum are often arranged in parallel stacks (Figure 13). The Golgi apparatus in granulosa lutein cells is extensive and prominent. Often several well-developed areas of Golgi apparatus are evident in a single profile. Numerous smooth and coated vesicles are associated with the Golgi cisternae as well as appearance of membranous cups with a dense material that aggregates at the peripheral portion of the cup, and these cups are associated with the Golgi apparatus (Figure 14). These structures are interpreted as Golgi saccules that were packaging a dense material. Presumably some of this dense material, still surrounded by membrane, is separated from the peripheral lip of the cup to form a membrane-limited granule. These granules tend to cluster in the cytoplasm, and large numbers of them frequently appear near the plasmalemma. Many of these dense bodies have a structure suggestive of a thin peripheral cortex, while the

remainder are homogenous (Figure 15, 16). These dense bodies are
negative to the acid phosphatase reaction. In addition to the small
granules just described, a population of larger dense bodies is
present; each of these possesses a limiting membrane. Some of the
larger bodies have a pleomorphic internal structure. Only a few
of these are positive for acid phosphatase, thus indicating
lysosomal activity.

Thecal lutein cells are seen frequently at all stages in
corpora lutea from pregnant gilts and are similar to those found
during the estrous cycle (Cavazos *et al.*, 1969).

Granulosa Lutein Cells During Estrous Cycle as Compared with those During Pregnancy and After Hysterectomy

In contrast to the fine structure of granulosa lutein cells
during the estrous cycle, those cells during pregnancy and after
hysterectomy contain a larger and extensive Golgi apparatus, more
agranular endoplasmic reticulum organized in arrays of fenestrated
cisternae, more granular endoplasmic reticulum highly organized in
stacks, and an immensely larger number of membrane-bound dense bodies
that are not acid phosphatase positive. The presence of considerable
areas of granular endoplasmic reticulum in granulosa lutein cells from
corpora lutea of pregnancy and hysterectomized gilts suggests an
increased capacity for protein synthesis over that observed in the
estrous cycle; these structures are sparse during the estrous cycle.

The presence of a profusion of membrane-bound dense bodies,
similar in appearance to secretory granules of cell types that
synthesize a protein-containing secretory product, is distinctly
characteristic of luteal cells during pregnancy and after hysterectomy. The increase in quantity of granular endoplasmic reticulum
and the enlargement of the Golgi apparatus may be correlated with the
marked increase in granule population. The granules are not lipid
droplets because the latter are identifiable as larger structures
that do not possess a limiting membrane. Furthermore, these dense
bodies are not lysosomes since no positive acid phosphatase was
obtained.

Relaxin in Porcine Corpora Lutea During the Estrous Cycle, During Pregnancy, and After Hysterectomy

The corpus luteum of the pig is a rich source of biologically
active relaxin, especially during late stages of pregnancy (Hisaw
and Zarrow, 1948; Belt *et al.*, 1971). Relaxin activity was determined
in porcine corpora lutea during the estrous cycle, throughout pregnancy and the first two weeks of lactation, and in corpora lutea
maintained for prolonged periods after hysterectomy (Anderson *et al.*,

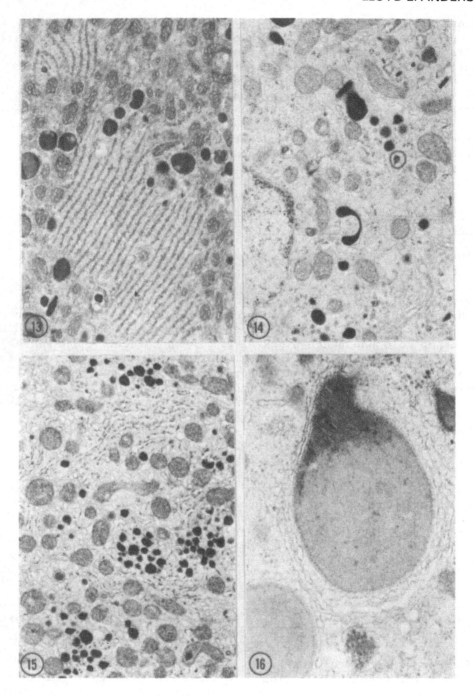

Figure 13.   *A portion of granulosa lutein cell from corpous luteum of 40-day hysterectomy. A well-developed stack of granular (rough) endoplasmic reticulum is adjacent to small electron-dense granules. X 22,500. From Belt et al. (1970).*

Figure 14.   *A portion of granulosa lutein cell from day 29 of pregnancy in the pig. Nucleus at lower left with filling Golgi succules (cup) to the right in meridional plane. Mitochondria are less dense than found in later states of pregnancy. X 40,000. From Belt et al. (1971).*

Figure 15.   *Granulosa lutein cell from day 29 of pregnancy in the pig. The cytoplasm contains abundant mitochondria, electron-dense granules, and images of the Golgi apparatus. X 12,200. From Belt et al. (1971).*

Figure 16.   *Granulosa lutein cell from 60-day hysterectomy. At top of larger granule is a specialized cortical region. The cortical material is tangential to the plane of section. X 49,900. From Belt et al. (1970).*

1973b).   Exogenous estrogen maintains corpora lutea in the unmated
pig, and relaxin levels were determined in these aged corpora lutea.
The ovaries were removed from 143 pigs during these different
reproductive stages, and luteal tissue from each pig was minced,
homogenized, and extracted twice in 3% hydrochloric acid at 5 C for
24 hours.   Sodium chloride (4%) was added before centrifugation, and
the combined supernatants were dialyzed against running tap water
24 hours and stored frozen for bioassay.   Relaxin activity was
measured by interpubic ligament formation in estrogen-primed mice
as described by Steinetz *et al.* (1960).   In this 6-point assay, 20
mice were used for each of the three dilutions of the NIH reference
relaxin and unknown test preparations.

Estrous Cycle

Relaxin remains extremely low throughout the estrous cycle,
even though corpora lutea are large and fully developed by days 8
and 14.   Relaxin concentrations (μg/g) in corpora lutea were 3 ± 1.5
at day 8, 2 ± 1.1 at day 14 and 1 ± 0.3 at day 18.

Pregnancy

The corpus luteum grows to maximal weight by day 14 and
remains large throughout pregnancy in the pig (Figure 7).   By the
last days of pregnancy (e.g., days 114, 115), the corpus attains its
maximum size, but with the onset of parturition and within a few
hours after delivery, the corpora lutea regress rapidly; their
weights decline by half (e.g., day 116).   By the second week of
lactation (day 128), the corpora albicantia regress to small masses
of connective tissue.

Relaxin levels in luteal tissue are extremely low by days 14
and 18 after mating; the concentrations are similar to those found
during the same days of the estrous cycle.   Between days 18 and 20-
29, there is a sevenfold increase in the level of relaxin.   This
hormone activity increases twofold between days 20-29 and 30-39.
By midgestation, relaxin levels are about 130 μg/g, and they continue
to increase to reach peak values by the last days of gestation
(days 100-115).   With the onset of parturition, relaxin levels drop
to extremely low levels (e.g., 12 μg/g) and remain low during the
first 2 weeks of lactation (day 128).

After Hysterectomy

In pigs hysterectomized during the luteal phase of the estrous
cycle or during early phases of pregnancy, the corpus luteum increases

from about 400 mg at <u>day 40</u> to maximum weights of >500 mg by day
100 (Figure 17). These corpora lutea remain large to <u>day 128</u>.

Relaxin levels in the corpora lutea increase to about 40 µg/g
and continue to increase sixfold by day 80. Between days 80 and 116,
there is considerable variability in relaxin activity, with maximal
values occuring at day 110. By day 128, there is a marked decrease in
relaxin levels even though the corpora remain large in these hysterectomized pigs.

Relaxin Activity in Corpora Lutea Maintained by Exogenous Estrogen

Corpora lutea are maintained more than 100 days in 5 of 6
pigs given injections of estradiol benzoate (total 30 mg) during the

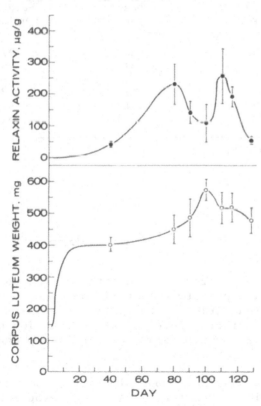

*Figure 17. Relaxin activity in NIH units and corpus luteum weight
after hysterectomy in pig. Hysterectomy was performed
at days 8-10. Mean ± SE. From Anderson et al. (1973b).*

luteal phase of the estrous cycle (Table 1). The corpora lutea (mean no. 10.4) remain large and similar to those found at the same stages during pregnancy and after hysterectomy.

Relaxin activity in corpora lutea from estrogen-treated pigs at days 110 and 116 is 110 $\pm$ 35 µg/g, which is significantly lower than found at the same days in hysterectomized pigs (222 $\pm$ 44 µg/g). By day 128, relaxin levels are similar in hysterectomized and estrogen-treated pigs (Figure 17, Table 1).

Table 1. RELAXIN IN PORCINE CORPORA LUTEA MAINTAINED BY EXOGENOUS ESTROGEN*

Pig no.	Days after estrus	Corpora lutea	
		Mean weight, mg	Relaxin in NIH units, µg/g
303	110	424	207
313	110	478	95
327	110	0	
317	116	471	98
319	116	514	42
323	128	515	51

*Anderson et al.(1973b).

Exogenous Oxytocin on Relaxin in Luteal Tissue and Ovarian Venous Plasma

The intravenous infusion of a total of 720 units of oxytocin for 6 hr does not induce premature parturition, but induces milk let-down during the infusion period. The levels of relaxin in the corpora lutea remain similar before and after infusion of oxytocin (Table 2) and comparable to similar stages of late pregnancy in other animals (Figure 7).

Relaxin levels in ovarian venous plasma increase approximately sevenfold after infusion of oxytocin. Although exogenous oxytocin has no acute affect on the morphology of the corpora lutea or levels of relaxin in them during late pregnancy, there is an abrupt release of high levels of relaxin into the ovarian venous blood.

Table 2.   *EFFECT OF EXOGENOUS OXYTOCIN ON RELAXIN ACTIVITY IN CORPORA*
              LUTEA AND OVARIAN VENOUS PLASMA DURING LATE PREGNANCY IN
              PIG*

| Pig no. | Day of pregnancy | Relaxin activity in NIH units | |
		Corpora lutea, µg/g	Ovarian vein plasma, ng/ml
61†	110	583	64
62†	110	237	76
61‡	111	587	431
62‡	111	164	425

*Anderson et al.(1973b).

†Before intravenous infusion of oxytocin (2 U) min for 6 hr

‡After infusion of oxytocin.

Relaxin in Residual Ovarian Tissue

Relaxin activity in residual ovarian tissue remains extremely low during pregnancy, lactation and after hysterectomy (Table 3). The follicular and interstitial tissues in porcine ovaries produce little, if any, relaxin. The hormone activity in residual ovarian tissue might indicate leakage of relaxin from adjacent corpora lutea in the ovary.

Progressive Changes in Cytoplasmic Organelles of Granulosa Lutein Cells During Pregnancy, Parturition, and Early Lactation

The most evident changes of fine structure of the granulosa lutein cell occur in the granule population, in the amount of granular endoplasmic reticulum, and in the organization of the agranular endoplasmic reticulum. To a lesser extent, the internal structure of mitochondria is altered, and the Golgi apparatus becomes more extensive.

Granules

At day 12 of pregnancy, granules are rarely observed; the granulosa lutein cell resembles that of the 12th day of the estrous cycle. Although a few granules are present by day 20 of pregnancy, they do not become a conspicuous cytoplasmic constituent until day

Table 3.   RELAXIN IN RESIDUAL OVARIAN TISSUE IN PIGS*

| | | Residual ovary | |
Pig no.	Day	Weight, g	Relaxin in NIH units, μg/g
3039	58 pregnancy	6.34	2.4
11	80 pregnancy	6.60	2.9
3003	110 pregnancy	3.75	4.7
23	128 pregnancy†	5.55	0.7
3031	110 hysterectomy	9.19	0.3

*Anderson et al.(1973b).

†After parturition.

28.   Their numbers continue to increase at days 40 to 60 (Figure 18, 19) and by days 105 to 110, the granule population is maximal (Figure 20). In 110- and 115-day cells, some granules appear with a central density and irregular outline, surrounded by a clear halo, but still enclosed by a membrane. These granules seem to be under- going solubilization. At 32 to 26 hours before parturition, some cells are nearly free of granules while adjacent cells still possess moderate numbers of granules. Within 6 hours of delivery, all gran- ulosa luteal cells are nearly free of granules (Figure 21). In spite of their relatively rapid disappearance, observations of exocytosis or granule extrusion are rare.

Granular Endoplasmic Reticulum

Although granular endoplasmic reticulum is a dominant organelle in early stages of luteinization, by day 12 of pregnancy only rare profiles of short strands are encountered. Occasional small arrays of cisternae are found at day 28; large stacks of cisternae often are present at days 40 and 60. The quantity of granular endo- plasmic reticulum diminishes to only occasional short strands by days 105 to 116.

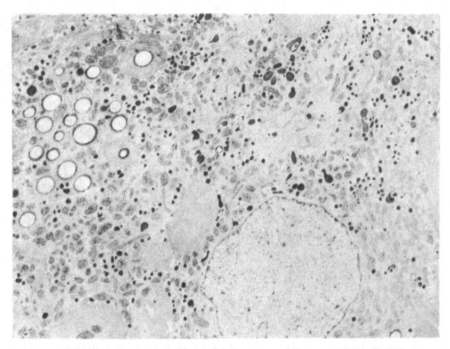

*Figure 18.   Granulosa lutein cell from 40-day hysterectomy in the
              pig.   Small electron-dense granules are beginning to
              accumulate in cytoplasm near images of Golgi apparatus.
              X 12,200.   From Belt et al. (1970).*

Agranular Endoplasmic Reticulum

The anastomotic system of tubules that characterizes steroid
secretory cells is well developed by day 12 of pregnancy. At days
16, 20 and 28, fenestrated cisternae form loose, parallel, and some-
times concentric arrays especially around lipid droplets. Arrays
of fenestrated cisternae of agranular endoplasmic reticulum become
progressively larger and better organized at days 40 to 60, but they
disappear by days 105 to 110.

Mitochondria

In early pregnancy, the matrix of the mitochondria is
relatively lucent, becomes more dense by day 28, and remains dense
throughout pregnancy (refer to Figure 9). Internal membranes are
tubular at day 12, and they appear as fenestrated lamelliform cristae
by days 40 to 60 (Figure 10). Near term, the mitochondrial cristae
become more nearly lamelliform with fewer fenestrae.

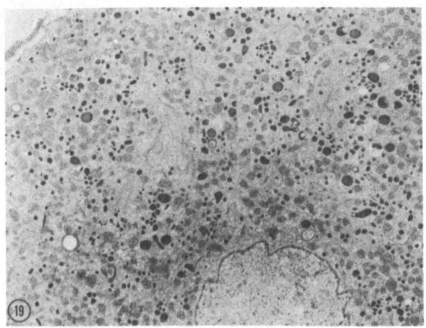

*Figure 19.   Granulosa lutein cell from day 60 of pregnancy.   The cyto-
             plasm contains abundant mitochondria, dense granules and
             multiple images of the Golgi apparatus. (G). X 12,200.
             From Belt et al. (1971).*

Golgi Apparatus

The Golgi apparatus is small and poorly defined at <u>day 12</u>
of pregnancy. A few short saccules are in array with associated
vesicles. As pregnancy progresses, the Golgi apparatus becomes increasingly well developed and prominent, often with arrays of saccules
containing dense material. These structures are evident from <u>days 28</u>
to <u>105</u> and are interpreted as stages of granule formation. The Golgi
apparatus remains well developed to term.

Relaxin Concentrations in Porcine Corpora Lutea and Ovarian Venous Plasma During Late Pregnancy

The levels of relaxin in corpora lutea are maximal at <u>days 105-
110</u> of pregnancy, but within 16 hr before parturition, these decline
to low levels (Table 4). Relaxin levels in ovarian venous plasma are
low between <u>days 105</u> and <u>110</u> and increase fourfold between 26 and
44 hr before parturition. Within 1 to 16 hr before delivery the
plasma relaxin drops to extremely low levels (Table 5).

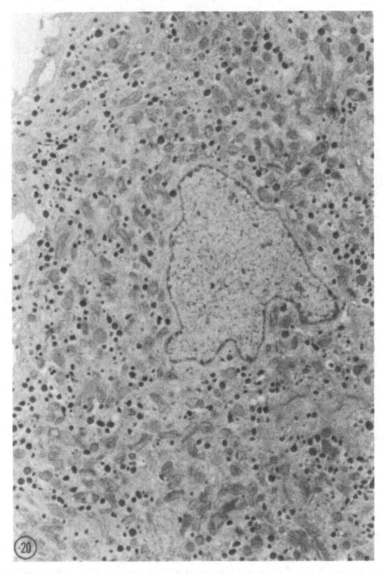

Figure 20.   A portion of a granulosa lutein cell at 110 days of
pregnancy in the pig.   The maximal granule content of the
cell is apparent; the Golgi apparatus is still well
developed.   Pig 69; 161 μg relaxin/g luteal tissue.
X 6,800.   From Belt et al. (1971).

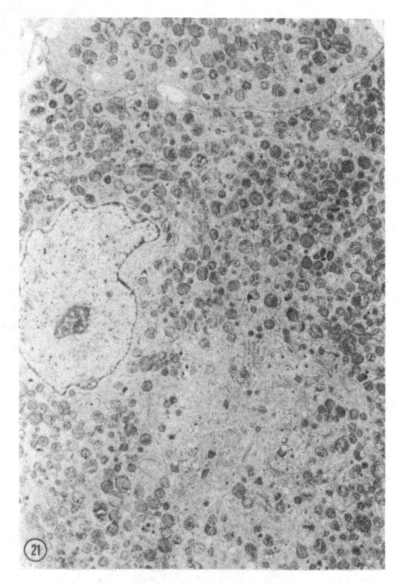

Figure 21. A portion of a granulosa lutein cell at 116 days of
            pregnancy, 6 hr before parturition. Granule depletion
            of the cell is nearly total. In spite of the imminence
            of farrowing, the cell does not appear degenerate. Pig
            92; relaxin was not detectable in luteal tissue. X 8,500.
            From Belt et al. (1971).

Table 4. *RELAXIN IN CORPORA LUTEA AND OVARIAN VENOUS PLASMA DURING LATE PREGNANCY IN THE PIG**

Pig no.	Day of pregnancy	Time to parturition§ (hr)	Relaxin activity in NIH units	
			Corpora lutea, μg/g	Ovarian vein plasma, μg/ml
63	80	abort	287	.104
90	105	abort	207	.126
91	105	abort	$-^a$	.003
70	105	abort	180	ND[c]
45	108	abort	245	.303
69	110	abort	161	.023
93	110	abort	298	.063
79	110	abort	248	ND[c]
61	110	abort	583	.064
94	110	abort	508	$-^b$
59	114	44	283	.264
95†	115	36	51	.351
64‡	115	32	102	.138
77†	116	26	128	.904
58‡	115	16	4	.034
92‡	116	6	ND[c]	$-^b$
56‡	114	2	10	.053
97‡	115	1	11	.038

*Data from Belt et al. (1971) and Anderson et al. (1973b).
†No milk let down.
‡Milk letdown.
§Parturition follows only when ovariectomy is performed within 36 hr of term.
[a]Tissue prepared for histology only.
[b]No blood collected.
[c]Not detectable. There was a significant ($F > 3.92$; 0.05 level) non-parallelism in dose response of standard and unknown preparations.

Table 5. *RELAXIN ACTIVITY IN CORPORA LUTEA AND OVARIAN VENOUS*
PLASMA DURING LATE PREGNANCY IN THE PIG*

No. of pigs	Day of pregnancy	Time to parturition† hr.	Relaxin activity in NIH units	
			corpora lutea, ug/g	Ovarian vein plasma, ng/ml
10	≤110	abort	301	76
4	≥114	44 to 26	141	414
4	≥114	16 to 1	6	42

*Data from Belt et al. (1971) and Anderson et al. (1973b).

†Parturition follows only when ovariectomy is performed within 36 hr of term.

Relation of Cytoplasmic Granules and Relaxin Levels in Porcine Corpora Lutea

In the fourth week of pregnancy, granular endoplasmic reticulum begins to increase in quantity, suggestive of protein or polypeptide synthesis. Clusters of granules, the results of such synthesis, are evident for the first time in moderate numbers. There is a parallel rise in relaxin in the corpora lutea by day 28, elevated also for the first time from the basal levels found during the estrous cycle (Figure 7). During midgestation, there are further increases in the quantity of granular endoplasmic reticulum and the Golgi apparatus. Indications of the lutein cell's protein synthetic capability are manifested by a continued increase in the population of granules, paralleled again by an increase in levels of relaxin. There is no evidence of significant granule release; therefore, the granule population continues to increase throughout most of pregnancy. As this accumulation continues, by days 105 to 110, the concentration of cytoplasmic granules reaches a peak, levels of relaxin in luteal tissue are maximal and the level of hormone is low in ovarian venous plasma (Figure 7 and 20; Table 5). After day 105, little synthesis is possible since, by this time, there is only a small quantity of endoplasmic reticulum. Between 44 and 26 hr before parturition, luteal tissue levels of relaxin decline to less than half peak values. The granule population diminishes, and simultaneously, an

increase in relaxin levels occurs in ovarian venous blood (Figure 21;
Table 5). These events indicate discharge of relaxin from .the luteal
cell into the blood stream. The mechanism of cellular release may
be solubilization of the granule and subsequent release of the hormone.
In the last day before delivery, the level of relaxin in corpora
lutea become minimal, the cells are depleted of cytoplasmic granules,
and the level of relaxin in ovarian venous plasma is low.

Relaxin in Peripheral Blood Plasma During Pregnancy

With the development of a radiommunoassay for porcine relaxin
incporated with tyrosine, Sherwood *et al.* (1975a, 1975b, 1978)
determined peripheral blood plasma levels throughout pregnancy and
at the time of parturition. Peripheral plasma levels of relaxin
remain low (range 0.1 to 2.0 ng/ml) during the first 100 days of
pregnancy and gradually increase to 12 ng/ml 3 days preceding
parturition. Relaxin reaches a maximum concentration (e.g., > 50 ng/
ml) 1 day before delivery and then decreases to 20 ng/ml on the day
of delivery and to < 1 ng/ml during the first few days of lactation.
Sequential bleeding at 4-hr intervals revealed that peak concentrations (e.g., 146 ng/ml) of relaxin occur 14 hr preceding delivery.
Peripheral plasma levels of relaxin during late pregnancy (days 90
to 110) are positively correlated with the number of corpora lutea
(Martin *et al.*, 1979). Pigs with fewer corpora lutea (e.g., 4 to
8) have lower plasma concentrations of relaxin in late gestation
than do those animals with > 13 corpora lutea.

Relaxin Activity in Isolated Fractions of Ovaries During Pregnancy in the Pig

Isolated fractions of porcine ovaries obtained during early,
middle and late pregnancy retain their biological activity, but the
total amount and relative proportions of relaxin in them change as
pregnancy advances (Oliver *et al.*, 1978). Polyacrylamide gel electrophoresis (PAGE) was used to separate three fractions with relaxin
activity from acid-acetone extracts (Griss *et al.*, 1967) of ovaries
from pigs at each of three stages of pregnancy, days 40, 70 and 100.
Relaxin activities in the fractions were determined by bioassays based
upon inhibition of spontaneous mouse uterine contractions *in vitro*
(Kroc *et al.*, 1959) and induction of interpubic ligament formation in
estrogen-primed mice (Steinetz *et al.*, 1960).

PAGE separated three cathodal bands (C1, C2, and C3) that
retain relaxin activity and probably represent different forms or
fractions of the hormone. All three bands induce interpubic ligament
formation and inhibit spontaneous uterine contractions. The amount
of cathodal band material per corpus luteum, as determined by
calculating the area under the peak of the scanning profile,

increased as pregnancy advanced (Figure 22). Although all three
bands are found at each stage of pregnancy, the relative amount of
cathodal material is directly proportional to specific activity
(Table 6).

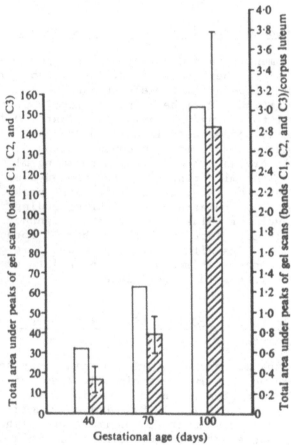

Gestational age (days)

*Figure 22.   Amount of cathodal bands in extracts of ovaries from days
40, 70 and 100 of pregnancy in the pig. Extracts from 5
animals were run for each period. Two milligrams of
extract were applied to each gel. Amount of cathodal band
material (cm²) was determined by measuring the areas under
scanning profiles. Hatched columns represent the total
amount of cathodal material from 5 sets of animals at each
stage of pregnancy. Open columns represent the total
amount of cathodal material from 5 animals per corpus
luteum. Vertical lines indicate ± SE. From Oliver et
al. (1978).*

Table 6. *UTERINE RELAXIN FACTOR (URF) AND MOUSE INTERPUBIC LIGAMENT (MIL) BIOASSAYS OF FRACTIONS ISOLATED BY POLYACRYLAMIDE GEL ELECTROPHORESIS OF EXTRACTS OF PORCINE OVARIES DURING EARLY PREGNANCY.*

Fraction	Specific activity (units/mg)	
	URF	MIL
WL1000†	1000	1000
C1	247	106
C2	840	369
C3	689	271

*Oliver et al., 1978.

†Porcine relaxin standard used in calculating specific activity.

These results indicate that PAGE-isolated fractions with relaxin activity increase as pregnancy advances and agree with findings of Anderson *et al.* (1973b) that relaxin levels increase in porcine corpora lutea during late pregnancy. Other investigators (Cohen, 1963a; Frieden, 1963; Frieden *et al.*, 1974; Sherwood and O'Bryne, 1974) also have reported relaxin activity in several fractions isolated from extracts of ovaries from pregnant pigs, but they did not relate biological activity of the fractions to stage of pregnancy.

Antibodies to porcine relaxin were generated in rabbits initially by Cohen (1963b). Antisera to porcine relaxin were produced in rabbits by injection of different fractions (C1, C2 and C3) separated by PAGE (Larkin *et al.*, 1977). In this series, antisera from one rabbit (R8) given fraction C2 bound biologically active porcine relaxin preparations. The R8 antiserum was tested for its ability to inhibit interpubic ligament formation in estrogen-primed mice (Figure 23). At a dilution of 1:4 or less, the R8 antiserum completely inhibited the effects of a standard dosage of porcine relaxin (WL150). When the R8 antiserum was absorbed with porcine relaxin (WL1000), there was no inhibiting effect on interpubic ligament formation in the relaxin-treated test mice (Figure 23). Although the specific activity of PAGE-isolated fractions is reduced in comparison with that in purified porcine relaxin standard (WL1000), these results indicate that the R8 antiserum inhibits the actions of relaxin *in vivo.*

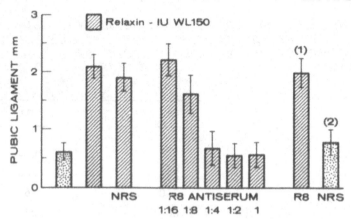

Figure 23.   Effect of rabbit antiserum on mouse interpubic ligament
formation.   Normal rabbit serum (NRS) or antiserum was
injected ip in volumes of 0.1 ml and 30 min before relaxin
(6.6 µg WL150).   Solid bars represent animals that did
not receive relaxin SC.   (1) R8 antiserum to which WL1000
had been added at concentration of 5 µg/ml of serum.
(2) NRS to which WL1000 had been added at concentration
of 5 µg/ml of serum.   At least 12 animals were used in
each group.   Mean ± SE.   From Larkin et al. (1977).

Immunocytochemical Localization of Relaxin in Porcine Granulosa Lutein Cells

Immunohistochemical techniques recently have been utilized in attempts to identify localization of relaxin within specific cell types in this species.   Immunofluorescent examination of sections of ovarian tissue, recovered from pigs on day 100 of pregnancy and reacted with a rabbit antiserum (R8), produced by an active fraction of porcine relaxin and indicated that only the corpus luteum exhibited specific fluorescence (Larkin *et al.*, 1977; Figure 24 and 25).   The majority of granulosa lutein cells fluoresce strongly at this late stage of pregnancy; no specific fluorescence is observed in the interstitium and other nonluteal tissue.   In corpora lutea recovered at day 40 of pregnancy, there was slight fluorescence, whereas by day 70, luteal cells were moderately fluroescent but not as intense as at day 100.   These results indicate that porcine relaxin is confined to the granulosa lutein cells of the corpus luteum.

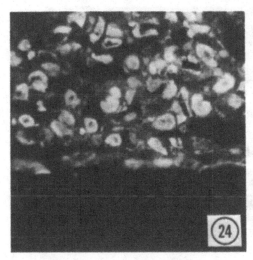

Figure 24.   *Low-power fluorescent micrograph of section of ovary from
sow on day 100 of pregnancy. Upper portion of micrograph
shows numerous fluorescing cells representing the corpus
luteum. The lower portion of the micrograph that shows
no fluroescing cells represents nonluteal tissue adjacent
to the corpus luteum. The majority of luteal cells
exhibit fluroescence; however, the intensity varies among
different cells. From Larkin et al. (1977).*

Limitations of the fluorescent antibody technique precluded identification of specific cytoplasmic organelles (granules) in granulosa
lutein cells as possible sites for relaxin storage. In a brief
report, Corteel *et al*. (1977) presented evidence for immunocytological
localization of relaxin during different stages of pregnancy in the
pig. Antirelaxin serum, produced in rabbits, was tested in ovaries
of pigs at <u>days 30</u>, <u>60</u> and <u>90</u> of pregnancy. Electron microscopy
revealed that the response to antirelaxin was localized in dense
bodies in granulosa lutein cells and that it changed from a weak to
a strong reaction with advancing stages of gestation. The presence
of relaxin in the corpus luteum of the rabbit (Zarrow and O'Conner,
1966) and rat (Anderson *et al.*, 1975) is indicated at the light microscopy level by fluorescent antibody techniques.

Convincing experimental evidence of immunocytochemical localization of relaxin in porcine granulosa lutein cells at the ultrastructural level has been presented by Kendall *et al*. (1978). Rabbit
antiserum used in the staining procedure was generated against highly
purified porcine relaxin. The primary criterion for specificity in

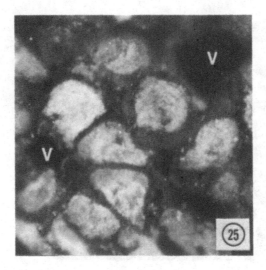

Figure 25.   Medium-power fluorescent micrograph of corpus luteum from
             sow ovary on day 100 of pregnancy. The fluorescent cells
             are ovoid to polyhedral. Blood vessels (V), smaller cells
             interspersed between the larger cells, and intercellular
             spaces do not exhibit fluorescence. X 1,200. From
             Larkin et al. (1977).

this investigation was the identification of a peroxidase-antiperoxi-
dase (PAP) complex and a reduction in staining intensity by prior
incubation with porcine relaxin. A 1:10,000 dilution of the antirelaxin serum incubated with luteal cells for 24 hr at room temperature
gave positive reactions. In granulosa lutein cells obtained from a
pig approximately 30 days pregnant, antirelaxin serum stained a
population of small granules, which ranged from 0.2 μm to 0.6 μm
diameter and included larger, heterogenous granules up to 1.0 μm
diameter. The smaller granules often appear in clusters within
the cytoplasm (Figure 26a) or near the plasmalemma (Figure 26b; 27a
and 27b). The larger irregular granules, however, often appeared
separated from the clusters. PAP molecules were recognized within
both the clustered and irregular granules and, to a slight extent,
within the cytoplasm. Larger granules, recognized previously as
lysosomes (Belt et al., 1971) did not stain. Prior absorption of
the antirelaxin serum with increasing amounts of relaxin reduced
staining in the granules (compare Figure 28 and 29) and cytoplasm,
whereas greater amounts abolished staining in these locations.
These results on immunocytochemical localization of relaxin agree
with those of Belt and colleagues (1971), who correlated changes
in the population of small cytoplasmic granules in porcine granulosa
lutein cells with relaxin concentrations in luteal tissue and ovarian

venous plasma during pregnancy. This sensitive and specific staining technique provides evidence for localization of relaxin in small cytoplasmic granules of porcine granulosa lutein cells at a time when endogenous levels of relaxin begin to increase in early pregnancy (refer to Figure 7), and the technique should be extended to later stages of pregnancy in this species.

Cow

The estrous cycle lasts about 21 days and pregnancy is approximately 283 days in cattle. Usually, only one ovulation occurs at each estrus. After ovulation, the newly developing corpus luteum is maintained to day 16 of the cycle or until parturition. It secretes progesterone throughout the luteal phase of these two reproductive states, as well as after hysterectomy (Anderson *et al.*, 1969). Fertilization occurs in the upper part of the oviduct, and the embryo enters the uterine horn on day 4. Attachment of the conceptus to the endometrium occurs about day 40 in the uterine horn ipsilateral to the ovary containing the corpus luteum.

Although histology and some histochemical reactions to the bovine ovary have been described by several investigators (refer to McNutt, 1924, 1927; Moss *et al.*, 1954; Foley and Greenstein, 1958; Rajakoski, 1960; Short, 1962), limited morphologic information is available on the fine structure of this tissue.

Estrous Cycle

Fine structural features of the largest graafian follicle and the corpus luteum from ovaries representing all stages of the estrous cycle were reported by Priedkalns and Weber (1968a, 1968b). Two cell types, large and small luteal cells, were described, with the most notable ultrastructural difference between the two types being presence of numerous large mitochondria in the larger luteal cells (30-40 μm diameter) and numerous lipid bodies in the smaller cells (15-20 μm diameter). The large luteal cells contain an abundance of agranular endoplasmic reticulum that is tubular and tortuous and an extensive Golgi apparatus. During luteinization, there is transformation in large mitochondria of plate-like cristae to tubular and villous forms as well as an accumulation of a dense material substance. In smaller mitochondria within the same luteal cell, typical features include lameliform cristae and tubular forms. The endoplasmic reticulum becomes agranular, tubular, and tortuous as well as very extensive during early stages of luteinization, but during luteal regression, the endoplasmic reticulum becomes vesicular. Lipid bodies are present to a moderate extent and located peripherally in the large luteal cells. Granules, assumed to be lipid pigment, accumulate during luteolysis. Lysosomes, membranous bodies, multi-

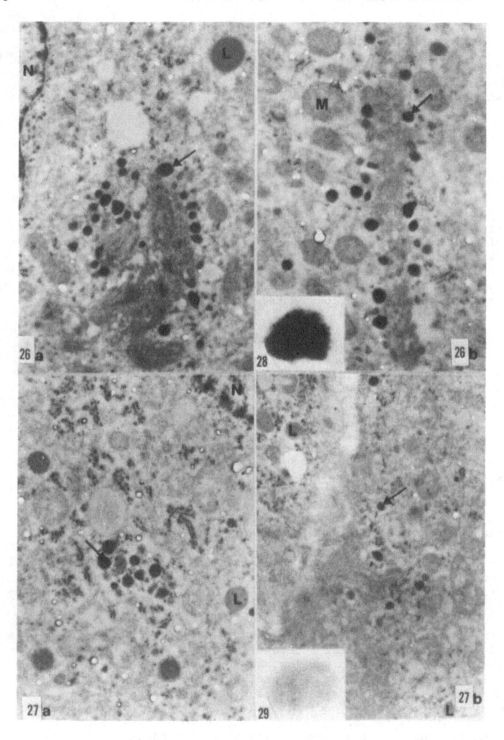

Figure 26a and 26b.   *Sections of granulosa lutein cells from a pig at 20 to 30 days of pregnancy. Stained with a 1:1000 dilution of antiserum to porcine relaxin and the PAP complex unlabeled antibody technique. Fixation 1 percent glutaraldehyde, embedding Araldite. After immunochemical staining the sections were floated on 4 percent OsO_4 for 15 min. No counterstain. Stain is on a population of granules (arrowed) distributed in clumps with the cytoplasm (a) or bordering the plasmalemma as can be observed in the two adjacent cells in (b). N = nucleus, L = lysosome, M = mitochondria. X 12,500. From Kendall et al. (1978).*

Figure 27a and 27b.   *Staining intensity in secretory granules (arrowed) incubated with antirelaxin serum is reduced by absorption with 5 ng of porcine relaxin (a). Control section (b) to that in Figure 26b. Normal rabbit serum (1:1000 dilution) was substituted for the antiserum. This section was run through the same immunochemical staining sequence as the grid in Figure 26b. N = nucleus, L = lysosome. X 12,500. From Kendall et al. (1978).*

Figure 28.   *The appearance of a secretory granule which has accumulated a large number of PAP molecules. X 56,000. From Kendall et al. (1978).*

Figure 29.   *The appearance of secretory granule stained as for Figure 28, but phosphate buffer was substituted for the PAP complex. X 56,000. From Kendall et al. (1978).*

vesicular bodies, and dense bodies are found in midcycle luteal cells
and are present in large numbers during luteal regression. Granulosa
lutein cells contain moderate amounts of granular endoplasmic reticulum and free ribosomes that are related to protein synthesis. Dense
granules associated with granular endoplasmic reticulum and Gogli
apparatus are not a prominent feature in these granulosa lutein cells
during a major part of the estrous cycle. Quantitative observations
reveal cyclic growth and regression of luteal cells during the estrous
cycle. There is an increase in cytoplasmic percentage volume of
mitochondria, an increase in the concentration of agranular cytoplasmic
membranes, and low levels of lipid bodies and lysosomes at times when
steroidogenesis and cell growth were maximal and were present in
large numbers during luteal regression.

Granulosa lutein cells contain moderate amounts of granular
endoplasmic reticulum and free ribosomes that would be related to
protein synthesis. Dense granules associated with granular endoplasmic reticulum and Golgi apparatus were not a prominent feature in
these granulosa lutein cells during a major part of the estrous cycle.

Pregnancy

Histological changes in the bovine corpus luteum during pregnancy
have been described by McNutt (1927), Foley and Greenstein (1958) and
Singh (1975). Granulosa lutein cells often are polyhedral and contain
periodic-acid-schiff positive glycogen granules. These cytoplasmic
PAS-positive granules increase in number with advancing stages of
pregnancy to at least day 240.

Fine-structural features in bovine lutein cells show an
abundance of mitochondria evenly distributed throughout the cytoplasm
(Singh, 1975). These mitochondria frequently appear as extremely
elongated and spherical forms with electron-dense inclusions within
their matrices. The dense body inclusions tend to increase in size
and frequency as pregnancy advances to 240 days. The endoplasmic
reticulum is primarily agranular, and whorls of agranular endoplasmic
reticulum frequently enwrap mitochondria and lipid droplets.
Spherical osmiophilic dense granules in the cytoplasm increase in size
and number to 240 days of gestation. Increased amounts of glycogen
accumulate in lutein cells during late pregnancy and may contribute
to protein synthesis. The abundant elongated mitochondria and
agranular endoplasmic reticulum in bovine lutein cells are features
typically found in steroid-secreting cells. Cytoplasmic dense granules
and lipid globules increase in size and number during late pregnancy.

Relaxin in Bovine Corpus Luteum and Placenta During Pregnancy

Wada and Yuhara (1960) attempted to extract relaxin from different tissues and reproductive organs in the cow. They found low
activities (< 0.5 GPU/mg) in extracts of whole ovaries and corpora
lutea by the interpubic ligament assay in mice as well as very little
uterine-relaxing activity in the rat. Placental extracts showed low
activity (0.2-0.3 GPU/mg), but large dosages of these extracts
inhibited spontaneous uterine contractions in the rat. They presented
the first experimental evidence of relaxin activity in extracts of
bovine placenta. Lesmeister (1975) attempted to isolate relaxin from
bovine corpora lutea and ovarian residual tissue. There was no significant interpubic ligament response in estrogen-primed mice to a
wide range of dosages of saline-ethanol extracts of corpora lutea
(5 μg to 10 mg) or residual ovarian tissue (33 μg).

Castro-Hernandez *et al.* (1976) observed that acid-acetone extracts
from bovine corpora lutea from the third trimester of pregnancy
inhibited contraction of mouse uterine strips *in vitro* to yield a
relative potency of 1.87 GPU/mg dessiccated crude extract, but these
extracts were ineffective in provoking interpubic ligament formation
in estrogen-primed mice. Further purification by isoelectric
precipitation and gel filtration revealed relaxin activity in two
fractions containing 176 and 16 GPU/mg by the *in vitro* mouse uterine
strip assay.

Do Valle (1970) attempted to isolate relaxin from bovine corpora
lutea by either acid-acetone or phosphate-buffer extraction procedures
and determine the relative potency of these extracts by the mouse
interpubic ligament assay. Ovaries from cows in late stages of
pregnancy were obtained from a local abbatoir. Stage of pregnancy was
determined by measuring fetal crown-rump length and estimating age
of fetus according to morphologic criteria of Swett *et al.* (1948).
Only corpora lutea from cows 210 to 260+ days gestation were used.
After removal of them from the animal, the ovaries were chilled on
ice, corpora lutea were enucleated and weighed, and luteal tissue
was prepared in a manner similar to that described by Griss *et al.*
(1967). A composite sample of corpora lutea from different animals
and representing the same stage of pregnancy, was minced, homogenized,
and extracted with 6 volumes of acetone-water-concentrated HCl
(5:2, 83:0.17 v/v) for 16 hours at 0-5°C. The extract was separated
from the insoluble tissue components by centrifugation at 2,700 rpm
for 20 minutes, and supernatant precipitated with 5 volumes of
acetone at -15°C for 2 to 3 hours. The resulting precipitate was
removed by centrifugation at 10,000 rpm for 20 minutes and washed
with acetone. The insoluble tissue was re-extracted with the same
volume of the extraction medium. The extracts were combined and
dried over $CaCl_2$, powdered, and stored at room temperature.

For phosphate-buffer extraction, a composite sample of corpora lutea from different animals was minced, homogenized, and extracted with 6 volumes of phosphate buffer solution (pH = 7.0) for 16 hours at 0-5°C. The extract was separated from the insoluble tissue components by centrifugation at 9,000 rpm for 20 minutes, dialyzed against tap water 24 hours, and lyophilized. The insoluble tissue was re-extracted with 5 volumes of the extraction medium. The extracts were combined and stored at room temperature in a desiccator containing $CaCl_2$.

Relaxin in standard and unknown preparations was based upon development of mouse interpubic ligament (MIL) according to the method described by Steinetz *et al.* (1960). Two strains of Swiss albino, virgin female mice, ICR and CF1, were used in these assays. The six-point balanced assay design included two unknown sample preparations run concomitantly with the standard. Twenty mice were used for each of three dilutions of standards and unknowns, and dose levels increased by twofold increments.

The mean quantity of acid-acetone extract obtained was 2.71 + 0.19 mg extract/g luteal tissue, with a range of 1.14 to 3.66 mg extract/g corpus luteum. Mean yields of phosphate buffer extracts were 21.13 + 4.92 mg/g corpus luteum, with a range of 14.06 to 35.16 mg/ g luteal tissue. Both the acid-acetone extracts and the phosphate buffer extracts were tested for relaxin activity. NIH porcine relaxin with an activity of 442 units/mg and purified relaxin (CM-B), also of porcine origin, with an activity of 3,000 units/mg were used as relaxin reference standards.

The results obtained by the MIL bioassay indicated that the relaxin activity in bovine luteal tissue was present at low concentrations (4.5×10^{-4} to 9.4 μg NIH-relaxin/g luteal tissue and 7.9×10^{-3} to 1.07×10^{-2} μg CM-B relaxin/g corpus luteum), and frequently relaxin activity was not detectable by this bioassay method.

Fields *et al.* (1979) isolated relaxin from bovine corpora lutea during late pregnancy and obtained three major active fractions yielding 30, 45 and 250 units/mg protein as compared with porcine fractions yielding 400, 2,500 and 2,760 units/mg protein. Acid-acetone extracts of luteal tissue were prepared by a modification of procedures described by Griss *et al.* (1967), and the precipitates subjected to gel filtration and isoelectric focusing. Biological activity of the fractions from the isoelectric focusing columns was tested by the mouse uterine motility inhibition assay and the mouse interpubic ligament assay. Bovine relaxin isolated by these procedures retained the following characteristics a) approximately 6,000 daltons, b) ability to inhibit spontaneous uterine contractions and induce formation of interpubic ligament in mice, c) several biologically active fractions with high isoelectric points, and d) a reaction of identity between porcine relaxin and bovine relaxin when assayed with an antiserum produced against porcine relaxin. Although bovine and porcine relaxin had similar biochemical characteristics, biological activity was less in bovine relaxin preparations.

Relaxin in Bovine Peripheral Blood

Wada and Yuhara (1955) used the guinea pig pubic symphysis palpation method to assay peripheral blood levels of relaxin in pregnant cows. They found 0.8 GPU/ml after the first month of pregnancy, with a gradual increase until the 7th month, when a plateau of 3.6 GPU/ml was reached and maintained throughout the remainder of pregnancy. After parturition, there was a rapid decline, and within one week after delivery, relaxin was not detectable. In a later report, Wada and Yuhara (1961), using the same assay procedures, indicated that relaxin activity increased from an average of 0.1 GPU/ml serum during the second trimester to an average of 0.3 GPU/ml during the last trimester of pregnancy. Relaxin activity decreased and was not detectable by 3 days post-partum.

Using a radioimmunoassay specific for porcine relaxin incor-porated with tyrosine, Sherwood et al. (1975a) found no high concen-trations of an immunoreactive substance in peripheral blood serum from cows in late stages of pregnancy. In three beef cows bled sequentially as early as 14 days before parturition and continuing 5 days into the postpartum period, immunoreactive serum concentrations of relaxin remained consistently low (Table 7). These serum levels of relaxin in beef cows were similar to those found in beef steers.

Cytoplasmic Granules and Hormone Secretion in Bovine Corpora Lutea

There is little information available on possible roles of cyto-plasmic granules in hormone secretion by bovine corpora lutea. Kramers et al. (1975) found small granules (0.2 μm diameter) that seem to be formed in the Golgi apparatus and transported to the cell membrane, where the contents are expelled by exocytosis. A particulate fraction, isolated from luteal tissue by subcellular fractionation and density-gradient centrifugation, contained a 10-fold enrichment of progesterone. Progesterone enriched fractions also contained large numbers of membrane-bound granules. They concluded that, in bovine corpora lutea, a steroid, progesterone, may be packaged and secreted by cellular processes typically described for protein hormones. At this time, there are no reports concerning any relation-ship of relaxin to cytoplasmic organelles in granulosa lutein cells in the cow.

*Table 7. IMMUNOACTIVE RELAXIN IN PERIPHAL BLOOD SERUM FROM COWS
           DURING LATE PREGNANCY**

Cow no.	Relaxin (pg/ml)[†]		
	Pre-partum	Delivery	Postpartum
130	147 (5)	75 (1)	107 (6)
310	187 (12)	77 (1)	132 (6)
0-318	184 (27)	182 (1)	198 (11)

*Lesmeister 1975).

[†]Radioimmunoassays by O. D. Sherwood with ^{131}I-labeled porcine relaxin as standard. Mean concentrations of relaxin with number of
serum samples indicated in parentheses.

COMPARATIVE ASPECTS OF RELAXIN PRODUCTION AND OVARIAN MORPHOLOGY

Experimental evidence on the relation of ovarian morphology to
hormone secretion will be considered in two other species, the rat
and sheep, to provide comparative aspects of relaxin production and
cell structure with the pig. The rat produces relaxin, but there is
not extensive evidence on relaxin secretion in sheep.

Rat

Relaxin in Ovarian Tissue and Peripheral Blood

Relaxin is present in ovaries of pregnant rats at days 13, 15
and 21 (Steinetz et al., 1959) as determined by interpubic ligament
formation in estrogen-primed mice and by presence of a uterine-
relaxin factor (Bloom et al., 1959). Relaxin was determined in rat
ovarian tissue by mouse interpubic ligament formation throughout
several reproductive stages: pregnancy, pseudopregnancy, pseudopregnancy in hysterectomized animals, and pseudopregnancy in rats
bearing deciduomata (Anderson et al., 1973a). Porcine relaxin was
used as the standard in these bioassays. Pseudopregnancy lasts about
13.5 days, whereas pseudopregnancy is extended to approximately 22
days after hysterectomy or induction of deciduomata and is a duration
similar to that of normal pregnancy. Relaxin in lyophilized ovarian

tissue remains consistently low (< 0.5 μg/mg) between <u>days</u> <u>6</u> and <u>13</u>
of pseudopregnancy. In pseudopregnant, hysterectomized rats or in
animals bearing deciduomata, the levels of relaxin remain low
(< 0.5 μg/mg) from <u>days</u> <u>6</u> to <u>21</u>. During normal pregnancy, they
remain consistently low through <u>day</u> <u>12</u>, and between <u>days</u> <u>14</u> and <u>20</u>,
relaxin increases to peak values (e.g., 5 μg/mg) by <u>day</u> <u>20</u>. From
<u>day</u> <u>20</u> to just before parturition, there is a marked decline to
a low level by <u>day</u> <u>1</u> of lactation and the level remains low throughout
the 18 days of lactation (Figure 30). Thus, relaxin in the rat
increases only during the later half of gestation. The levels of
relaxin seem unrelated to the age of the corpus luteum because the
diestrous interval is of about the same duration in hysterectomized
animals or rats with deciduomata as in pregnancy. Progesterone
concentrations in ovarian venous blood are less during pseudopregnancy,
after hysterectomy, and in animals bearing deciduomata than those
during the later half of pregnancy (Hashimoto *et al.*, 1968). Thus,

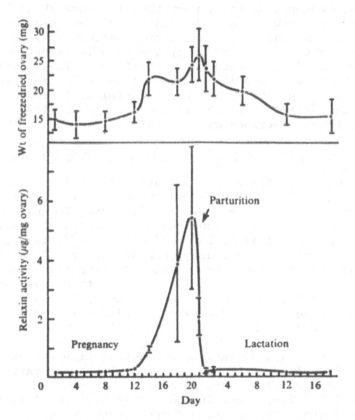

*Figure 30. Relaxin activity and ovarian weight changes during dif-
ferent reproductive stages in the rat. Mean ± SE.
From Anderson et al. (1973a).*

the conceptuses stimulate the ovaries to increase, not only progesterone production and size of granulosa lutein cells, but also relaxin
production during late pregnancy. In nongravid rats with prolonged
diestrous intervals, progesterone synthesis seems unrelated to minimal
relaxin production by the ovaries.

     With recent production of highly purified forms of rat relaxin
(Sherwood, 1979) and development of an homologous radioimmunoassay
for rat relaxin (Sherwood and Crnekovic, 1979), concentrations of
the hormone have been determined in fresh ovarian tissue and in
peripheral blood serum throughout pregnancy. Radioimmunoassay of
rat relaxin in ovarian tissue indicated that hormone levels begin to
increase at day 16 to peak values by day 20, decrease during the last
2 days of pregnancy, and drop precipitously after parturition. These
results are in close agreement with the occurrence and relative levels
of ovarian relaxin biological activity reported by Anderson et al.,
(1973a). Peripheral serum levels of rat relaxin are consistently low
until 2 days preceding parturition, when they increase abruptly but
then drop soon after parturition. The profile of rat relaxin levels
in peripheral blood indicates that the hormone accumulates in ovarian
tissue during the last week of pregnancy and then is abruptly
released into the blood just preceding parturition. These profiles
of relaxin accumulation in ovarian tissue and secretion into peripheral blood during pregnancy in the rat are similar to those described for the pig (Belt et al., 1971; Anderson et al., 1973b;
Sherwood et al., 1975b; Sherwood et al., 1978).

Fine Structure of the Corpus Luteum During Pregnancy in the Rat

     The corpus luteum in the rat is essential for the successful
maintenance of pregnancy and is the primary source of progesterone
(Fajer and Baraclough, 1967; Hashimoto et al., 1968; Uchida et al.,
1970; Morishige et al., 1973). Granulosa lutein cells at day 2
of pregnancy are approximately 12-15 μm diameter and contain a
spherical nucleus, numerous lipid droplets, and spherical mitochondria with tubular and vesicular cristae. During the later half
of pregnancy, the granulosa lutein cells increase to maximal diameters
of 28 to 32 μm, primarily in response to increasing levels of chorionic
mammotropin. The corpus luteum decreases in diameter after delivery,
and numerous lipid droplets accumulate.

     Long (1973) presents a definitive account of fine structural
changes in the corpus luteum throughout pregnancy in the rat. During
early pregnancy, the granulosa lutein cells have features typical
of steroid-secreting cells; these include large numbers of mitochondria and lipid droplets, well-developed agranular endoplasmic
reticulum, and a prominent Golgi apparatus. A few irregularly
shaped, membrane-bound, electron-dense granules are seen near the
Golgi apparatus. These granules are about 500 μm in diameter and
are categorized as type I granules. By days 7-10, the lutein cells
have enlarged, and the number of lipid inclusions declines. The

amount of agranular endoplasmic reticulum greatly increases. By
day 12, the most significant cytoplasmic changes are the increasing
amounts of agranular endoplasmic reticulum and the formation of
stacks of granular endoplasmic reticulum.

By day 17, granulosa lutein cells have reached maximum size,
primarily as a result of the proliferation of agranular endoplasmic
reticulum (Figure 31). Furthermore, a second population of electron-
dense, membrane-bound granules, first observed at day 14, are not
abundant (Figure 31 and 32). These granules are categorized as type
II granules and they usually are smaller ($\sim$ 270 μm in diameter),
more uniform in size, and more electron-dense than the type I
granules. The type II granules also are present at day 20. After
parturition, the corpus luteum regresses rapidly; ovulations and
the corpora lutea of lactation soon are formed. By the third day
of lactation, the granulosa lutein cells of the old corpora lutea
of pregnancy contain numerous lipid droplets, and there results a
decline in agranular endoplasmic reticulum and disappearance of the
type II granules (Figure 33 and 34).

Histochemical characteristics of the larger granules (type I),
initially found early in pregnancy, indicate that they are lysosomes
as evidenced by their positive acid phosphatase and aryl sulfatase
reactions. The type II granules do not show a positive reaction of
either enzyme, and they presumably are not lysosomes.

Thus, during pregnancy in the rat, a striking feature in
granulosa lutein cells is presence of two types of membrane-bound
dense granules. The larger type I granules contain lysosomal enzymes
and are observed at all stages of gestation, whereas the smaller type
II granules are found during late stages of pregnancy and do not
contain lysosomal enzymes. Long (1973) concluded that these type
II granules in granulosa lutein cells of the rat are possible sites
for storage of relaxin.

Agranular endoplasmic reticulum is implicated in synthesis
of steroid hormones, and the increasing amounts of agranular endoplasmic reticulum in lutein cells correlate with increased production
of progesterone, especially during the latter half of gestation in
this species. The decline in the number of lipid droplets is compatible with an increase in progesterone secretion during pregnancy;
precursors of progestin synthesis, cholesterol and cholesterol
esters, are stored in lipid and utilized in hormone production.
The agranular endoplasmic reticulum becomes disorganized as progesterone levels decline in late pregnancy. Mitochondria become
elongate and lamellar as pregnancy advances, and the cristae in them
appear with tubules and vesicles; cholesterol side-chain cleavage
enzymes are found in rat lutein cells. Finally, the Golgi apparatus
increases in size during pregnancy, implicating an increase in the
synthesis of cytoplasmic proteins.

Figure 31.   *Rat granulosa lutein cell from day 17 of pregnancy. There is an abundance of smooth endoplasmic reticulum throughout the cytoplasm. Two classes of granules may be distinguished: type I (1) granules are larger, more variable in shape, and less electron-dense than the type II granules (arrows), which may be sites of storage for relaxin. X 9,000. From Long (1973).*

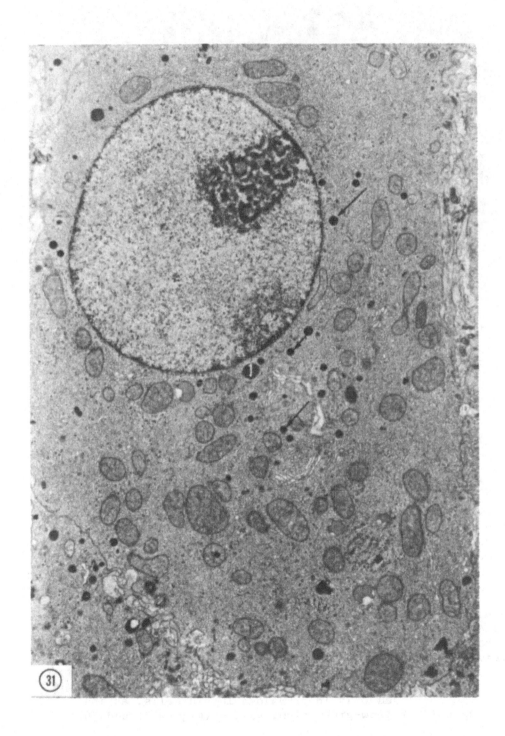

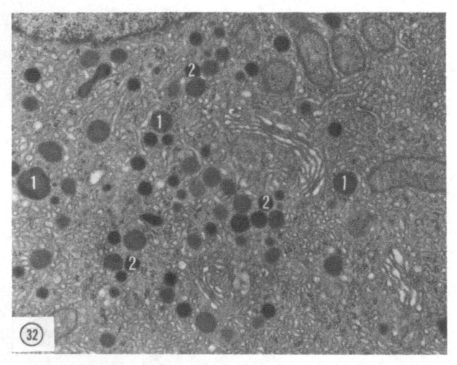

*Figure 32.   Higher-magnification view of Golgi region in a day 17
               rat granulosa lutein cell. Representative type I and II
               granules are labeled 1 and 2, respectively. X 18,000.
               From Long (1973).*

Localization of Relaxin in Rat Corpus Luteum

Cytological evidence for the presence of relaxin in granulosa
lutein cells during late pregnancy in the rat has been examined by
fluorescent antibody techniques and by determining relaxin activity
in tissue extracts and subcellular fractions of ovarian tissue.

By utilizing indirect fluorescent antibody techniques, Anderson
et al. (1975) have demonstrated presence of relaxin in granulosa
lutein cells. Antiserum to porcine relaxin was produced in New
Zealand rabbits, and the indirect fluorescent antibody method used
was that described by Glass (1971). The best antisera yielded
positive hemagglutination to dilutions of 1:4000.

In paraffin sections of ovaries from <u>day 17</u> pregnant rats,
relaxin is localized only in granulosa lutein cells, as indicated
by the specific yellow-green fluorescence (Figure 35 and 36). The

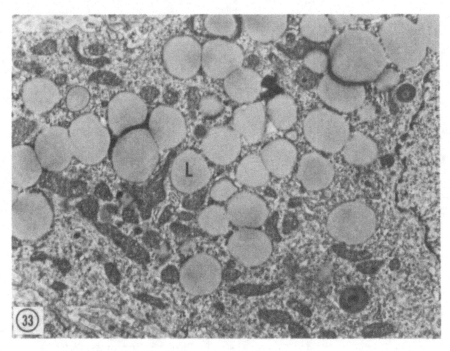

*Figure 33.   Low-magnification view of lutein cell of pregnancy removed
3 days after parturition in the rat.   Note the absence
of type II granules and the marked accumulation of lipid
(L) in this cell.   X 6,300.   From Long (1973).*

specific fluorescence seems to involve most of the cytoplasm of
the lutein cell, with the strongest fluorescence in a juxtanuclear
position presumably over the Golgi apparatus (Figure 35), but not
all luteal cells fluoresce. Ovarian follicles and interstitial cells
do not display any specific fluorescence for relaxin. Frozen
sections of rat ovaries, fixed according to the method of Zarrow and
O'Conner (1966), also reveal localization of fluorescent label in
granulosa lutein cells at this stage of pregnancy, but staining also
appears in intercellular spaces as a result of hormone diffusion from
the luteal cells. Thus, the indirect fluorescent-antibody method
clearly demonstrates the greatest concentrations of relaxin in the
juxtanuclear area of luteal cells in this species.

Further attempts on localization of relaxin were investigated
by preparing tissue extracts of rat luteal cells, remaining (residual)
ovarian tissue, and subcellular fractions of luteal cells and bio-
assaying them for relaxin activity (Anderson and Long, 1978). The
bioassay method was based upon the ability of relaxin to inhibit
spontaneous contractions of uterine segments from virgin, estrogen-

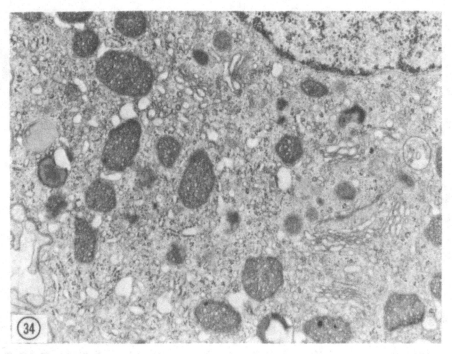

*Figure 34.   A portion of a lutein cell from the corpus luteum of
lactation taken 3 days after parturition in the rat.
No type II granules are present, but type I granules are
abundant.   X 16,200.   From Long (1973).*

primed rats (Griss *et al.*, 1967; Wiqvist and Paul, 1958).   Tissue
extracts of corpora lutea and residual ovarian tissue were obtained
from <u>day 17</u> pregnant rats and prepared as described by Bloom *et al.*
(1958).   For cell-fractionation studies, corpora lutea, dissected
free from other ovarian tissue, were homogenized in 0.5 M sucrose
containing 5 x 10^{-4} EDTA and subjected to differential centrifugation.
The initial homogenate was centrifuged (270 x g) to remove the
nuclear fraction.   The supernatant was diluted with sucrose-EDTA
and centrifuged at 7,000 x g, with the resulting pellet designated
as the mitochondrial fraction.   The original supernatant and washes
of the pellet fraction were centrifuged at 15,000 x g to yield a
granular fraction.   Supernatant fluids and washings then were
centrifuged at 10,000 x g to sediment a microsomal fraction.
All fractions were resuspended in saline for bioassay of relaxin and
for examination of subcellular components by electron microscopy.

The minimal quantity of porcine relaxin required to produce
total inhibition of uterine contractions in this bioassay system was
a concentration of 0.027 GPU/ml.   Extracts of corpora lutea from

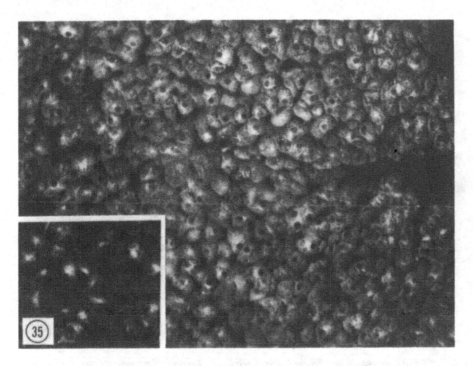

Figure 35.   Fluorescent photomicrograph.   Paraffin section of a portion
of a corpus luteum from an ovary at day 17 of pregnancy
in the rat.   Stained with rabbit antirelaxin serum and
fluorescein labeled antirabbit gammaglobulin. Note the
juxtanuclear location of the fluorescent label for
relaxin in the luteal cells (inset).   Not all the
cells seem to possess relaxin.   X 138.   Inset X 173.
From Anderson et al. (1975).

day 17 of pregnancy, yield total inhibition at a chamber concentration of 3.2 µg/ml (dry-weight basis), whereas only partial uterine
inhibition results in the case of two extracts of residual ovarian
tissue at concentrations of 7 and 24 µg/ml.   The granular fraction
of lutein cells results in the greatest relaxin activity.   Electron
micrographs of this fraction reveal the presence of granules and
some mitochondria (Figure 37).   The mitochondrial fractions
demonstrate 1/3 to 1/4 the specific relaxin activity of the granular
fraction.   The microsomal fraction consists of smooth-surfaced and
ribosome-studded membranous vesicles and contains little relaxin
activity.

Electron micrographs of the granular fraction show both mitochondria and a heterogenous population of granules, similar in
appearance to the type I and type II granules of intact granulosa

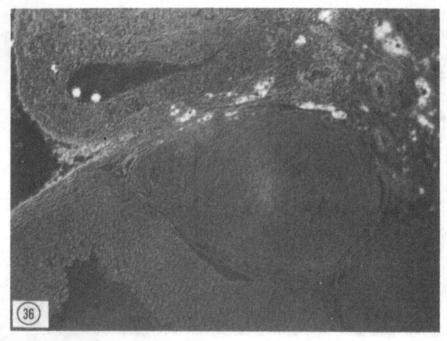

*Figure 36. Fluroescent photomicrograph. Paraffin section of an
ovary at day 17 of pregnancy in the rat. Saline control.
There is a low background in the luteal cells of the
corpus luteum (center) and in the follicle (lower left).
Note autofluoresence of the interstitial cells. X 150.
From Anderson et al. (1975).*

lutein cells described by Long (1973). On the basis of bioassay and
cell fractionation studies, Anderson and Long (1978) concluded that
the subcellular component that stores relaxin is either the granules
or the mitochondria. Mitochondria are abundant in luteal cells
throughout pregnancy in the rat and are not known to be sites of
storage for hormones. The larger type I granule population
described by Long (1973) is lysosomal, as demonstrated by their
content of acid phosphatase and aryl sulfatase; the smaller type
II granules do not contain these hydrolytic enzymes. Thus, the
previous fine-structural studies by Long (1973) on the appearance
of type II granules during the last week of pregnancy and the
disappearance of them at parturition parallel the increase in
relaxin activity in the ovaries of rats the last week of pregnancy
and the precipitous decline in relaxin near parturition (Anderson
et al., 1973a). This and other correlative evidence obtained by
cell fractionation of lutein cells by differential centrifugation
suggest that the type II granules are storage sites for relaxin in
this species.

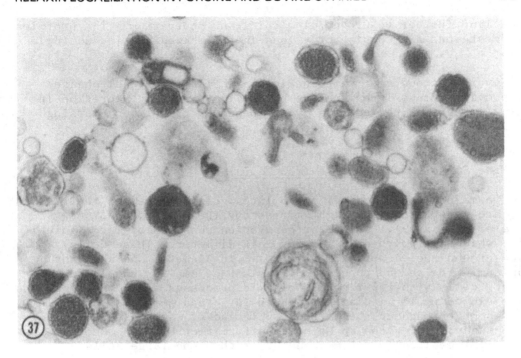

*Figure 37.   Electron micrograph of rat granule fraction isolated by
differential centrifugation.   X 36,000.   From Anderson
and Long (1978).*

Sheep

The estrous cycle in the ewe is about 16.5 days, and pregnancy
lasts approximately 150 days. The endocrine activity of ovine
corpora lutea throughout the estrous cycle is indicated by progesterone concentrations in luteal tissue (Stormshak *et al.*, 1963;
Deane *et al.*, 1966), in ovarian venous blood plasma (Short, 1964) and
peripheral blood plasma (Thorburn *et al.*, 1969). Progesterone in
peripheral plasma remains low (< 0.3 ng/ml) from days 0 to 3,
increases to mean concentrations of 1.5-2.5 ng/ml between days 4
and 9, and declines rapidly on days 14 and 15 to reach extremely
low levels (0.1 ng/ml) at onset of estrus.

During pregnancy, in ewes carrying twin fetuses, there is
a gradual increase in peripheral plasma concentrations from 1.0
to 5.0 ng/ml from weeks 1 to 10, a steady rise from 5.0 to 9.0 ng/
ml from weeks 10 to 17, and then an abrupt increase to peak levels
of 16 ng/ml by week 19 (Stabenfeldt *et al.*, 1972). Thereafter,
progesterone levels decrease precipitously to onset of parturition
at week 21. Progesterone levels are about 2 ng/ml at parturition

and decline further to 0.8 ng/ml within 1 hr postpartum. The profiles
of progesterone are consistently less in those ewes bearing a single
fetus.

Several accounts of histochemical and fine structural changes
in the ovine corpus luteum relate primarily to steroid secretion in
terminal stages of the estrous cycle (Deane *et al.*, 1966; Bjersing
et al., 1970; Gemell *et al.*, 1974).

Fine Structure of Ovine Luteal Cells

Two major populations of ovine luteal cells, based on their cell
size, are recognizable by light microscopy (Deane *et al.*, 1966;
O'Shea *et al.*, 1979). The first population consists of large luteal
cells, which are polyhedral, 25-50 μm in diameter. These cells
possess round nuclei approximately 10 μm in diameter and abundant
cytoplasm. The second population consists of smaller angular or
elongate cells with tapering cytoplasmic processes and with dimensions
seldom exceeding 15 μm diameter. Both large and small luteal cells
are present throughout the estrous cycle and at days 15 to 140
of pregnancy; there seem to be no transformation between them.
The small luteal cells are more numerous than the large cells.

The major cytoplasmic organelles in the small luteal cells are
abundant agranular endoplasmic reticulum and endoplasmic reticulum
of tubular form associated with clusters of attached ribosomes.
Mitochondria in these small cells are of variable size and contain
tubular and lamellar cristae; electron-dense matrix granules are
found within them. Small numbers of dense, membrane-bounded granules
(0.4-1.0 μm in diameter) are scattered throughout the cytoplasm.
Lipid droplets are present in small numbers in these cells but they
increase during luteal regression, a time when there also is an
increase in lysosome-like granules. These small luteal cells
possess the $\Delta^5$3 -hydroxysteroid dehydrogenase and, thus, steroid
synthetic function.

The population of larger polyhedral lutein cells of the ovine
corpus luteum has been described extensively by Deane *et al.*, 1966;
Bjersing *et al.*, 1970; Gemell *et al.*, 1974). From days 10 to 14
of the estrous cycle, histological features of these cells consist
of a finely granular cytoplasm and a vesicular nucleus containing
1 or 2 nucleoli. Initial histological signs of luteal regression
occur on day 15 when nuclei of the lutein cells begin to degenerate.
As regression proceeds, lutein cells become shrunken and more
densely stained, and cytoplasmic vacuoles develop (Deane *et al.*,
1966). Between days 10 and 14, $\Delta^5$3 -hydroxsteroid dehydrogenase
(DHA) activity is high throughout the luteal cells, whereas by
day 15, there is a reduction in the number of reactive cells. After
incubation with $NADH_2$, the lutein cells stain darkly, and the intensity

of this diaphorase reaction in these cells closely parallels the DHA patterns.

Typical fine-structural features in the cytoplasm of the <u>larger lutein cells</u> at <u>days</u> 2 and 3 of the estrous cycle are an abundance of ribosomes, granular endoplasmic reticulum, and mitochondria. Several Golgi regions are evident as well as a few small electron-dense granules 0. 2 μm in diameter. By <u>days</u> 4 and <u>6</u>, the amount of granular endoplasmic reticulum diminishes while there is an increase in agranular endoplasmic reticulum. The dense granules often appear at the periphery of the cell and in extracellular space near the cytoplasmic membrane, and the population of them increases at <u>days</u> 7 and <u>8</u>. From <u>days</u> <u>10</u> to <u>14</u>, these parenchymal cells of the fully functional ovine corpus luteum have abundant mitochondria, clumps of stacked Golgi lamellae and numerous dense membrane-bound granules. There is a slow accumulation of lipid droplets within membranous sacs and an overall increase in size of the mitochondria as well as a gradual rarefication of the mitochondrial matrix and some swelling of the cytoplasmic vacuoles during this time. By <u>day</u> 15, the granulosa lutein cells are smaller, and there is disorganization of the Golgi apparatus, degeneration of the agranular endoplasmic reticulum, and further accumulation of lipid droplets. Lysosomes are present at all stages of the cycle, and there is little further increase in their numbers at <u>day</u> 15, a time of marked cellular degeneration.

During pregnancy, changes in the small luteal cells are less marked than those in the large ones during the last third of gestation (O'Shea *et al.*, 1979). In the large lutein cells, there is a marked increase in lipid droplets and numbers of lysosome-like granules. The cells become smaller, and their cytoplasmic processes appear withdrawn. Furthermore, the mitochondria are tightly packed, and large granules often exceeding 1.0 μm in diameter are found in the mitochondrial matrix. Small cytoplasmic granules of approximately 0.2 μm diameter are progressively less numerous during late pregnancy in the population of large luteal cells.

Cytoplasmic Granules in Ovine Luteal Cells

The small, electron-dense membrane-bounded granules, are found predominantly in the large rather than small ovine luteal cells. These granules show no acid phosphatase activity at any stage of the estrous cycle; thus, they likely are not lysosomes. Accumulation of the cytoplasmic granules occurs early in the luteal phase of the cycle, and both granule formation and discharge of them increases to <u>day</u> 11; thereafter, secretion of the granules declines, with no evidence of secretion by <u>day</u> 15. As granule secretory activity gradually declines, it is accompanied by marked degenerative changes of cytoplasmic organelles at <u>day</u> 15, which include autophagocytic bodies containing hydrolytic enzymes and an abundance of lipid bodies

(Gemmell *et al.*, 1974). The coarse lipid droplets in the corpus
albicans prevail at least 15 days (Deane *et al.*, 1966).

The possible role of decreased ovarian blood flow as initiating
the decline in progesterone secretion and the demise of the functional
cytology of ovine granulosa lutein cells remains undefined (Niswender
et al., 1975; Nett *et al.*, 1976). Decreasing concentrations of
progesterone in luteal tissue or peripheral blood occur before extensive cellular changes in ovine corpora lutea (Bjersing *et al.*,
1970).

Morphological evidence for progesterone secretion via granules
in luteal cells of the sheep was suggested on the basis that the
hormone is sequestered into the secretory granules by a binding
protein and then released by an exocytotic mechanism; protein and
progesterone are presumed to be secreted together (Sawyer *et al.*,
1977; Abel *et al.*, 1977). When slices of ovine granulosa lutein
tissue are incubated in the presence of luteinizing hormone (LH) and
(or) calcium ionophore, an increase in progesterone secretion results
at the same time that the contents of numerous Golgi-derived
secretory granules are released into extracellular spaces (Sawyer
et al., 1979). The structural appearance and location of these
cytoplasmic granules frequently found near the lateral aspects of
the Golgi cisternae may represent immature granules in various
degrees of formation. The addition of colchicine has no effect on
basal progesterone secretion of incubated luteal slices, but when it
is added at least 30 minutes before the addition of LH, LH-stimulated
progesterone secretion is reduced. These *in vitro* results suggest
qualitatively that colchicine blocks formation of granules at the
level of the Golgi apparatus, but has little effect on the release of
preformed granules. Sawyer *et al.* (1979) further suggest a possible
sequence of events that a progesterone-carrier protein may be
packaged into secretory granules at the level of the Golgi apparatus,
that these granules accumulate progesterone from tubular elements of
the agranular endoplasmic reticulum as they migrate toward the cell
surface, and that the contents of these granules are released into
the extracellular space via exocytosis.

Relaxin Activity During Different Reproductive States in the Ewe

The experimental evidence for relaxin activity in sheep is based
upon its immunoactivity with antiporcine relaxin. According to
Bryant, ovine plasma crossreacts in a porcine relaxin radioimmunoassay system (Bryant, 1972; Bryant and Stelmasiak, 1975) and this
system has been utilized to determine relaxin activity every second
hour during 4-day periods throughout the ovine estrous cycle
(Chamley *et al.*, 1975). Sequential bleedings reveal that immunoreactive relaxin is secreted episodically at approximately 12.00 h

and 24.00 h throughout most of the estrous cycle. Bursts of hormone
release, ranging from 600 to 3,000 ng/ml, occur during periods of
2 to 4 hr. These bursts are followed by a rapid decline in relaxin
that results in a hormone half-life of approximately 8 minutes. These
profiles of relaxin levels in peripheral plasma yield little relationship to luteal function and progesterone secretion during the
estrous cycle in this species. Relaxin is elevated before the pre-
ovulatory release of LH, and thus may be associated with follicular
growth and maturation. The source of relaxin immunoactivity,
whether ovine or uterine, during the ovine estrous cycle is unknown.

An immunofluorescence technique developed by Kruip *et al.* (1976)
indicated that theca interna cells of tertiary follicles exhibit
immunofluorescence in pregnant ewes from days 18 to 140. They also
found positive immunofluorescence reactions in luteal tissue of
pregnant ewes from days 80 to 140. The antisera for this investigation were produced in rabbits against porcine relaxin and used at
dilutions of 1:50. Sections of ovarian tissue were incubated
initially with antirelaxin serum and then fluorescent sheep anti-
rabbit-γ-globulin serum.

Both relaxin and prolactin immunoactivities, measured at days
45 and 110 of pregnancy, indicate that prolactin, but not relaxin,
increases in the later part of the gestation in this species
(Chamley *et al.*, 1976). Near the time of parturition, both prolactin
and relaxin rise and are significantly correlated during the period
of expulsion of the lamb.

In lactating ewes, there is an abrupt rise in peripheral blood
plasma levels of both relaxin and prolactin within 1.5 minutes after
initiation of machine milking (Chamley *et al.*, 1976). After 2
minutes, relaxin immunoactivity drops to premilking levels, whereas
prolactin remains elevated. Teat stimulation of lactating ewes
also causes a peak release of relaxin within 2 minutes, but a more
gradual elevation in prolactin to maximal levels by 6 minutes.
Relaxin drops within 3 minutes after initiation of the suckling
stimulus and remains extremely low at a time when prolactin levels
are maximal. The infusion of oxytocin also elicits release of relaxin
within 5 minutes in some anestrous ewes pretreated with estrogen
and progesterone, but the response may not be comparable to
appropriate stimuli in lactating ewes. The infusion of oxytocin also
induces release of relaxin during late pregnancy in the pig
(Anderson *et al.*, 1973b). These results in lactating ewes indicate
that the suckling or milking stimulus precipitates release of relaxin
immunoactivity, but the physiological significance of this response
is unclear. Furthermore, the endogenous source of relaxin in
lactating ewes is unknown. Corpora lutea are completely regressed,
and ovarian follicular growth is inhibited during lactation in
this species.

CONCLUSIONS

Relaxin is a polypeptide hormone produced primarily by the
ovaries in several mammalian species. The hormone is produced in
largest amounts during pregnancy. Experimental evidence is reviewed
on the production and localization of relaxin, primarily in the
porcine and bovine ovary, but with reference to findings in a few other
domestic and laboratory species. The granulosa lutein cells in the
corpus luteum are a rich source of biologically active relaxin in the
pig during pregnancy and after hysterectomy, but not during the
estrous cycle. Changes in histochemical and fine-structural features
of the granulosa lutein cell throughout different reproductive states
are described in this species and in cattle, as well as in the rat
and sheep.

Two populations of small and large granulosa lutein cells are
found in porcine, bovine, and ovine corpora lutea. These two sizes
of lutein cells are present throughout the estrous cycle and pregnancy.
Relaxin concentrations in porcine granulosa lutein cells begin to
increase steadily from the fourth week of gestation and reach peak
values just before parturition. Relaxin levels in luteal tissue
drop near onset of delivery and remain low during lactation. The
appearance and accumulation of electron-dense membrane-bounded
granules in the cytoplasm of these lutein cells in early and midgestation and their disappearance in the last days of pregnancy
parallel the rise and fall of relaxin in corpora lutea. Profiles of
relaxin in ovarian venous blood and peripheral blood also suggest
that the porcine corpora lutea accumulate relaxin and then secrete
the hormone during late stages of pregnancy. Immunofluorescent
techniques based upon fluorescence reaction to antirelaxin serum,
reveal that relaxin is confined to the porcine granulosa lutein cell.
Immunocytochemical localization of relaxin at the ultrastructural
level indicates that the hormone is contained in the small electron-
dense granules of these granulosa lutein cells. Although both relaxin
and progesterone are produced by the corpus luteum in the pig,
profiles of secretion of these two hormones, a polypeptide and a
steroid, are markedly different during the estrous cycle and
pregnancy.

In cattle, relaxin activity has been isolated in corpora lutea
from late stages of pregnancy. The hormone activity is much less
than found in the pig on the basis of assays that utilize porcine
relaxin as the standard. There is as yet no evidence on the identification of cytoplasmic organelles associated with the production of
relaxin within granulosa lutein cells in this species.

There is convincing evidence for localization of relaxin in
electron-dense, membrane bounded granules of granulosa lutein cells
during late pregnancy in the rat. The accumulation and disappearance
of these granules correlate with ovarian relaxin content and
peripheral blood levels.

REFERENCES

Abel, J. H., Jr., McClelland, M. C., Sawyer, H. R., Schmitz, M., Niswender, G. D. and Nau, E. (1977). Synthesis and release of secretory protein from lutein cells. J. Cell Biol. 75:374a. Abstract.

Anderson, L. L. (1973). Effects of hysterectomy and other factors on luteal function. In: Handbook of Physiology (R. O. Greep and E. B. Astwood, eds.). Vol. 2, Sect. 7, Part II. American Physiological Society. Washington, D.C. pp. 69-86.

Anderson, L. L. (1978). Growth, protein content and distribution of early pig embryos. Anat. Record. 190:143-154.

Anderson, L. L., Bast, J. D. and Melampy, R. M. (1973a). Relaxin in ovarian tissue during different reproductive stages in the rat. J. Endocrinol. 59:371-372.

Anderson, L. L., Bland, K. P. and Melampy, R. M. (1969). Comparative aspects of uterine-luteal relationships. Recent Progr. Hormone Res. 25:57-104.

Anderson, L. L., Butcher, R. L. and Melampy, R. M. (1963). Uterus and occurrence of oestrus in pigs. Nature (Lond.) 198:311-312.

Anderson, L. L., Ford, J. J., Melampy, R. M. and Cox, D. F. (1973b). Relaxin in porcine corpora lutea during pregnancy and after hysterectomy. Am. J. Physiol. 225:1215-1219.

Anderson, L. L., Hard, D. L. and Kertiles, L. P. (1979). Progesterone secretion and fetal development during prolonged starvation in the pig. Am. J. Physiol. 236:E335-E341.

Anderson, M. L., Long, J. A. and Hayashida, T. (1975). Immunofluorescence studies on the localization of relaxin in the corpus luteum of the pregnant rat. Biol. Reprod. 13:499-504.

Anderson, M. L. and Long, J. A. (1978). Localization of relaxin in the pregnant rat. Bioassay of tissue extracts and cell fractionation studies. Biol. Reprod. 18:110-117.

Belt, W. D., Anderson, L. L., Cavazos, L. F. and Melampy, R. M. (1971). Cytoplasmic granules and relaxin levels in porcine corpora lutea. Endocrinology 89:1-10.

Belt, W. D., Cavazos, L. F., Anderson, L. L. and Kraeling, R. R. (1970). Fine structure and progesterone levels in the corpus luteum of the pig during pregnancy and after hysterectomy. Biol. Reprod. 2:98-113.

Belt, W. D. and Pease, D. C. (1956). Mitochondrial structure in sites of steroid secretion. J. Biophys. Biochem. Cytol. 2:Suppl. 369-374.

Bjersing, L. (1967). On the ultrastructure of granulosa lutein cells in porcine corpus luteum. Z. Zellforsch. 82:187-211.

Bjersing, L., Hay, M. F., Moor, R. M., Short, R. V. and Deane, H. W. (1970). Endocrine activity, histochemistry and ultrastructure of ovine corpora lutea. Z. Zellforsch. 111:437-457.

Bloom, G., Paul, K. G. and Wiqvist, N. (1958). A uterine-relaxing factor in the pregnant rat. Acta Endocrinol. 28:112-118.

Bryant, G. D. (1972). The detection of relaxin in porcine; ovine and human plasma by radioimmunoassay. Endocrinology 91:1113-1117.

Bryant, G. D. and Stelmasiak, T. (1975). The specificity of a radioimmunoassay for relaxin. Endocr. Res. Commun. 1:415-433.

Castro-Hernandez, A., Larkin, L. H., Warnick, A. C. and Fields, M. J. (1976). Isolation of bovine relaxin. J. Anim. Sci. 43:277-278. Abstract.

Cavazos, L. F., Anderson, L. L., Belt, W. D., Henricks, D. M., Kraeling, R. R. and Melampy, R. M. (1969). Fine structure and progesterone levels in the corpus luteum of the pig during the estrous cycle. Biol. Reprod. 1:83-106.

Chamley, W. A., Stelmasiak, T. and Bryant, G. D. (1975). Plasma relaxin immunoactivity during the oestrous cycle of the ewe. J. Reprod. Fertil. 45:455-461.

Chamley, W. A., Hooley, R. D. and Bryant, G. D. (1976). The relationship between relaxin and prolactin immunoactivities in various reproductive states: radioimmunoassay using porcine relaxin. In: Growth Hormone and Related Peptides (A. Pecile and E. E. Muller, ed.), Excerpta Medica Int. Congr. Ser. 381, Amsterdam, pp. 407-413.

Christensen, A. K. and Gillim, S. M. (1969). The correlation of the fine structure and function in steroid-secreting cells, with emphasis on those of the gonads. In: The Gonads (K. W. McKerns, ed), Appleton-Century-Crofts, New York, pp. 415-488.

Cohen, H. (1963b). Immunologic inhibition of the biological effects of relaxin. Endocrinology 72:164-166.

Corner, G. W. (1915). The corpus luteum of pregnancy, as it is in swine. Carnegie Instr. Contr. Embryol. 5:69-94.

Corner, G. W. (1919). On the origin of the corpus lutuem of the sow from both granulosa and theca interna. Am. J. Anat. 26:117-183.

Corteel, M., Lemon, M. and Dubois, M. (1977). Evolution de la reactio immunocytologique du corps jaune de Truie au cours de la gestation. J. Physiol. (Paris) 73:63-64A Abstract.

Deane, H. W., Hay, M. F., Moor, R. M., Rowson, L. E. A. and Short, R. V. (1966). The corpus luteum of the sheep relationships between morphology and function during the estrous cycle. Acta Endocrinol. 51:245-263.

Do Valle, E. R. (1978). Relaxin in bovine ovarian tissue during late pregnancy. M.S. Thesis. Iowa State University Library. pp. 1-88.

Dubois, M. P. and Dacheux, J. L. (1978). Relaxin, a male hormone? Cell. Tiss. Res. 187:201-214.

du Mesnil du Buisson, F., and Dauzier, L. (1957). Influence de l'ovariectomie chez la truie pendant la gestation. C. R. Soc. Biol. 151:311-313.

Enders, A. C. (1973). Cytology of the corpus luteum. Biol. Reprod. 8:158-182.

Fajer, A. B. and Barraclough, C. A. (1967). Ovarian section of progesterone and 20 α-hydroxypregn-4-en-3-one during pseudopregnancy and pregnancy in rats. Endocrinology 81:617-622.

Fawcett, D. W., Long, J. A. and Jones, A. L. (1969). The ultrastructure of endocrine glands. Recent Progr. Hormone Res. 25:315-380.

Fevold, H. L., Hisaw, F. L. and Meyer, R. K. (1930). The relaxative hormone of the corpus luteum: its purification and concentration. J. Am. Chem. Soc. 52:3340-3348.

Fields, M. J., Fields, P. A., Castro-Hernandez, A. and Larkin, L. H. (1979). Isolation of relaxin from corpora lutea of late pregnant cows. Endocrinology (in press).

Foley, R. C. and Greenstein, J. S. (1958). Cytological changes in the bovine corpus luteum during early pregnancy. IIIrd Reprod. Infertil. Symp. Pergamon, New York. pp. 88-96.

Frieden, E. H. (1963). Purification and electrophoretic properties of relaxin preparations. Trans. N.Y. Acad. Sci. 25:331-336.

Frieden, E. H., Chen, S. and Rawitch, A. B. (1974). Isolation and partial characterization of two peptides with relaxin activity. Fed. Proc. 33:1358. Abstract.

Frieden, E. H. and Hisaw, F. L. (1953). The biochemistry of relaxin. Recent Progr. Hormone Res. 8:333-378.

Gemmell, R. T., Stacy, B. D. and Thorburn, G. D. (1974). Ultrastructural study of secretory granules in the corpus luteum of the sheep during the estrous cycle. Biol. Reprod. 11:447-462.

Class, L. E. (1971). Fluorescent antibody methods. In: Methods in Mammalian Embryology. (J. C. Daniel, Jr., ed). W. H. Freeman and Co., San Francisco, pp. 355-377.

Goodman, P., Latta, J. S., Wilson, R. B. and Kadis, B. (1968). The fine structure of sow lutein cells. Anat. Record. 161: 77-90.

Griss, G., Keck, J., Engelhorn, R. and Tuppy, H. (1967). The isolation and purification of an ovarian polypeptide with uterine relaxin activity. Biochem. Biophys. Acta. 140:45-54.

Guthrie, H. D., Henricks, D. M. and Handlin, D. L. (1972). Plasma estrogen, progesterone and luteinizing hormone prior to estrus and during early pregnancy in pigs. Endocrinology 91:675-679.

Hard, D. L. and Anderson, L. L. (1979). Maternal starvation, progesterone secretion, litter size and growth in the pig. Am. J. Physiol. 237:E273-E278.

Hashimoto, I., Henricks, D. M., Anderson, L. L. and Melampy, R. M. (1968). Progesterone and pregn-4-en-20 α-ol-3-one in ovarian venous blood during various reproductive states in the rat. Endocrinology 82:333-341.

Hisaw, F. L. (1925). The influence of the ovary on the resorption of the pubic bones of the pocket gopher, Geomys Bursarius (Shaw). J. Exp. Zool. 42:411-441.

Hisaw, F. L. (1926). Experimental relaxation of the pubic ligament of the guinea pig. Proc. Soc. Exp. Biol. Med. 23:661-663.

Hisaw, F. L. and Zarrow, M. X. (1948). Relaxin in the ovary of
    the domestic sow (*Sus scrofa, L.*). Proc. Soc. Exp. Biol. Med.
    69:395-398.
Hisaw, F. L. and Zarrow, M. X. (1950). The physiology of relaxin.
    Vitam. Horm. 8:151-178.
Hisaw, F. L., Zarrow, M. X., Money, W. L., Talmage, R. V. and
    Abramovitz, A. A. (1944). Importance of the female reproductive
    tract in the formation of relaxin. Endocrinology 34:122-134.
James, R., Niall, H., Kwok, S. and Bryant-Greenwood, G. (1977).
    Primary structure of porcine relaxin: homology with insulin
    and related growth factors. Nature (Lond.) 267:544-546.
Jamieson, J. D. and Palade, G. E. (1971a). Condensing vacuole
    conversion and zymogen granule discharge in pancreatic enxocrine
    cells: metabolic studies. J. Cell Biol. 48:503-522.
Jamieson, J. D. and Palade, G. E. (1971b). Synthesis, intracellular
    transport and discharge of secretory proteins in stimulated
    pancreatic exocrine cells. J. Cell Biol. 50:135-158.
Kendall, J. Z., Plopper, C. G. and Bryant-Greenwood, G. D. (1978).
    Ultrastructural immunoperoxidate demonstration of relaxin in
    corpora lutea from a pregnant sow. Biol. Reprod. 18:94-98.
Kertiles, L. P. and Anderson, L. L. (1979). Effect of relaxin on
    cervical dilatation, parturition and lactation in the pig.
    Biol. Reprod. 21:57-68.
Kramers, M. T. C., Sheppard, B. L. and Thorburn, G. (1975). Evidence
    in favour of progesterone secretory granules in the bovine
    corpus luteum. Acta Endocrinol. Suppl. 199:277. Abstract.
Kroc, R. L., Steinetz, B. G. and Beach, V. L. (1959). The effects
    of estrogens, progestagens, and relaxin in pregnant and non-
    pregnant laboratory rodents. Ann. N.Y. Acad. Sci. 75:942-980.
Kruip, T. A. M., Taverne, M. A. M. and Beneden, T. H. (1976).
    Demonstration of relaxin in the ovary of pregnant sheep by
    immunofluorescence. Proc. VIIIth Intr. Congr. Anim. Reprod.
    Artificial Insem., Krakow 3:375-377.
Larkin, L. H., Fields, P. A. and Oliver, R. M. (1977). Production
    of antisera against electrophoretically separated relaxin and
    immunofluorescent localization of relaxin in the porcine corpus
    luteum. Endocrinology 101:679-685.
Lemon, M. and Loir, M. (1977). Steroid release *in vitro* by two
    luteal cell types in the corpus luteum of the pregnant sow.
    J. Endocrinol. 72:351-358.
Lesmeister, J. L. (1975). Hormonal effects of pelvic development
    and calving difficulty in beef cattle. Ph.D. Dissertation
    University of Nebraska, Lincoln, pp. 1-188.
Long, J. A. (1973). Corpus luteum of pregnancy in the rat--
    ultrastructural and cytochemical observations. Biol. Reprod.
    8:87-93.
Martin, P. A., Sherwood, O. D. and Dziuk, P. J. (1979). Effect of
    CL number on relaxin levels in pregnant pigs. Society for
    the Study of Reproduction, 12th Annual Meeting, Laval Univ.
    Quebec, p. 17a Abstract.

Masuda, H., Anderson, L. L., Henricks, D. M. and Melampy, R. M. (1967). Progesterone in ovarian venous plasma and corpora lutea of the pig. Endocrinology   80:240-246.

McNutt, G. W. (1924). The corpus luteum of the ox ovary in relation to the estrous cycle. J. Am. Vet. Med. Assoc.   65: 556-597.

McNutt, G. W. (1927). The corpus luteum of pregnancy in the domestic cow (Bos taurus) and a brief discussion of cyclicial ovarian changes. J. Am. Vet. Med. Assoc. 72:286-299.

Morishige, W. K., Pepe, G. J. and Rothchild, I. (1973). Serum luteinizing hormone, prolactin and progesterone levels during pregnancy in the rat. Endocrinology 92:1527-1530.

Moss, S., Wrenn, T. R. and Sykes, J. F. (1954). Some histological and histochemical observations of the bovine ovary during the estrous cycle. Anat. Record 120:409-434.

Nett, T. M., McClellan, M. C. and Niswender, G. D. (1976). Effects of prostaglandins on the ovine corpus luteum: blood flow, secretion of progesterone and morphology. Biol. Reprod. 15:66-78.

Niswender, G. D., Reimers, T. J., Diekman, M. A. and Nett, T. M. (1975). Blood flow: A mediator of ovarian function. Biol. Reprod. 14:64-81.

Oliver, R. M., Fields, P. A. and Larkin, L. H. (1978). Separation of relaxin activities in extracts of ovaries of pregnant sows by polyacrylamide gel electrophoresis. J. Endocrinol. 76:517-525.

O'Shea, J. D., Cran, D. G. and Hay, M. F. (1979). The small luteal cell of the sheep. J. Anat. 128:239-251.

Palade, G. (1975). Intracellular aspects of the process of protein secretion. Science 189:347-358.

Parvizi, N., Elsaesser, F., Smidt, D. and Ellendorff, F. (1976). Plasma luteinizing hormone and progesterone in the adult female pig during the oestrous cycle, late pregnancy and lactation, and after ovariectomy and pentobarbitone treatment. J. Endocrinol. 69:193-203.

Priedkalns, J. and Weber, A. F. (1968a). Ultrastructural studies of the bovine graafian follicle and corpus luteum. Z. Zellforsch. 91:554-573.

Priedkalns, J. and Weber, A. F. (1968b). Quantitative ultrastructural analysis of the follicular and luteal cells of the bovine ovary. Z. Zellforsch. 91:574-585.

Rajakoski, E. (1960). The ovarian follicular system in sexually mature heifers with special reference to seasonal, cyclical and left-right variations. Acta Endocrinol. 34:Suppl. 52:1-68.

Robertson, H. A. and King, G. J. (1974). Plasma concentrations of progesterone, oestrone, oestradiol-17β and of oestrone sulphate in the pig at implantation, during pregnancy and at parturition. J. Reprod. Fertil. 40:133-138.

Sawyer, H. R., Abel, J. H., Jr., McClellan, M. C., Schmitz, M. and
    Niswender, G. D. (1979). Secretory granules and progesterone
    secretion by ovine corpora lutea *in vitro*. Endocrinology
    104:476-486.
Sawyer, H. R., McClellan, M. C., Abel, J. H., Jr., Chen, T. C. and
    Niswender, G. D. (1977). Cellular mechanism involved in the
    packaging and secretion of a secretory protein from ovarian
    granulosa lutein cells. Anat. Record   187:706. Abstract.
Schwabe, C. and McDonald, J. K. (1977). Relaxin: a disulfide
    homolog of insulin. Science 197:914-915.
Schwabe, C., McDonald, J. K. and Steinetz, B. G. (1976). Primary
    structure of the A chain of porcine relaxin. Biochem. Biophys.
    Res. Commun. 75:503-510.
Schwabe, C., Steinetz, B., Weiss, G., Segaloff, A., McDonald, J. K.,
    O'Bryne, E., Hochman, J., Carriere, B. and Goldsmith, L. (1978).
    Relaxin. Recent Progr. Hormone Res. 34:123-211.
Sherwood, O. D. (1979). Purification and characterization of rat
    relaxin. Endocrinology 104:886-892.
Sherwood, O. D., Chang, C. C., Bevier, G. W. and Dziuk, P. J. (1975b).
    Radioimmunoassay of plasma relaxin levels throughout pregnancy
    and parturition in the pig. Endocrinology 97:834-837.
Sherwood, O. D. and Crnekovic, V. E. (1979). Development of a
    homologous radioimmunoassay for rat relaxin. Endocrinology
    104:893-897.
Sherwood, O. D. and O'Bryne, E. M. (1974). Purification and
    characterization of porcine relaxin. Arch. Biochem. Biophys.
    160:185-196.
Sherwood, O. D., Rosentreter, K. R. and Birkhimer, M. L. (1975a).
    Development of a radioimmunoassay for porcine relaxin using
    ^{125}I-labeled polytyrosyl-relaxin. Endocrinology 96:1106-1113.
Sherwood, O. D., Wilson, M. E., Edgerton, L. A. and Chang, C. C.
    (1978). Serum relaxin concentrations in pigs with parturition
    delayed by progesterone administration. Endocrinolgoy
    102:471-475.
Short, R. V. (1962). Steroid concentrations in normal follicular
    fluid and ovarian cyst fluid from cows. J. Reprod. Fertil. 4:
    27-45.
Short, R. V. (1964). Ovarian steroid synthesis and secretion *in
    vivo*. Recent Progr. Hormone Res. 20:303-340.
Singh, U. B. (1975). Structural changes in the granulosa lutein
    cells of pregnant cows between 60 and 245 days. Acta Anat.
    93:447-457.
Stabenfeldt, G. H., Drost, M. and Franti, C. E. (1972). Peripheral
    plasma progesterone levels in the ewe during pregnancy and
    parturition. Endocrinology 90:144-150.
Steinetz, B. G., Beach, V. L.and Kroc, R. L. (1959). The physiology
    of relaxin in laboratory animals. In: Recent Progress in
    the Endocrinology of Reproduction (C. W. Lloyd, ed),
    Academic Press, New York. pp. 389-427.

Steinetz, B. G., Beach, V. L., Kroc, R. L., Stasilli, N. R.,
    Nussbaum, R. E., Nemith, P. J. and Dun, R. K. (1960). Bioassay
    of relaxin using a reference standard: a simple and reliable
    method utilizing direct measurement of interpubic ligament
    formation in mice. Endocrinology 67:102-115.
Stormshak, F., Inskeep, E. K., Lynn, J. E., Pope, A. L. and Casida,
    L. E. (1963). Progesterone levels in corpora lutea and
    ovarian effluent blood of the ewe. J. Anim. Sci. 22:1021-1026.
Swett, W. W., Matthews, C. A. and Fohrman, M. H. (1948). Development
    of the fetus in the dairy cow. U. S. Dept. Agric. Tech. Bull.
    964.
Thorburn, G. D., Bassett, J. M. and Smith, I. D. (1969). Proges-
    terone concentration in the peripheral plasma of sheep during
    the oestrous cycle. J. Endocrinol. 45:459-469.
Uchida, K., Kadowaki, M., Nomura, Y., Miyata, K. and Miyake, T.
    (1970). Relationship between ovarian progestin secretion
    and corpora lutea function in pregnant rats. Endocrinol.
    Jpn. 17:499-507.
Wada, H. and Yuhara, M. (1955). Studies on relaxin in ruminants.
    2. Relaxin content of the blood serum of pregnant and post-
    partum cows of the Japanese black breed of cattle. Sci. Rep.
    Fac. Agric. Okayama Univ. 7:22.
Wada, H. and Yuhara, M. (1960). Extraction of relaxin from sow
    ovary and cow tissues. Jpn. J. Zootech. Sci. 31:237.
Wada, H. and Yuhara, M. (1961). Concentration of relaxin in the
    blood serum of pregnant cow and cow with ovarian cyst. Proc.
    Silver Jubilee, Laboratory of Animal Husbandry, Kyoto University,
    pp. 61-66.
Wiqvist, N. and Paul, K. G. (1958). Inhibition of the spontaneous
    uterine motility *in vitro* as a bioassay of relaxin. Acta
    Endocrinol. 29:135-146.
Zarrow, M. X. and O'Conner, W. B. (1966). Localization of relaxin
    in the corpus luteum of the rabbit. Proc. Soc. Exp. Biol.
    Med. 121:612-614.

DISCUSSION FOLLOWING DR. L. L. ANDERSONS' PAPER

Dr. Ralph R. Anderson
    Thank you for that excellent presentation on the source of
relaxin, Dr. Anderson. This paper is now open for discussion.

Dr. Gast
    (Washington Univ., St. Louis). Dr. Anderson, I notice that
you didn't talk about the generation of the rough endoplasmic
reticulum cross-pregnancy in these animals. We might expect a
tremendous proliferation of rough ER if a protein hormone was being
elaborated intercellularly throughout pregnancy. Has there been any
work that distinguishes the presence or the growth of the amounts of
rough endoplasmic reticulum in any of the animals that you discussed?

Dr. L. L. Anderson
    Yes. I didn't allude to that. The rough endoplasmic reticulum
is abundant as pregnancy advances. However, during late stages of
pregnancy only very short stacks of rough endoplasmic reticulum are
found in the cytoplasm. At a time when the relaxin is about at
terminal stages of synthesis, we do not see much of this, just patches
of RER in the cytoplasm. Of course, we have an abundance of smooth
endoplasmic reticulum in the cytoplasm of luteal cells throughout the
whole pregnancy.

    Of course, you would presume that the rough endoplasmic reticulum
is implicated in the synthesis of dense membrane-bound granules.

Dr. Greenwood
    (Dr. Greenwood, University of Hawaii).

    I think in your '73 paper you presented some evidence for a very
small amount of release of relaxin from granules. There were very few
examples of those granules fusing and showing the release. Is that
still true?

Dr. L. L. Anderson
    We have seen little evidence of fusion of the granule to the
cytoplasmic membrane, and then release of it into the intercellular
space. Obviously, this should be examined if, indeed, these granules
are being dropped out into the intercellular spaces all at once.
Only rarely did we see ultrastructural evidence of it.

Dr. Greenwood
    That is despite a maintenance of a blood level through pregnancy?

Dr. L. L. Anderson
    No, the blood levels are relatively low during the major part
of pregnancy.

Dr. Greenwood

No the blood levels, in fact, are high. They are 2,000 picograms/ ml. It is a question of how you express the result. You quoted a figure of .322 ng/ml through pregnancy in the pig. That's a lot of picograms which are being produced per minute in a volume of distribution of 2-4 liters in the pig with a short half-life. I think my point is, it represents a massive biosynthesis of relaxin and its release throughout pregnancy in the pig. I think we're overly fascinated by the granule population. From our ovarian perfusion studies I would regard the biosynthesis in the ovaries as being directed to the release of relaxin and the maintenance of blood levels, and the granule population is almost a side point.

Dr. L. L. Anderson

During the whole of pregnancy, from early on until day 100, peripheral blood levels of relaxin, according to Dr. Sherwood's results, are around .2 of a nanogram to one nanogram, which I presume to be low in comparison to the massive release of relaxin at or near parturition.

Now, you might argue that this is indeed high during the whole of pregnancy. I do not know whether it is high or not, but it is markedly lower than what you find at the end of pregnancy.

Maybe Dr. Sherwood would like to comment.

Dr. Sherwood

Peripheral plasma relaxin immunoactivity levels which were determined at 10-day intervals throughout the first 100 days of gestation ranged from 0.1 to 2 ng per ml (Sherwood *et al.*, Endocrinology 97:834, 1975). To my knowledge the physiological significance, if any, of the relatively low levels of relaxin found within the peripheral plasma during the first 100 days of pregnancy is not known. It is clear that relaxin immunoactivity levels generally range from 5 to 10 ng per ml from days 105 to 110 of gestation and increase to levels generally exceeding 100 ng per ml during the day preceeding parturition. It is my expectation that it will soon be appreciated that the relatively high plasma levels of relaxin experienced by the pig during late pregnancy make a major contribution to the preparation of the uterus for parturition.

Dr. Kendall

(University of Texas): If you have the values for half life, can you give us some information on the secretion of relaxin?

Do you have values for relaxin secretion at different stages of pregnancy?

Dr. Greenwood
   If you take ovaries throughout pregnancy and perfuse them, then you get maximum perfusion.

Dr. Kendall
   This is *in vitro*?

Dr. Greenwood
   Yes.

Dr. Steinetz
   (Ciba-Geigy): Perhaps you have some indirect evidence, Lloyd, in some of the recent work that you did with your graduate student, Mr. Kertiles. You showed that injected purified porcine CM relaxin was active in the sow in really very low doses. I think it was something like 600 micrograms a day required to dilate the uterine cervix in the pregnant sow prior to the normal time.

Dr. Greenwood
   Yes, a beautiful experiment.

Dr. Steinetz
   Then, based on that experiment the endogenous levels of relaxin must be extremely low during pregnancy or you wouldn't see any effect of these low doses on the cervix much before normal softening occurs.

Dr. L. L. Anderson
   Yes, I agree. However, we have a series of events in the uterine cervix that are occurring in late pregnancy that are not equivocable in earlier stages of pregnancy. I do not say that we could move back to day 50 or day 30 of pregnancy and by giving relaxin, demonstrate that the cervix is capable of responding by marked cervical dilation. We have not tried this.

Dr. Steinetz
   But you can dilate the cervix with low doses of exogenous relaxin before the expected time?

Dr. L. L. Anderson
   Yes, a few days before expected parturition of luteectomized gilts, exogenous relaxin can cause cervical dilatation, whereas in the saline injected-luteectomized controls, one does not get cervical dilatation, but abortion occurs with expulsion of the conceptuses.

Dr. Steinetz
   So I think if you calculate the distribution of 600 micrograms of injected relaxin in an entire pregnant sow, the blood concentration is going to be extremely low.

Dr. Bryant-Greenwood
(University of Hawaii): Dr. Geoffrey Thorburn of the University
of Brisbane, Australia has done some interesting work with the sheep,
and he says that the granules he sees within the granulosa cells
contain progesterone. Have you any comments on that?

Dr. L. L. Anderson
I would have presented some results on the sheep during this
presentation if I had more time.

I am not too familiar with the sheep work other than what you
have presented, and what Dr. Thorburn has presented on progesterone
and its relation to granule population in luteal cells.

My only comment is that, in comparison with the other two species,
such as the rat and the pig, we do not see a coincidence of relaxin
secretion and progesterone secretion in the same way at all during
pregnancy.

For example, in the pig during pregnancy, progesterone is
secreted at maximal levels early and secretion levels are maintained
throughout the whole of pregnancy, and then progesterone drops toward
the end, whereas measurable blood levels of relaxin are extremely
low throughout that major part of pregnancy and then relaxin levels
increase at the time near onset of parturition.

We assume that these two hormones, progesterone and relaxin, are
being produced by the same granulosa lutein cell. We have no
evidence to the contrary. These two hormones, a steroid and a protein,
apparently are being secreted at markedly different rates at different
times during pregnancy in the pig and rat. There is recent *in vitro*
evidence on ovine luteal cells implicating the fact that progesterone
may actually be bound by some protein associated with the granule
population of the granulosa lutein cell. Then this binding protein
presumably carries along the progesterone to the outer cytoplasmic
membrane and then extrudes the progesterone plus part of the granule
out into the intercellular space.

Now, this is largely conjecture. It is based on *in vitro*
progesterone synthesis, and the effects of LH stimulation *in vitro*
on ovine luteal cells by Sawyers, Niswender and Strubb (Colorado State
University) and on the fact that you can get discharge of both progesterone and pre-formed granules with such protein inhibitors as colchicine in this medium. The colchicine stops, of course, further
formation of granular material. These may be associated events:
The expulsion of the pre-formed granule, whether it is progesterone
or a protein associated with progesterone.

In the sheep, I do not know of other evidence that would possibly
suggest progesterone association with the granule and as a mechanism

for release.

In the pig we do not have good evidence that granules are being exocytosed in large numbers during the course of pregnancy. We have not seen this in electron micographs in several stages of pregnancy. And if, indeed, progesterone depends on getting out of the cell by tagging onto a granule, then we certainly should be looking for this event during the estrous cycle when progesterone concentrations are high but relaxin levels are low.

We have not observed many instances of exocytosis of granules in the very late pregnancy, at a time when there is very marked dispersion and solubilization of these granules in luteal cells.

Dr. Greenwood
Dr. Steinetz, can I beg a question and make a point? Six hundred micrograms injected into a volume of distribution of four liters would produce a blood level, similar to that shown by Dr. Sherwood, of 150 ng/ml just before parturition. Do you know if this is correct?

Dr. Steinetz
No, I don't. I was going to ask you if you had actually measured the half life in the pigs by an injected amount of relaxin?

Dr. Greenwood
No, but one can calculate a half-life from the switchoff of endogenous relaxin, which although an underestimate, approximates 1-2 minutes.

Dr. Steinetz
O.K. But then the single injection of 600 micrograms is only going to last, what, a minute?

Dr. Greenwood
150 ng/ml at time 0, 75 ng/ml at time 0 plus 2 minutes, etc., in the blood.

Dr. Steinetz
For how long?

Dr. Greenwood
By 10 minutes the blood levels would be about 2 ng/ml. Then, of course, you need data on the half life of relaxin on a receptor. But I think that that is enough to dilate a cervix. It is certainly more than you would need to calm down a uterus.

Dr. L. L. Anderson
Would you then presume relaxin has this role during pregnancy in the pig?

Dr. Greenwood
     I think I am led to that conclusion on the basis of these
assumptions of the half life and the rate of synthesis in pregnancy.
Why is there so much synthesis and release both *in vivo* and *in vitro*?
In fact, there may be a small amount of storage!

Dr. Boime (St. Louis)
     Fred, could you please explain how you calculate
the half life? I don't understand how you do that; what do you mean
by switch-off?

Dr. Greenwood
     In, say, lactation or in parturition, you get a short burst of
secretion of the hormone out into the plasma and then a rapid return
to base line level. One then assumes that this is an accurate release
of the hormone. With any hormone, you can then by repeat measurements
on the down part of that curve, assuming there is no more secretion
represents the decay curve as the clearance of the endogenous hormone
from plasma similar to a decay curve of exogenous injected labeled
hormone.

     To my mind, the decay curve, the switchoff of endogenous hormone,
in fact, is more physiological than injecting a battered labeled
hormone into an animal. The assumption is that there is no more
secretion. If that is not true, and some more hormone is being
secreted, it would distort the curve and make the apparent $t\frac{1}{2}$ longer.

Dr. Ralph R. Anderson
     I am wondering whether or not you have any evidence that
prostaglandins stimulate the synthesis and/or release of relaxin?

Dr. L. L. Anderson
     We have evidence that prostaglandins are involved in this
process, but we have not looked at it in that light. We have examined
the effects of oxytocin which effectively release relaxin in a very
dramatic fashion during a very few hours from granulosa lutein cells
in late pregnancy. We have not looked at the effects of exogenous
PGF_2 alpha to determine whether this would discharge pre-formed
relaxin from these cells.

     I think one curious phenomenon is that aged corpora lutea,
whether maintained by estrogen or maintained by hysterectomy in the
pig, are morphologically rather normal but they lose their ability
to produce much relaxin. Relaxin concentrations eventually decline
in these aged porcine corpora lutea (> 130 days old).

Dr. Bryant-Greenwood
     I would like to ask you about your infusion of oxytocin. Where
do you think the relaxin you see in ovarian vein blood is coming from?

Dr. L. L. Anderson
In that experiment, the animals, as I recall, were day 110 of
pregnancy, a time when one would find large amounts of relaxin in
luteal tissue. We infused the oxytocin for a period of six hours,
two units per minute. The low pre-infusion levels of relaxin
increased seven times during the prolonged infusion period of relaxin.

Now, we do not have evidence where that relaxin was coming from
a source other than the ovaries as indicated by ovarian vein plasma
concentrations of relaxin in those particular animals.

Dr. Bryant-Greenwood
Did you do it on postpartum animals?

Dr. L. L. Anderson
No, we have not. This was done during pregnancy, when one would
expect to find a lot of relaxin in the luteal tissue.

Dr. Bryant-Greenwood
Yes, but postpartum you'd expect to have an oxytocin release,
would you not?

Dr. L. L. Anderson
Yes, you would. Now, may I ask you a question in relation to
that?

In the sheep Dr. Chamley and others in your group have demonstrated immunoreactive relaxin that is released in certain amounts at
the time of delivery in the ewe or in response to a suckling stimulus
by the lamb or manual teat stimulation.

In ewes the corpora lutea would regress at the end of parturition
and the ovaries would contain essentially old corpora albicantia and
perhaps some small follicles. Yet you obtain massive releases of
relaxin that occur as a marked response initially to teat stimulation
and later decline with further teat stimulation.

My question is: Where do you think this relaxin is coming from?

Dr. Bryant Greenwood
Thank you very much for asking the question. It give me an
opportunity to answer. We've just done the similar experiments in the
pig using the homologous porcine radioimmunoassay. We find also very
acute rise of relaxin in suckling. This work has just appeared the
last month or two.

There are acute releases throughout the period of expulsion of
each of the fetuses and whether this is due to actual uterine contraction or not, we don't know.

It's a very interesting thought where this relaxin is coming from, and I have two candidates at the moment. I have just completed a series of work with Dr. R. Seamark in Adelaide, South Australia, and it appears that relaxin is also produced by the granulosa cell prior to luteinization, that is, by the follicle. Therefore, the small follicles which are present could be the source of relaxin. However, in the pig, the rises on suckling are acute and the half life is very short, the levels are surprisingly high, in terms of the prepartum release. That is, they are in the order of 8 ng/ml. Therefore, I suggest another source of relaxin in the pig is the uterus.

Has anybody looked at the lactation uterus in the sow as a source of relaxin?

Dr. Frieden
(Kent State University): I don't know if this really applies, but quite a long time ago Zarrow showed that the uterus could serve as a source of relaxin, at least in the guinea pig. That was long before anybody thought of looking for it in the rat or even before any effects on the mouse were obtained. So it would not be too surprising if the uterus turned out to be a source of relaxin.

Dr. Greenwood
Dr. Rae Nagao in Dr. Bryant's lab recently did some studies on the pregnant guinea pig uterus and could detect immunoreactive relaxin in the uterus. We would go for isolation, but this would take too many animals. As I recall, the final fractions had radio-receptor activity in Dr. Mercado-Simmen's assay. I certainly think the uterus is a prime candidate.

Dr. Kendall
I just want to change the direction of the discussion a little bit. You showed a granulosa cell, I forget whether it was during pregnancy of the cycle, with a parallel arrangement of rough endoplasmic reticulum. Is that something you see consistently or can you put a marker on the time of change during pregnancy? The reason why I'm asking this question is because we find that very characteristically in placenta.

It occurs in the rabbit, for example, and I don't yet know what the stimulus is, but it is at a very specific stage of gestation. Have you noted this?

Dr. L. L. Anderson
The RER does show up in stacks during pregnancy. This starts to appear in abundance around day 30 and during later stages of pregnancy. As pregnancy advances to term, we see less rough endoplasmic reticulum and find primarily short stacks or groups of it.

We do not see a time specifically, as you mentioned for the rabbit.

Dr. Kendall
Again, I thought you made a specific point about the parallel nature.

Dr. L. L. Anderson
Well, it is typical of rough ER in luteal cells.

Dr. Wixon
(University of Missouri): Would the possibility be that the uterus is a source of relaxin--I'll ask the question and maybe someone knows. Is there any possibility that the placenta would make relaxin?

I'm thinking of that long, growing list of peptide hormones produced by the placenta.

Dr. Gast
(Washington University): We've looked at messenger RNA in cell populations encoding relaxin, and we're going to look at them a little bit more later. In those studies, we looked at placenta, not, unfortunately porcine placenta. We looked at endometrium; but unfortunately, not porcine endometrium, and in neither of those tissues did we detect messenger RNA, encoding our relaxin-containing proteins.

So in light of the heterologous nature of the systems, I think that you have to approach that kind of data with caution. But in both first trimester placenta and term placenta and in human endometrium, we didn't see anything that looked like a relaxin-producing product.

Dr. Greenwood
We have evidence that you can isolate a relaxin-like peptide with biological activity from the human placenta.

Dr. Steinetz
I'll be very interested in hearing that because we have tried to do that ourselves and have not been able to find any biological activity other than that which could be explained by the blood levels of the hormone in term placenta.

Regarding the presence of relaxin in the uterus, this is really old work by Hisaw and his colleagues, who showed that in the pregnant guinea pig and in the pregnant rabbit, one could find reasonably high levels of biologically active guinea pig pubic symphysis-relaxin in the uterus and placenta.

In our own labs, when we were looking for sources of the hormone, we did look carefully at the pregnant sow uterus and placenta, and there was no detectable relaxin bioactivity. We did not investigate the lactating animals. But my question was going to be: If you find levels in the several nanogram range in the pig uterus, I wonder why Dr. Sherwood doesn't see it with his radioimmunoassay, which is sensitive down to the picogram range, I think, 50 or so picograms?

Dr. Greenwood
    So you didn't see it in the pregnant sow uterus?

Dr. Steinetz
    We didn't see it in the pregnant sow uterus or placenta. I said I have no evidence regarding lactation; however, I wonder why Dr. Sherwood does not find measurable relaxin in his radioimmunoassay.

Dr. Bryant-Greenwood
    Could I comment on this?

We have used the pregnant sow uterus for isolation studies; there appear to be low levels of relaxin present. I don't know about lactation yet. I would suggest that we see it, whereas Dr. Sherwood didn't, because of our use of protease inhibitors throughout the isolation procedure, so that the small amounts of relaxin present are virtually chewed up during his isolation.

BIOASSAY METHODS FOR RELAXIN:

USES AND PITFALLS

B. G. Steinetz[1,2], E. M. O'Byrne[1,3], G. Weiss[2]
and C. Schwabe[4]

[1]CIBA-GEIGY CORPORATION, ARDSLEY, NY, [2]New York
University School of Medicine, New York, NY.,
[3]New York Medical College, Valhalla, NY., [4]Medical
University of South Carolina, Charleston, SC.

INTRODUCTION

The ability of aqueous extracts of porcine corpora lutea of
pregnancy to "relax" the pubic symphysis of the estrogen-primed
ovariectomized guinea pig was first described by Hisaw (1926).
Subsequent work showed that porcine luteal extracts which contained
guinea pig pubic symphysis-relaxing activity could inhibit contractions
of uterine myometrium of rats *in vitro* (Sawyer *et al.*, 1953) and
guinea pigs *in vivo* (Krantz *et al.*, 1950). Around the same time,
it was reported that crude extracts of sow corpora lutea induced
interpubic ligament formation in estrogen primed mice (Hall and
Newton, 1946; Kliman *et al.*, 1953). These basic observations led
to the development of numerous bioassay methods for relaxin which
have been amply documented in previous reviews (Frieden and Hisaw,
1953; Hall, 1960; Steinetz *et al.*, 1969). The present paper will,
therefore, be devoted primarily to a discussion of the uses (and
abuses!) of the various assay methods, the pitfalls which may be
encountered in assaying relaxin activity in impure extracts and the
growing realization that relaxin activity may be associated with a
family of related polypeptides. Of special interest are recent
observations which suggest that relaxin-like hormones obtained from
different species may not be equally effective in the classical bioassay methods.

HISTORICAL SURVEY OF RELAXIN BIOASSAYS

Guinea Pig Pubic Symphysis Palpation Assays

The first quantitative assay for relaxin activity was reported by
Abramowitz et al. (1944). The method employed ovariectomized estrogen
primed guinea pigs and defined a "guinea pig unit" (GPU) as the
dose of relaxin required to induce unmistakable mobility ("relaxation")
of the pubic symphysis of two-thirds of a group of twelve animals
(Abramowitz et al., 1944). The flexibility of the pubic symphysis
was determined subjectively by manual palpation, and scored on an
"all or none" basis. A graded scoring system was proposed by Frieden
and Hisaw (1950) and Talmadge and Hurst (1950) described a method
which combined subjectively determined palpation scores and x-ray
measurement of the interpubic distance. (We, ourselves, were unable
to correlate palpation scores and interpubic distance as determined
by x-ray (see Steinetz et al., 1969). Kroc and co-workers (1959)
later described a balanced guinea pig assay design in which pubic
symphysis responses to two or more doses of an unknown preparation
were compared with those to graded doses of a reference standard in
estrogen primed intact guinea pigs. The most important features of
the assay were the use of a scoring system of 0-6 (no detectable
to extreme flexibility of the pubic symphysis), treatment and palpation under rigid double blind conditions and independent scoring by
two or more operators (see Steinetz et al., 1969 for review). The
variability of responses of groups of 10-20 guinea pigs each to the
original Warner-Lambert Standard (150 gpu/mg) and the 95% confidence
limits are shown in Figure 1. This method though cumbersome, proved
to be reproducible and reasonably accurate, and provided potency
estimated with limits of error of less than $\pm$ 50% when 20 guinea
pigs were used at each of two or more doses of standard and unknown
(Steinetz et al., 1969).

The guinea pig pubic symphysis palpation assay may yet be
of more than historical interest. Recent work has demonstrated that
extracts of shark ovaries markedly "relax" the guinea pig pubic
symphysis but are inactive in the mouse pubic symphysis and mouse
uterine motility inhibition assays as will be described later.

Mouse Pubic Symphysis Bioassays of Relaxin

Histologic (Hall, 1956; Crelin, 1954; Storey, 1957) and roengteno-
graphic (Hall and Newton, 1947; Hall, 1948; Dorfman, 1953; Kliman
et al., 1953; Kliman and Greep, 1958) techniques have demonstrated
beyond a doubt that the pubic symphysis of the estrogen primed mouse
responds to relaxin-containing extracts with a highly specific and
dose-dependent formation of a long interpubic ligament. Kliman and
Greep (1958) discovered that a repository vehicle (Beeswax-oil)
markedly enhanced the effects of the hormone in the mouse and this

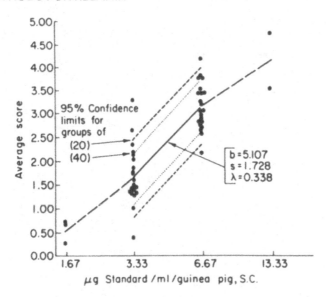

*Figure 1. Variability of guinea pig pubic symphysis palpation assay
in response to graded doses of a reference standard (W1164-
A, lot 8) over a period of 3 months. The 95% confidence
limits for different size groups of guinea pigs are shown.
Black dots indicate mean values for groups of 20 guinea
pigs each. Reproduced with permission from Steinetz et
al., 1969.*

principle was confirmed and extended by numerous investigators (Hall,
1957; Horn, 1958; Kroc *et al.*, 1959; Steinetz *et al.*, 1960). In the
popular version of the mouse assay benzopurpurine 4B is used as the
vehicle. This vehicle enhances the activity of porcine relaxin some
300 fold when compared with saline solutions of the hormone (Steinetz
et al., 1960). The mouse assay because of its simplicity, accuracy
and reproducibility, has been instrumental in the development of
superior methods for isolation and purification of relaxin from
porcine ovaries. Typical mouse bioassay results are shown in Figure
2 and the good agreement between mouse and guinea pig pubic symphysis
is illustrated in Table 1.

The mouse method has turned out not to be a panacea, for relaxin
extracts of ovaries of species other than the pig may not always
stimulate interpubic ligament formation in mice. Whether these
aberrant results are due to deficiencies in the benzopurpurine vehicle
or to an idiosyncracy of the mouse is not at all clear at present.
These problems will be discussed in a later section.

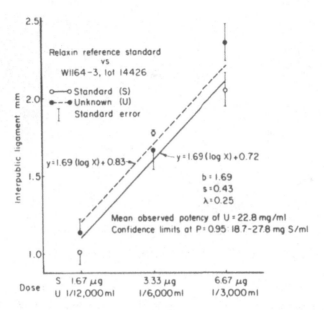

*Figure 2.   Mouse interpubic ligament bioassay of an unkown sample vs.
reference standard W1164-A, lot 8.   The unknown was made
up to an estimated concentration of 20 mg. Std/ml.
Reproduced with permission from Steinetz et al., 1960.*

Uterine Motility Assays for Relaxin

Numerous investigators reported in the 1950's that extracts of
swine corpora lutea inhibited myometrial contractions *in vivo* and
in vitro (Krantz *et al.*, 1950; Sawyer *et al.*, 1953; Felton *et al.*,
1953; Wada and Yuhara, 1956; Miller *et al.*, 1957; Wiquist and Paul,
1958; Wiquist, 1959a,b). Krantz *et al.* (1950) and Felton and
colleagues (1953) measured uterine contractility *in situ* in
anesthetized guinea pigs which had been primed for variable periods
of time with massive doses of estradiol benzoate. Aqueous extracts
of swine corpora lutea were injected i.v. and the uterine relaxin
factor ("URF") unit was defined as the dose required to induce a
90% reduction in isotonically recorded contractile amplitude. No
reference standards were employed.

Wiqvist and Paul (1958) proposed a quantal assay based on *in
vitro* inhibition of contractions of segments of uteri obtained from
estrogen-primed ovariectomized rats. Assay variables were carefully
investigated and two dose levels each of standard and unknown were
tested on segment of the same uterus. Responses to single additions
to the baths were scored visually according to the scheme illustrated
in Figure 3. A sample four-point assay is shown in Table 2.

Table 1. *COMPARISON OF BIOASSAY RESULTS ON SEVERAL IMPURE RELAXIN SAMPLES USING THE GUINEA PIG AND MOUSE PUBIC SYMPHYSIS BIOASSAY METHODS WITH RELAXIN REFERENCE STANDARD W1164A-LOT 8. REPRODUCED WITH PERMISSION FROM STEINETZ et al. (1969).*

Material and method of bioassay	Total animals (S + U)	Potency of U (mg S/ml) or mg)	Limits of error at $P = 0.95$ (%)	λ
Vialed sterile solutions				
Lot 016 (prepared from S)				
Guinea pig	120	17.4	73–137	0.40
Mouse	120	21.6	79–127	0.28
Lot 017				
Guinea pig	80	19.0	73–138	0.41
Mouse	97	22.2	78–128	0.26
Lot 14296				
Guinea pig	108	17.1	70–142	0.40
Mouse	117	17.2	76–132	0.32
Lot 14286				
Guinea pig	88	18.7	70–142	0.36
Mouse	107	14.5	82–122	0.22
Lot 018 (low potent control)				
Guinea pig	60	1.72	70–144	0.40
Mouse	140	1.70	76–132	0.30
Powders				
M30-31				
Guinea pig	85	0.74	77–131	0.27
Mouse	107	0.74	78–128	0.26
M66				
Guinea pig	120	1.06	76–131	0.33
Mouse	140	0.99	72–140	0.33
M36 (low potent control)				
Guinea pig	110	0.07	66–151	0.47
Mouse	69	0.07	81–123	0.21

Kroc *et al.* (1959) described a somewhat similar method employing uterine segments obtained from estrous mice. Again relaxin standards and unknowns were tested on segments of the same uterus. However, in this version, the test preparations were added to the baths at 5 minute intervals in doses which doubled the concentration until a similar degree of inhibition of motility was observed (e.g. 50, 75, or 100%). A typical assay is shown in Figure 4.

Numerous other investigators have studied the effects of relaxin on myometrial contractions since these early reports (Wiqvist, 1959c; Rudzik and Miller, 1962a,b; Paterson, 1965; Naagai, 1966; Khalig, 1968; Porter, 1972, 1974; Porter and Challis, 1974, 1979), and these studies have done much to elucidate the mechanism of the

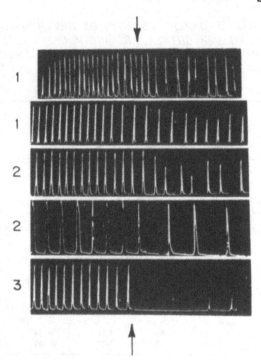

Figure 3. *Rat uterine motility inhibition scoring system of Wiqvist*
and Paul (1958). Responses to single additions of hormones
in vitro are assigned subjective scores of 0 (no effect)
to 3 (total inhibition). Reproduced with permission.

inhibitory effects. Chamley (1978) has reported a modified bioassay
method in which CM relaxin was compared with other relaxin preparations
for effects on motility of uterine segments of estrogen primed rats.
Chamley found that (according to the nomenclature of Sherwood and
O'Byrne, 1974) porcine relaxin CM-a[1] was much more potent than CM-B
or CM-a (Figure 5). Unfortunately, the preparations may have been
tested on different days on uterine segments obtained from different
rats (see Schwabe *et al.*, 1978, p. 209). In view of our own experience
and that of Wiqvist (1959a,b,c) the variability in response of segments of different uteri to relaxin is great. The inevitable day-
to-day variations in conditions of any bioassay raise further doubts
about Chamley's findings. In our own experience, utilizing estrous
mouse uterine segments (method of Kroc *et al.*, 1959), CM-a, CM-a[1]
and CM-B exert approximately equipotent inhibitory effects on
mymetrial contractility (Figure 6, Table 3). Also, Fields *et al.*
(1980) found that mouse uterine motility-inhibiting and mouse pubic
symphysis-relaxin activities of their porcine relaxin fractions
(labeled C1, C2 and C3) were in reasonable agreement. However, a
rat/mouse species difference in myometrial contraction-inhibiting
activities of porcine relaxin fractions cannot be excluded at this

Table 2. *SAMPLE RAT UTERINE MOTILITY INHIBITION ASSAY OF WIQVIST*
AND PAUL (1958). OBSERVATIONS ARE VISUAL SCORES OF
RESPONSE AS ILLUSTRATED IN FIGURE 3. REPRODUCED WITH
PERMISSION FROM WIQVIST AND PAUL (1958).

Animal No.	Standard preparation No. 3 Dose (μg)		Test preparation No. 4 Dose (μg)		Totals
	2	4	32	64	
1	0.5	1.0	0	1.5	3.0
2	0	1.0	1.5	1.0	3.5
3	1.0	2.0	3.0	3.0	9.0
4	0.5	2.0	0.5	1.0	4.0
5	0.5	2.5	0	2.5	5.5
6	2.0	2.5	1.0	2.5	8.0
7	0.5	0.5	0	0.5	1.5
8	1.5	3.0	2.0	2.0	8.5
Totals	6.5	14.5	8.0	14.0	43.0
No. of curves	8	8	8	8	32
Means	0.81	1.81	1.0	1.75	—

time, and the very important question of a highly specific uterine
relaxant variety of relaxin remains open.

RELAXIN STANDARDS

In the days when impure relaxin extracts were being studied,
bioassay reference standards were indispensible. Early standards
included porcine relaxin preparations Warner-Lambert W1164-A, lot
8 (150 GPU/mg) and Warner-Lambert W1164, 48E-2103a (1000 GPU/mg).
Subsequently the NIH purchased from the Warner-Lambert Corporation
and offered to investigators a porcine preparation similar in
electrophoretic properties to 48E- 2103a. This was designated NIH-R-P
1 and assayed 443 GPU/mg. Each of these standard preparations contained guinea pig pubic symphysis, mouse pubic symphysis and mouse
uterine motility-inhibiting properties in a ratio which did not
differ significantly from 1:1:1 when calibrated against an original
guinea pig pubic symphysis standard curve of many years experience
(Steinetz *et al.*, 1969). Essentially "pure" porcine relaxin has
assayed in the range of 1500-3000 "guinea pig units" per mg against
the impure standards by the mouse and guinea pig pubic symphysis

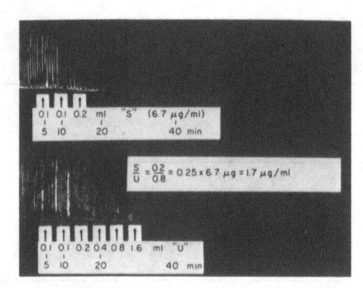

Figure 4. *Kymographic tracing of paired segments of a mouse uterus*
treated with concentration-doubling increments of standard
(S) and unknown (U) relaxin preparations. Potency ratio
was estimated from the 50% inhibitory concentrations of S
and U. Reproduced with permission from Kroc et al., 1959.

methods (Blythe *et al.*, 1965; Griss *et al.*, 1967; Sherwood and O'Byrne,
1974; Schwabe *et al.*, 1976; Frieden and Yeh, 1977). Whether or not
these preparations all possess similar myometrial contraction-
inhibiting properties has not been finally answered (see previous
section on uterine motility assays). However, hitherto unpublished
data of Turner and colleagues at Warner-Lambert suggests that highly
purified porcine relaxin peptides (isolated by starch gel electrophoresis) exhibit pubic symphysis-relaxin and uterine motility-
inhibiting activities in the expected ratios when assayed against
the same reference standard. Their data are reproduced in Table 4.
The various bio-activities of relaxin-like peptides obtained from
other species is another matter, and will be discussed in subsequent
sections.

PITFALLS IN THE BIOASSAY OF RELAXIN

Under rigidly controlled conditions, and utilizing the same
reference standard, mouse and guinea pig pubic symphysis assays
yield similar potency estimates of porcine ovarian extracts (see

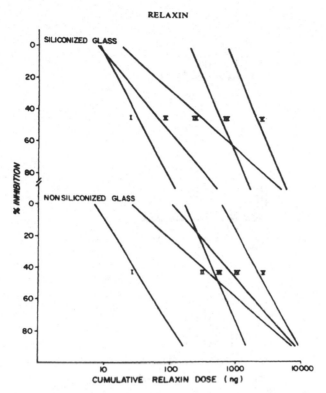

*Figure 5. Summary of rat uterine motility assays of carboxymethyl
cellulose relaxin fractions CM-a, CM-a¹ and CM-B. I =
CMa¹, II = CM-B, III = CMa, IV = NIH-R-Pl, V = W1164-3.
Reproduced with permission from Chamley, 1978.*

Table 1). However, the guinea pig assay historically has led to
serious interlaboratory differences, particularly when "guinea
pig units" based on response criteria are employed. Thus, when
results reported by five different laboratories were compared with
those obtained in our laboratory on the identical preparations assayed
double blind against a common reference standard, the "guinea pig
unit" became almost meaningless, varying up to nearly 100-fold
(Table 5).

The mouse pubic-ligament assay likewise becomes less reliable
when end-point units or "experience curves rather than concomitant
reference standards are employed. Thus, when several strains of

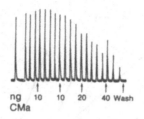

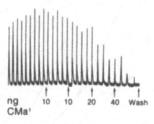

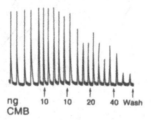

Figure 6.   Effects of increasing concentrations of carboxymethyl
cellulose-isolated (CM) relaxin peptides on spontaneous
motility of estrous mouse uterine segment in vitro.   CM
relaxin nomenclature according to Sherwood and O'Byrne
(1974).   Additions were made at 5 minute intervals to
the baths containing uterine segments in Krebs-Ringer,
bicarbonate-buffered medium (pH 7.4), aerated with O_2/CO_2,
95%/5%.   Isotonic contractions; load 1 g.

Table 3.   MOUSE UTERINE SEGMENT ASSAYS OF CM RELAXINS

Preparation (U)	No. Assays	(S)	S/U (± SE)
CMa'	5	CMa	1.0 ± 0.0
CMB	6	CMa	1.17± 0.17
CMB	4	CMa'	1.13± 0.31

Table 4. COMPARISON OF RESULTS OF MOUSE PUBIC SYMPHYSIS BIOASSAYS
AND MOUSE UTERINE MOTILITY INHIBITION ASSAYS OF RELAXIN
PEPTIDES PREPARED ACCORDING TO THE METHOD OF BLYTHE et al.
(1965).

		Uterine Motility Inhibition Assay (units/mg)			Mouse Pubic Symphysis Assay (Units/mg)	
Preparation	N	Average	Range at p=0.95	N	Average	Range at p=0.95
Standard: W1164A, lot 8	6	150		84	150	
Starch Gel Fractions:						
C-1	4	2500	1000–4100	30	2219	1660–3006
C-2	5	2500	1000–4100	30	1813	1345–2429
C-3	5	630	210–1000	30	appr. 351	–
A-5	3	30	19–38	30	appr. 29	–
A-3	3	45	24–59	–	–	–
A-1	2	50	30–69	30	206	163–272

STARCH GEL ELECTROPHORETIC PATTERN OF RELAXIN AT pH·7.3

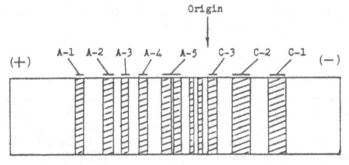

Unpublished data of Turner, Doczi and Blythe (1965) on file at Warner–Lambert
Research Institute, Morris Plains, N.J.

Table 5. *RELATIVE "SIZE" OF THE GUINEA PIG UNIT (GPU) IN 5 DIFFERENT*
LABORATORIES, WHEN ASSAYED AGAINST THE SAME REFERENCE
STANDARD. REPRODUCED WITH PERMISSION FROM STEINETZ (1963).

Laboratory	A	B	C	D	E
Sample designation	Lot No. 017	Control No. 136891	RXP 82/91	R-1	Sample "B"
Labeled potency (gpu)	3000/ml	4000/ml	600–800/ mg	1000/mg	200/mg
Potency *vs.* W1164-A, lot 8 (gpu)	3200/ml	47/ml	267/mg	196/mg	6.1/mg
Range of potency at $P = 0.95$	2550–4000	33–68	219–326	162–236	4.3–8.7
Relative "size" of gpu $\dfrac{\text{assay potency}}{\text{labeled potency}}$	1.07	0.012	0.382	0.196	0.030

mice were studied over a period of years, their sensitivity to relaxin
was found to vary markedly, and a hypothetical "mouse unit" ranged
from 2.5 to 5 µg of the relaxin reference standard (Figure 7).
Glucocorticoids and ACTH inhibit the response of the mouse pubic
symphysis to relaxin (Steinetz *et al.*, 1959) and thus stress can
have an unfavorable effect on the assay. Sudden drops in temperature,
rough animal handling and excessive noise all may reduce the
sensitivity of mice to injected relaxin.

Of greater consequence, relaxin preparations from species other
than the pig may not induce ligament formation in mice. Sherwood
(1979) observed an impaired dose response to purified rat relaxin
in mice (Figure 8). It is not clear if this is an idiosyncrasy of
the mice or of the benzopurpurine vehicle. However, relaxin isolated
from the ovaries of pregnant sharks does not cause significant
elongation of the interpubic ligament in mice (Schwabe *et al.*, 1980).
We injected the shark hormone in benzopurpurine and also in 5%
beeswax in peanut oil, a mechanical retardant vehicle. In neither
case was a significant pubic symphysis response obtained (Figure 9).
However, shark relaxin elicited a dose-dependent relaxation of the
guinea pig pubic symphysis and this was parallel to that obtained
with relaxin (Figure 10).

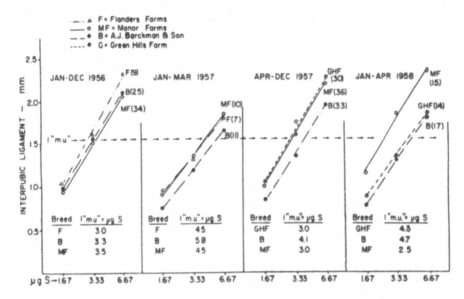

Figure 7. Seasonal variations in pubic ligament response of various
strains of mice to relaxin reference standard W1164-A, lot
8. Numbers in parentheses refer to number of assays in
each time period. Approximately 60 mice were employed for
each assay and the total number of mice representing each
curve can be derived by multiplying the number in parenthesis
by 60. Approximate limits of error at P = 0.95 are
± 15% for 308 mice, ± 10% with 686 mice and ± 5% with
2745 mice. Data on approximately 14,400 mice are shown in
the figure. "M.U." refers to a hypothetical mouse unit
or the dose of relaxin necessary to produce a mean
ligament length of 1.55 mm (midpoint of curve, January,
1956). Reproduced with permission from Steinetz et al.
(1960).

These species differences were also evident when we studied the
myometrial-inhibiting properties of purified shark relaxin (Schwabe
et al., 1980). This hormone failed to inhibit contractions of
estrous mouse uteri *in vitro* in high concentrations (Figure 11), but
was about 4% as active as porcine relaxin in inhibiting myometrial
activity of segments of estrogen-primed guinea pig uteri under
identical conditions (Figure 11). The shark hormone thus appears
to affect two major target organs of relaxin (pubic symphysis, uterus)
in guinea pigs, but not in mice (Schwabe *et al.*, 1980).

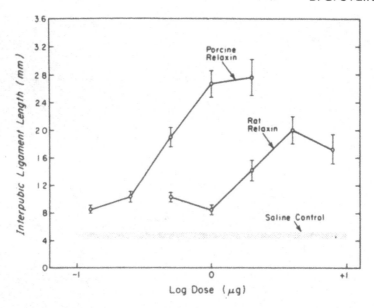

Figure 8.   A comparison of the mouse interpubic ligament responses
             to graded doses of highly purified porcine and rat relaxin.
             Twenty estrogen primed mice were used at each dose level.
             Note lack of parallelism and qualitative failure of rat
             relaxin to induce a maximal response.   Reproduced with
             permission from Sherwood (1979).

USES OF RELAXIN BIOASSAYS

      From the foregoing it is apparent that bioassays are still
required for the elucidation of the biological activities of peptides
related to porcine relaxin.   In addition, bioassays should be used
to support results obtained with radioimmunoassays (RIA's).   In
most species, peripheral blood levels of relaxin are too low to be
detected by bioassay.   However, relaxin levels in ovarian venous
blood or luteal tissue may be high enough for a bioassay.   If biological activity in such tissues correlates well with immunoactivity
in peripheral plasma as determined by RIA a strong case can be made
for secretion and circulation of the active hormone.   The best
studied animal in this regard is the pig in late pregnancy.   Anderson
and coworkers (Anderson *et al.*, 1973; Belt *et al.*, 1971) have
determined by mouse bioassay, the relaxin levels in porcine corpora
lutea and ovarian venous blood over the last several weeks of
pregnancy.   These determinations correlate well with the RIA data
of Sherwood *et al.* (1975) on peripheral plasma levels of immunoactive
relaxin over the same time course (Figure 12).   In addition, both

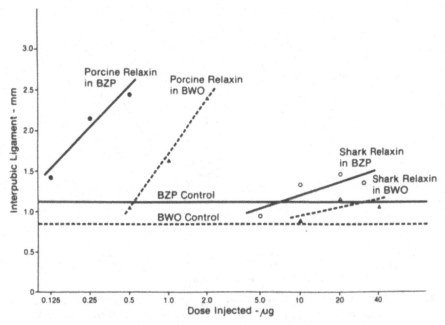

Figure 9. A comparison of the mouse interpubic ligament responses to
graded doses of highly purified porcine and shark relaxin.
Twenty estrogen primed mice were used at each dose level.
BZP = benzopurpurine vehicle. BWO = 5% beeswax in peanut
oil vehicle. None of the responses to shark relaxin were
significantly greater than control. Reproduced with
permission from Schwabe et al., 1980.

sets of data also correlate with the increase in cervical diameter
observed during this time by Kertile and Anderson (1979; Figure 12).
Thus a strong case can be made that during the last 10 days of
pregnancy in the pig luteal synthesis of relaxin increases; the
active hormone is secreted via the ovarian vein in increasing
quantities to elevate peripheral plasma levels which in turn include
softening of the uterine cervix (Figure 12).

Peripheral plasma levels of relaxin are likewise too low for
biological determination during human pregnancy. Human corpora
lutea of pregnancy contain sufficient relaxin to induce a response
in the guinea pig pubic symphysis assay (Figure 13), but the amounts
are so low that isolation and purification of the human hormone do
not seem feasible at this time. However, human luteal extracts do
cross react with rabbit anti-porcine relaxin antiserum (Figure 14)
and this finding led to the development of a heterologous RIA

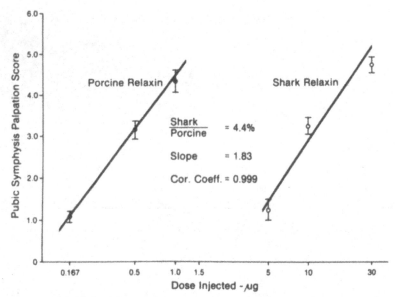

Figure 10. *A comparison of the guinea pig pubic symphysis responses*
graded doses of porcine and shark relaxin. Shark
relaxin was highly active in the guinea pig in doses which
were completely negative in the mouse assay (see Figure
9). Each point represents the mean value for 25 guinea
pigs except the 30 μg shark dose where 6 were used.
Reproduced with permission from Schwabe et al. (1980).

(O'Byrne and Steinetz, 1976; Weiss *et al.*, 1976; O'Byrne *et al.*,
1978a,b). The immunological crossreactivity appeared to be due to
a specific interaction between rabbit anti-porcine relaxin antibody
and relaxin-like substances in the human luteal extracts. Thus, the
anti-porcine relaxin antiserum partially neutralized the pubic-
symphysis-relaxing activity of the human luteal extracts in guinea
pigs (Szlachter *et al.*, 1979; Figure 15). This method has been used
to elucidate the pattern of secretion of relaxin during pregnancy
(O'Byrne *et al.*, 1978b; Quagliarello *et al.*, 1979) and to identify
the corpus luteum as the source of the immunoactive hormone
(Weiss *et al.*, 1976, 1977, 1978). A comparison of the results
obtained with the guinea pig bioassay and the heterologous RIA of
several extracts of human corpora lutea of pregnancy shows the
methods to be in reasonable agreement (Table 6). The RIA tends to
underestimate relaxin levels, as one might anticipate with a
heterologous system, but the relative amounts appear to be consistent.

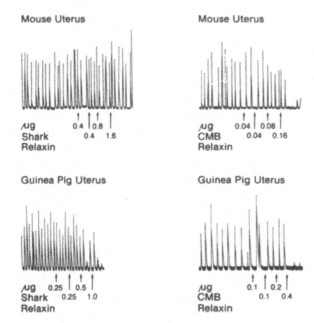

Figure 11.   *A comparison of the responses of guinea pig and mouse*
uterine segments to additions of shark and porcine (CMB)
relaxin in vitro.   Note that shark relaxin did not inhibit
motility of the mouse uterus in concentrations 10 times
those required for complete inhibition by porcine (CMB)
relaxin.   The shark hormone was about 40% as active as
the porcine hormone in inhibiting contractions of the
guinea pig uterus.   Reproduced with permission from
Schwabe et al. (1980).

<u>*CONCLUSIONS:*</u>

We conclude that the mouse pubic ligament bioassay is the
method of choice for porcine relaxin fractions but may not be as
useful for relaxin of other species (e.g. shark, rat).   The guinea
pig pubic symphysis palpation assay, with all of its obvious faults
may be preferable to the mouse method for assaying peptides with
relaxin activity from species other than the pig.

Uterine motility inhibition assays, while they offer greater
sensitivity than the pubic symphysis assays do not offer the same
degree of specificity and should only be used with purified extracts.
Crude homogenates may contain other uterine-relaxing substances
(e.g. progesterone) and/or myometrial stimulants (e.g. serotonin)
which could mask the effects of relaxin (see paper by Fields
et al. elsewhere in this publication).   There may also be marked

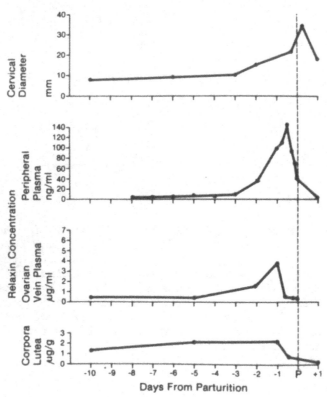

Figure 12.   Changes in the concentration of relaxin in corpora lutea,
ovarian vein and peripheral plasma and increased
dilabability of the uterine cervix in pre-parturient
pigs.   Relaxin concentrations in corpora lutea and
ovarian vein plasma were measured by mouse pubic
symphysis bioassay, and in peripheral plasma by RIA.
Composite figure redrawn from data of Anderson et al.
(1973), Belt et al. (1971), Sherwood et al. (1975) and
Kertiles and Anderson (1979).

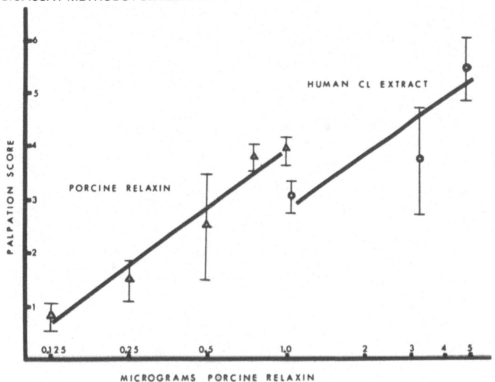

Figure 13. Guinea pig pubic symphysis palpation assay of extracts of corpora lutea obtained from women at caesarean section versus porcine CM relaxin standard. Reproduced with permission from O'Byrne et al. (1978).

differences in uterine response to relaxins of different species (e.g. shark).

Each of the bioassay methods for relaxin should employ a suitable reference standard. When this is done, potency estimates obtained with the guinea pig and mouse pubic symphysis and uterine motility inhibition bioassays are in close agreement, at least when the relaxin preparations are of porcine origin. In the case of relaxins extracted from other than porcine tissues, it is obviously important to characterize the hormonal activity on as many target tissues as possible.

We hope that recent work on the molecular biology of relaxin will eventually lead to the development of better, highly specific and more sensitive biological assays for relaxin.

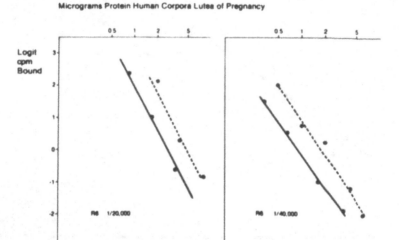

Figure 14. *Radioimmunoassay of extract of human corpora lutea of pregnancy using the heterologous porcine RIA of O'Byrne et al. (1978) at 2 different dilutions of rabbit anti-porcine relaxin antiserum R_6. Reproduced with permission from O'Byrne et al. (1978).*

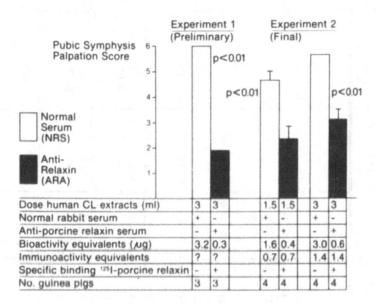

	Experiment 1 (Preliminary)			Experiment 2 (Final)				
Dose human CL extracts (ml)	3	3		1.5	1.5		3	3
Normal rabbit serum	+	–		+	–		+	–
Anti-porcine relaxin serum	–	+		–	+		–	+
Bioactivity equivalents (μg)	3.2	0.3		1.6	0.4		3.0	0.6
Immunoactivity equivalents	?	?		0.7	0.7		1.4	1.4
Specific binding ¹²⁵I-porcine relaxin	–	+		–	+		–	+
No. guinea pigs	3	3		4	4		4	4

*Figure 15. Inhibition of guinea pig pubic symphysis-relaxing activity
of human pregnancy luteal extracts by a specific antiserum to porcine relaxin. Acetone dried luteal tissue
was taken up in buffer and mixed with either rabbit-
antiporcine relaxin antiserum or normal rabbit serum
(3 ml/100 mg). Antibody excess was proven by specific
binding of [^{125}I] polytyrosyl relaxin. Note that
bioactivity was reduced 75-89% relative to the reference
standard curve (not shown). Reproduced with permission
from Szlachter et al. (1979).*

Table 6. *BIOLOGICAL VERSUS IMMUNOLOGICAL ACTIVITY OF EXTRACTS OF HUMAN CORPORA LUTEA AS DETERMINED BY GUINEA PIG SYMPHYSIS PALPATION ASSAY AND HETEROLOGOUS RIA. REPRODUCED WITH PERMISSION FROM O'BYRNE ET AL. (1978).*

Preparation	Description	Dose mg Protein	Dose RIA Relaxin ug purified porcine relaxin immunoactivity equivalents	Number guinea pigs per dose	Palpation Score ± S.E.	ug purified porcine relaxin bioactivity equivalents per mg protein	ug purified porcine relaxin immunoactivity equivalents per mg protein	Bioactivity Immunoactivity Ratio
W 1164-48E2103a	Porcine Relaxin Bioassay Reference Standard	0.0005 0.0015		38 40	1.79 ± 0.16 3.41 ± 0.13			
18-28CMA+B	Purified Porcine Relaxin RIA Standard	0.000125 0.00025 0.00050 0.00075 0.00100		6 15 17 11 29	0.77 ± 0.24 1.55 ± 0.28 2.49 ± 1.00 3.75 ± 0.21 3.90 ± 0.22			
Human CL of Pregnancy #1	Homogenate of acetone dried tissue 8 CLs	45	0.585	4	3.73 ± 0.25	0.020	0.013	1.53
Human CL of Pregnancy #2	Water soluble extract 10 CLs	9.0	0.252- 0.684	5	4.08 ± 0.38	0.124	0.028- 0.076	1.63- 4.43
Human CL of Pregnancy #3	Water soluble extract 3 CLs	1.1 3.3 4.95	0.21 0.64 0.96	4 4 2	3.00 ± 0.29 3.70 ± 1.0 5.40 ± 0.60	0.513 0.266 0.518	0.200 0.200	2.57 1.33 2.59
Human CL of Cycle #1	Water soluble extract 6 CLs	3.0 11.0	<0.0012 <0.0044	4 5	0.95 ± 0.22 1.00 ± 0.22	<0.015	<0.0004	No observed biological activity

REFERENCES

Abramowitz, A. A., Money, W. L., Zarrow, M. X., Talmage, R. V.,
     Kleinholtz, L. H. and Hisaw, F. L. (1944). Preparation, bio-
     logical assay and properties of relaxin. Endocrinology 34:103.
Anderson, L. L., Ford, J. J., Melampy, R. M. and Cox, D. F. (1973).
     Relaxin in corpora lutea during pregnancy and after hysterectomy.
     American Journal Physiol. 225:1215.
Belt, W. D., Anderson, L. L., Cavazos, L. F. and Melampy, R. M.
     (1971). Cytoplasmic granules and relaxin in corpora lutea.
     Endocrinology 89:1.
Blythe, R., Doczi, J., Palumbo, G., Phillips, G. and Turner, J.
     (1965). Isolation of relaxin peptides from a partially
     purified preparation and their characterization. Annual
     Meeting of the American Chemical Society. Abstract 57c.
Chamley, W. (1978). Discussion of paper entitled, "Relaxin",
     Rec. Progr. Horm. Res. 34:206.
Crelin, E. S. (1954). The effects of androgen, estrogen and
     relaxin on intact and transplanted pelvis in mice. American
     Journal Anatomy 95:47.
Dorfman, R. I., Marsters, R. W. and Dinerstein, J. (1953). Bio-
     assay of relaxin. Endocrinology 52:204.
Felton, L. C., Frieden, E. H. and Bryant, H. H. (1953). The effects
     of ovarian extracts upon activity of the guinea pig uterus
     in situ. J. Pharmacol. Exper. Therap. 107:160.
Fields, M. J., Fields, P. A. and Larkin, L. H. (1981). Chemistry
     of bovine relaxin. 15th Midwest Conference on Endocrinology
     and Metabolism--Relaxin. Ralph R. Anderson, ed. Plenum Press,
     publishers.
Frieden, E.H. and Hisaw, F.L. (1950). Purification and
     properties of relaxin. Arch. Biochem. 29:166.
Frieden, E. H. and Hisaw, F. L. (1953). The biochemistry of
     relaxin. Rec. Progr. Horm. Res. 8:333.
Frieden, E. H. and Yeh, L. A. (1977). Evidence for a prorelaxin.
     Proc. Soc. Exper. Biol. Med. 154:407.
Griss, G., Keck, J., Engelhorn, P. and Tuppy, H. (1967). The iso-
     lation and purification of an ovarian polypeptide with uterine-
     relaxin activity. Biochem. Biophys. Acta 140:45.
Hall, K. (1948). Further notes on the action of oestrone and
     relaxin on the pelvis of the spayed mouse, including a single
     dose of potency of relaxin. J. Endocrinol. 5:314.
Hall, K. (1957). The effect of relaxin extracts, progesterone
     and oestradiol on maintenance of pregnancy, parturition and
     rearing of young after ovariectomy in mice. J. Endocrinol.,
     15:508.
Hall, K. (1960). Relaxin. J. Reprod. Fertil. 1:368.
Hall, K. and Newton, W. H. (1946). The action of "relaxin" in the
     mouse. Lancet 1:54.

Hall, K., and Newton, W. H. (1947). The effect of oestrone and
    relaxin on the x-ray appearance of the pelvis of the mouse.
    J. Physiol. 106:18.
Hisaw, F. L. (1926). Experimental relaxation of the pubic ligament
    of the guinea pig. Proc. Soc. Exper. Biol. Med. 23:661.
Horn, E. (1958). Effects of feeding thiouracil and/or thyroid powder
    upon pubic symphyseal separation in female mice. Endocrinology
    63:481.
Kertiles, L.P. and Anderson, L. L. (1979). Effect of relaxin on
    cervical dilatation, parturition and lactation in the pig.
    Biol. Reprod. 21:57.
Khalig, H. (1968). Inhibition by relaxin of spontaneous contractions
    of the uterus of the hamster *in vitro*. J. Endocrinol. 40:125.
Kliman, B. and Greep, R. O. (1958). The enhancement of relaxin-
    induced growth of the pubic ligament in mice. Endocrinology
    63:586.
Kliman, B., Salhanick, H. and Zarrow, M. X. (1953). The response
    of the pubic symphysis of the mouse to extracts of pregnant
    rabbit serum and pregnant sow ovaries and its application as an
    assay method. Endocrinology 53:391.
Krantz, J. C., Bryant, H. H. and Carr, C. J. (1950). The action of
    aqueous corpus luteum extract upon uterine activity. Surg.
    Gynec. Obst. 90:372.
Kroc, R. L., Steinetz, B. G. and Beach, V. L. (1959). The effects
    of estrogens, progestogens and relaxin in pregnant and non-
    pregnant laboratory rodents. Ann. N.Y. Acad. Sci. 75:942.
Miller, J. H., Kesley, A. and Murray, W. J. (1957). The effects of
    relaxin-containing ovarian extracts on various types of smooth
    muscle. J. Pharm. Exper. Therap. 120:426.
Nagai, S. (1966). Regulation of relaxin secretion. Tohuku J.
    Exptl. Med. 90:219.
O'Byrne, E. M., Carriere, B. T., Sorenson, L., Segaloff, A., Schwabe,
    C., and Steinetz, B. (1978b). Plasma immunoreactive relaxin
    levels in pregnant and nonpregnant women. J. Clin. Endocrinol.
    Metab. 47:1106.
O'Byrne, E. M., Flitcraft, J., Sawyer, W. K., Hochman, J., Weiss,
    G. and Steinetz, B. G. (1979a). Relaxin bioactivity and
    immunoactivity in human corpora lutea. Endocrinology 102:1641.
O'Byrne, E. M. and Steinetz, B. G. (1976). Radioimmunoasay (RIA)
    of relaxin in sera of various species using an antiserum to
    porcine relaxin. Proc. Soc. Exper. Biol. Med. 152:272.
Porter, D. G. (1972). Myometrium of the pregnant guinea pig. The
    probable importance of relaxin. Biol. Reprod. 7:458.
Porter, D. G. (1974). Inhibition of myometrial activity in the
    pregnant rabbit: evidence for a "new" factor. Biol. Reprod.
    10:54.
Porter, D. G. and Challis, J. (1974). Failure of high uterine con-
    centrations of progesterone to inhibit myometrial activity
    in vivo in the postpartum rat. J. Reprod. Fertil. 39:157.

Paterson, G.   (1965).   The nature of the inhibition of the rat uterus
     by relaxin.   J. Pharm. Pharmacol.   17:262.
Quagliarello, J., Szlachter, N., Steinetz, B., Goldsmith, L., and
     Weiss, G.   (1979).   Serial relaxin concentrations in human
     pregnancy.   Am. Journal Obstet. Gynecol.   135:43.
Rudzik, A. and Miller, J.   (1962a).   The mechanisms of uterine
     inhibitory action of relaxin-containing ovarian extracts.
     J. Pharmacol. Exper. Therap.   138:82.
Rudzik, A. and Miller, J.   (1962b).   The effect of altering the
     catecholamine content of the uterus on the rate of contractions
     and the sensitivity of the myometrium to relaxin.   J. Pharmacol.
     Exper. Therap.   138:88.
Sanborn, B., Kuo, H., Weisbrodt, N. and Sherwood, O. D.   (1979).
     Effect of relaxin on uterine cyclic AMP levels and contractile
     activity.   Program of the 61st Annual Meeting of the Endocrine
     Society.   June 13-15.   Abstract #848.
Sawyer, W. H., Frieden, E. H. and Martin, A. C.   (1953).   *In vitro*
     inhibition of uterine contractions of the rat uterus by relaxin-
     containing extracts of sow ovaries.   Amer. J. Physiol.   172:547.
Sherwood, O. D.   (1979).   Purification and characterization of rat
     relaxin.   Endocrinology 104:886.
Sherwood, O. D., Chang, C. C., Bevier, G. W. and Dziuk, P. J.   (1975).
     Radioimmunoassay of plasma relaxin levels throughout pregnancy
     and at parturition in the pig.   Endocrinology 97:834.
Sherwood, O. D. and O'Byrne, E. M.   (1974).   Purification and
     characterization of porcine relaxin.   Arch. Biochem. Biophys.
     160:185.
Schwabe, C., McDonald, J. K. and Steinetz, B.   (1976).   Primary
     structure of the A chain of porcine relaxin.   Bioch. Biophys.
     Res. Comm.   70:397.
Schwabe, C., McDonald, J. K., O'Byrne, E. M. and Steinetz, B. G.
     (1980).   Chemical and biological properties of shark relaxin.
     Endocrinology in press.
Schwabe, C., Steinetz, B., Weiss, G., Segaloff, A., McDonald, J. K.,
     O'Byrne, E. M., Hochman, J., Cariere, B. and Goldsmith, L.
     (1978).   Relaxin.   Rec. Progr. Horm. Res.   34:123.
Steinetz, B. G.   (1963).   Relaxin assay.   Trans. N. Y. Acad. Sci.
     25:307.
Steinetz, B., Kroc, R. L., and Beach, V. L.   (1959).   The physiology
     of relaxin in laboratory animals.   In: The Endocrinology of
     Reproduction.   C. H. Lloyd, ed.   Academic Press, New York.
Steinetz, B. G., Beach, V. L. and Kroc, R. L.   (1969).   Bioassay
     of relaxin.   In: Methods in Hormone Research.   Vol. IIA,
     R. I. Dorfman, ed.   Academic Press, New York.
Steinetz, B. G., Beach, B. L., Kroc, R. L., Stasilli, N. R., Nussbaum,
     R. E., Nemith, P. J. and Dun, R. K.   (1960).   Bioassay of
     relaxin using a reference standard: a simple and reliable method
     utilizing interpubic ligament formation in mice.   Endocrinology
     67:102.

Storey, E. (1957). Relaxation in the pubic symphysis of the mouse during pregnancy and after relaxin administration, with special reference to the behavior of collagen. J. Path. Bact. 74:147.

Szlachter, N., O'Byrne, E. M., Goldmsith, L., Steinetz, B. and Weiss, G. (1979). Myometrial-inhibiting activity of relaxin-containing extracts of human corpora lutea of pregnancy. Program of the 61st Annual Meeting of the Endocrine Society, Anaheim, CA Abstract No. 574.

Talmage, R. V. and Hurst, W. R. (1950). Variability in the response of the symphysis pubic of the guinea pig to relaxin. J. Endocrinol. 7:24.

Wada, H. and Yuhara, M. (1956). Inhibitory effect of relaxin preparation upon spontaneous uterine contractions of the rat and the guinea pig in vitro. Sci. Rept. Facult. Agr. Okayama Univ. 9:11.

Weiss, G., O'Byrne, E. and Steinetz, B. (1976). Relaxin: a product of the human corpus luteum and pregnancy. Science 194:948.

Weiss, G., O'Bryne, E. M., Hochman, J., Goldsmith, L., Rifkin, I., and Steinetz, B. G. (1977). Secretion of progesterone and relaxin by the human corpus luteum at midpregnancy and at term. Obstet. Gynecol. 50:679

Weiss, G., O'Byrne, E. M., Hochman, J., Steinetz, B. G., Goldsmith, L., and Flitcraft, J. (1978). Distribution of relaxin in women during pregnancy. Obstet. Gynecol. 52:569.

Wiqvist, N. (1959a). Effects of relaxin on uterine motility and tonus in vitro and in vivo following treatment with oestradiol and progesterone. Acta Endocr. 31:391.

Wiqvist, N. (1959b). Desensitizing effect of exo- and endogenous relaxin on the immediate uterine response to relaxin. Acta Endocr. Suppl. 46:3.

Wiqvist, N. (1959c). The effect of prolonged administration of relaxin on some functional properties of the non-pregnant mouse and rat uterus. Acta Endocr. Suppl. 46:15.

Wiqvist, N. and Paul, K. G. (1958). Inhibition of the spontaneous uterine motility in vitro as a bioassay of relaxin. Acta Endocr. 29:135.

DISCUSSION FOLLOWING DR. B. G. STEINETZ'S TALK

Dr. Ralph R. Anderson
     Thank you very much for that fine presentation, Dr. Steinetz.
Dr. Steinetz's paper is now open for discussion.

Dr. Bryant-Greenwood
     As you asked me to comment, I feel as though I really ought to.
Those of you who know Wayne Chamley realize that I didn't have to
hold his hand while he was carrying out his work. But the statistics
of that was gone over very thoroughly by Dr. Finney from the University of Edinburgh, who is an expert on the statistics of bioassay,
so I have confidence that the statistics were O.K.

     One thing which I should point out and perhaps was important
why you didn't obtain the same results as we did, the preparations
in CMa, CMa^1, and CMB that we used weren't the ones directly taken
from the CM cellulose column of the second purification step of the
Sherwood and O'Byrne procedure. We were at that time interested with
Dr. Niall in the sequence differences between those three preparations
and found that CMa and CMa^1 certainly had tremendous amounts of
contamination, one with the other. So we did a further purification
step on those preparations. So, this may be a reason for the difference.

Dr. Steinetz
     I wonder if it is proper to call them CMa, CMa^1, and CMB if they
are not prepared according to the Sherwood procedure.

Dr. Bryant-Greenwood
     They were prepared according to the Sherwood procedure; they
are just superpurified.

Dr. Kendall
     Can you tell us how they were superpurified?

Dr. Bryant-Greenwood
     They were just rerun on carboxymethyl cellulose columns.

Dr. Kendall
     Using the same gradient?

Dr. Bryant-Greenwood
     Yes.

Dr. Frieden
     I don't think I'll take the time to show the slides now, but
perhaps I can do so in connection with a later presentation. I do

have some gel electrophoretic patterns of CMa, CMa[1] and CMB provided
to me by Dr. Steinetz, compared with some of our preparations. There
is some cross-contamination indicated there.

It is not too difficult, though, I think, to clean them up. We
didn't try it, but we do have preparations that are quite similar
and quite clean.

Dr. Schwabe
(University of South Carolina): On that topic, we have reported
during the Laurentian Hormone Conference on the purification of the
CM relaxin fractions and have given an example.

In fact, Bernie, under a code name, you have assayed the other
fractions, which were similarly purified and you have recorded the
same specific activity for all samples.

Dr. Steinetz
Yes. I would have to ask what is the order of contamination
we're talking about, really? I mean, is it 2 percent, 5 percent,
10 percent? Would it be significant? Would it be significantly high
enough to affect the bioassay?

Dr. Bradshaw
You talked about the CMa, CMa' and CMb relaxins in terms of the
uterine assay. What about other assays, particularly the pubic
synthesis assay?

Dr. Steinetz
Yes. We have assayed all three in each of the assays, and we
get essentially similar potencies in the range of 2,000 to 3,000
units per milligram, with no real difference between them. I would
say a mean value is 2,500.

Dr. Bradshaw
You don't see any difference between these three forms in any
of your assays?

Dr. Steinetz
No, we don't, nor in the RIA.

I think this question is really important concerning the effects
on uterine motility, because it is bad enough to have species differences such as the mouse not reacting to shark relaxin or getting
a bizarre reaction of mice to rat relaxin, but if different preparations from the same species then have different effects on a given
endpoint like uterine motility, it's going to be very difficult to
know where we are.

Dr. Schwabe

I recall a famous controversy in the history of biochemistry between Drs. Racker and Green on the subject of the efficiency of phosphorylation and this problem was finally solved when one of the two went to the lab of the other and they found that their difference was an artifact caused by a lack of CO_2 absorbing base in the vessel of one.

I wonder whether we should not go to that same extent and have, say, Hawaii visit in New York and have these preparations assayed under one and the same condition, because I, too, feel, with Dr. Steinetz, that the answer to that question is so important that we shouldn't let it hang in the air. It is holding us all up at every step of what we are doing in terms of relaxin in different species and so on.

Dr. Steinetz

I certainly agree with you, Chris. I would just suggest that maybe we should hold this meeting in Hawaii, though.

Dr. Greenwood

First of all, I would agree wholeheartedly with your thesis that bioassay is not dead. Even the usefulness of the radioreceptor assay is, I think, under question in our lab, that Dr. Rosalia Mercado-Simmen has developed. We still feel that we have to have formal recourse to bioassay.

The answer to your last question, Bernie, is that we actually have, with Dr. Hugh Niall, a grant application in to the NSF with the Australian government to hold an Australian-USA meeting in Hawaii, in fact, next June.

Dr. Steinetz

My prayers have been answered.

Dr. Greenwood

Ours will be, if they fund it.

Dr. Schwabe

Fred, just to follow up my previous comment, I would like to hear the answer from the Hawaiian group to my suggestion, i.e., if we couldn't get together on that subject.

Dr. Greenwood

The trouble is, Dr. Schwabe, that the technique was set up by Dr. Bryant-Greenwood and an undergraduate student, Marlene Basoro. Dr. Chamley came, took over the assay and the assay was discontinued when Dr. Chamley left.

It is not a technique which I am particulary endeared with, having spent some time on it in Australia. I don't really want to

get in the position--and I don't think Gill does either--in resetting
up that assay. I don't know whether it is a moot point now or not
because I don't think it is a crucial point. We have a number of
relaxins with minor sequence differences, and that I'm prepared to
accept. I think Dr. Steinetz's data is on the more fundamental
in vivo bioassays. I don't think we should be sitting here wasting
our time arguing on an *in vitro* bioassay.

Dr. Schwabe
     At the danger of seeming stubborn about this--which I am not,
I assure you--I do see an increasing number of papers referring to
Chamley's assay and I think I differ with you on the importance of
that particular point. I think it's possibly an important physio-
ogical activity in some species. Whether we like to get into assays
or not, I believe it is a very, very important problem that
Relaxinologists ought to solve for their own curiosity as well as
for those who depend on us for that information.

Dr. Greenwood
     One very important and significant point: None of this data has
actually ever seen the light of day.

Dr. Schwabe
     It is in the proceedings of the Laurentian Hormone Conference.

Dr. Greenwood
     That was a nonreviewed publication. It's the only place that we
have been allowed to get this data anywhere out for people to look
at in detail. *Endocrinology* held that data up for a year before they
rejected the paper. What can we do? We can't publish the data.
(We have asked Dr. Chamley to submit the data to a non-American
journal).

Dr. Schwabe
     You're in an admirable position that you are getting publicity
without seeking it.

Dr. Greenwood
     Absolutely. I agree with you wholeheartedly. We have no
intention of repeating it, I can assure you.

Dr. Kendall
     Is the *in vitro* data really going to be relevant to the *in vivo*
situation?

Dr. Steinetz
     Yes, I think it is extremely relevant, or potentially so. If
you have been following the work of Porter in England, he seems to
be making a fairly good case that a relaxin-like hormone, and not

progesterone, may be responsible for maintenance of pregnancy in the guinea pig.

Dr. Kendall
    Dr. Porter's experiments are done *in vivo*?

Dr. Steinetz
    Yes. These are cross-circulation experiments.

Dr. Kendall
    The questions I am really referring to Dr. Schwabe are: How much emphasis should be put on this *in vitro* assay that Dr. Greenwood doesn't like and doesn't want to persist in? Should the experiments be going more into the *in vivo* situation?

    The technical difficulties in trying to establish a potency ratio with an *in vivo* uterine motility method are horrendous. You cannot necessarily use the same animal for standard and unknown because of the tachyphylaxis problem. This means you have to use huge groups of animals and the technology is really very difficult. For reliable potency estimates, you have to use several dose levels each (standard and unknown), with 5 to 10 animals per dose. Most of the papers on *in vivo* studies of uterine motility might contain a total of 10 animals. It is difficult. Whereas, with *in vitro* methods, which seem to show the same bioactivity, one can use the segments obtained from the same uterus on the same day and use the same preparation of medium.

Dr. Fields
    (University of Florida): We have ongoing bioassays that you covered today, including the guinea pig bioassay, but right now we do have the *in vitro* uterine strip bioassays you described by Kowk and the interpubic ligament bioassay that your program has developed. In terms of mutual ground, we would like to extend an invitation to the group to resolve this particular problem at the University of Florida with Dr. Lynn Larkin and Dr. Phillip Fields and myself.

    Now, regarding CM, carboxylmethyl cellulose, eluded relaxin, we are not working with carobxylmethyl cellulose. However, with the Bio-Gel P-10 separation with Sephadex G-50, with Sephadex G-25, going to isoelectric focusing, where we are isolating three fractions with bioactivity, there is a very distinct difference in the bio-activity of these three fractions. Again, this is not CM relaxin, but, in our hands, by isoelectric focusing, we are seeing some differences.

Dr. Steinetz
    Do you mean differences in the uterine motility tests?

Dr. Fields
    In the uterine motility bioassay that is confirmed by the inter-
pubic ligament bioassay.

Dr. Steinetz
    They agree, then, in this case?

Dr. Fields
    Yes, they agree, but the biological activity is always lower
in the interpubic ligament bioassay in our hands.

Dr. Steinetz
    Even when assayed against the same standards?

Dr. Fields
    Even when assayed against the same standard, which we are a
bit puzzled about in terms of trying to relate this to Dr. Chamley's
comment in the recent review that Dr. Schwabe and others published.

Dr. Frieden
    Maybe I ought to say a little bit about these other preparations.
We have also isolated from, starting with NIH relaxin, three electrophoretically distinct relaxins from this material, each of which is
electrophoretically homogenous and which have been assayed in a
variety of ways by, among others, the guinea pig assay in our own
laboratory, the mouse assay in Dr. Steinetz's laboratory, and by
the uterine strip assay by Dr. Chamley.

    One of these preparations is quite interesting. It has the
lowest electrophoretic mobility toward the cathode at pH 5. It
has a distinctly lower guinea pig pubic symphysis activity as
compared to the other two, which have about the same as CMa and CMa[1]
or CMb. But in Dr. Chamley's hands, at any rate, it was the most
active uterine relaxin activity or had the most active or the
greatest uterine relaxin activity of any preparation he had assayed,
being somewhere in the neighborhood of 40 times that of the standard,
which was NIH relaxin.

    In the mouse, this was rather peculiar. We don't have very
much data, as Bernie knows, but it behaved a little bit like the
shark relaxin, as I remember it. It would elongate the symphysis
pubis of the mouse, but only to a certain point. And then beyond
that, it just sort of flattened out.

    So, I think there are some peculiar things about these. Now,
it is possible--and we ought to be cautious about this--in NIH
relaxin preparations that we isolated this from RP1. It had been
around for a long time. It is possible that this particular fraction
was an artifact either of storage or of isolation, which doesn't
detract, as far as I'm concerned, from its intrinsic biological or

biochemical interest. But we are sensitive to this and are now looking for this particular material in extracts of fresh ovaries.

Dr. Steinetz
        May I ask a question? I have forgotten at the moment, how did the potency in your guinea pig assay compare with Chamley's uterine motility result?

Dr. Frieden
        In the guinea pig assay, this material was about half the activity of CMa or CMb. That is our most active fraction purified from NIH relaxin.

        Well, all right. Let's put it on the basis of the activity of our RP1, which is a good basis, and which, in our hands, is about 400 to 450 guinea pig units per milligram. But that's our standard. This stuff was about twice as active. The other purified fractions were from four to six times as active as RP1. So statistically, it was significantly different and lower.

        But in Chamley's assay, it was considerably more active than either of ours, more than RP1. Does that answer you question?

Dr. Steinetz
        I guess it does. It just fortifies, I think, what Chris and I have been saying; this sounds like a very real problem.

Dr. Frieden
        You know, I would have to put myself on the side of those who think the whole question of the *in vitro* assay on the uterus is an important thing. I guess in a sense I have a self-interest in this, because it was two of my colleagues and I who first reported this with respect to the rat. So I have, I guess you might say, a vested interest in it. But nevertheless, it does seem to me to be one of the ways in which an important significant physiological function of the rat can, in fact, be established. And I hope, like others, that we can arrange this conference in Hawaii.

Dr. Niall
        (Florey Institute, University of Melbourne): I would just like to point out that perhaps it would be nice, as I am sure we all realize, to start talking about defined chemical entities rather than peaks from carboxymethyl cellulose columns or substances obtained by other fractionation procedures. I don't want to preempt this afternoon's meeting, but we have now sequenced the different fractions in CMa, CMa[1] and CMB and I will present our results this afternoon.

Dr. Greenwood
        On Dr. Frieden I'm very pleased, and I certainly accept the data. I'm glad to see that Dr. Chamley has confirmed those observations.

But what I want to make a point on is these two target tissues. The
pubic symphysis, on our perceptions is a target tissue of fibroblast
and epithelial cells, whereas in the uterus, we're talking about
myometrial receptors. This may represent the difference between
these two bioassays.

We're not talking about a common target tissue, are we, Bernie?

Dr. Steinetz
No. I couldn't agree more. I just think that the way things
are going, we're confusing the literature again. This has happened
in the past more than a few times with relaxin. I think it would be
desirable to clarify it.

Dr. Greenwood
I'm thoroughly confused myself! I mean to ask you about human
myometrial concentrations *in vitro*. Are you saying that purified
porcine relaxin doesn't affect the human uterus?

Dr. Steinetz
That's correct.

Dr. Greenwood
Where was that uterus from?

Dr. Steinetz
These are both proliferative and luteal phase myometrial strips.
Actually, this has been known for many years. Even relatively crude
porcine extracts were reported by McGoy and others back in the '50's
not to affect human myometrial strips *in vitro*.

Dr. Greenwood
I see. This is very important from our point of view, because
obviously we're interested in looking at receptors for purified porcine relaxin in the human uterus.

Dr. Steinetz
I wouldn't look in the human uterus.

Dr. Greenwood
Thank you very much. Maybe we should!

Dr. Frieden
You might, however, look in the human cervix. There is a fair
amount of data that porcine relaxin will cause dilatation in the
human cervix.

Dr. Greenwood

That is useful, because certainly the human cervix does respond to porcine relaxin. We'll show the data this afternoon.

Dr. Ralph R. Anderson

Any other questions or comments? If not, we certainly appreciate the fine discussion we have had.

ISOLATION AND CHARACTERIZATION OF

PORCINE AND RAT RELAXIN

O. D. Sherwood[1]

School of Basic Medical Science and Department of
Physiology and Biophysics, University of Illinois
Urbana, IL   61801

INTRODUCTION

Hisaw (1926) first reported that experimentally induced
"relaxation" of the pubic ligament in guinea pigs was controlled by
hormones. In 1930 Fevold, Hisaw, and Meyer (1930) showed that an
aqueous extract of sow corpora lutea caused relaxation of the pubic
ligament in estrogen-primed, ovariectomized guinea pigs. They
named the active substance relaxin. Essentially all subsequent
efforts to isolate relaxin employed ovaries obtained from pigs
during late pregnancy since this source of relaxin is known to have
a high content of relaxin activity and is relatively easy to acquire.
Progress toward the isolation of porcine relaxin was slow. It was not
until the 1950's and early 1960's when new techniques for the
isolation and characterization of proteins, as well as improved methods
for relaxin bioassay (Steinetz *et al.*, 1960, 1969), became available
that well documented advancement was made in relaxin purification
efforts.

During the 1960's, three laboratories (Cohen, 1963; Frieden *et
al.*, 1960; Griss *et al.*, 1967) reported procedures whereby they
obtained preparations of porcine relaxin which contained high biological activity. However, the amino acid compositions of the
preparations of Cohen (1963) and Frieden *et al.* (1960) were not in
agreement with the amino acid composition of highly purified porcine
relaxin which is now available (Sherwood and O'Byrne, 1974); and

[1]Research originating from the author's laboratory was
 supported by NIH Grant 08700.

therefore, it appears likely that these preparations contained con-
taminating proteins. The porcine relaxin preparation of Griss
et al. (1967) displayed no evidence of contamination when examined by
chromatographic and electrophoretic procedures. However, the amino
acid composition of that preparation (Griss *et al.*, 1967) was not
reported; and, therefore, its homogeneity was not clearly established.
Although the physicochemical properties of porcine relaxin were not
precisely described by these workers, it is important to acknowledge
that they correctly indicated that porcine relaxin (a) is a protein
with a molecular weight between 4,000 and 10,000 (Cohen, 1963;
Frieden *et al.*, 1960; Griss *et al.*, 1967), (b) has a basic isoelectric
point (Cohen, 1963; Griss *et al.*, 1967) and (c) contains disulfide
bonds which are essential for biological activity (Cohen, 1963;
Frieden and Hisaw, 1953). Additionally, Frieden and his coworkers
reported that multiple components containing relaxin activity were
obtained when porcine relaxin was subjected to counter-current
distribution (Frieden *et al.*, 1960) and starch gel electrophoresis
(Frieden, 1963).

In 1974 we reported an isolation procedure whereby highly
purified porcine relaxin was obtained in high yields and also
described many of the physicochemical properties of the relaxin
isolated by that method (Sherwood and O'Byrne, 1974). Recently, we
reported the isolation and characterization of relaxin from a second
species--the rat (Sherwood, 1979). The present discussion will be
confined to a description of the isolation methods and characterization
studies we have conducted with porcine and rat relaxin. In order
to retain focus on principal findings, many of the experimental
details found in our original reports describing the isolation and
characterization of porcine relaxin (Sherwood and O'Byrne, 1974)
and rat relaxin (Sherwood, 1979) are omitted from this chapter.

PORCINE RELAXIN

Isolation of Porcine Relaxin

Our objective was to develop a simple procedure for the isolation
of highly purified porcine relaxin in sufficient yields to permit
rigorous chemical and physiological characterization of this hormone.
Ovaries collected from pregnant sows which contained fetuses with a
crown-rump length of 10 cm or greater were obtained from Geo A.
Hormel and Company, Austin, Minnesota, and stored at -35°C until
extracted. Our initial goal was to select a procedure for the
extraction of relaxin from porcine ovaries. Frozen whole sow
ovaries were finely ground in a meat grinder and extracted with
either (a) 40% ethanol--0.15 M sodium acetate, pH 5.5 according to
the procedure described by Koenig and King (1950) for the extraction
of gonadotropins from sheep pituitary glands, (b) an aqueous
extraction solvent which consisted of 0.2 M sodium acetate, pH 5.0,

or (c) 70% acetone -0.15 N HCl according to the procedure described
by Doczi (1963) for the extraction of relaxin from sow ovaries.
Relaxin activity within each of the three ovarian extracts, as well as
subsequent preparations obtained throughout the isolation procedure,
was determined by direct measurement mouse interpubic ligament bioassay (Steinetz et al., 1960). Table 1 shows that the acid-acetone
extract contained the least protein, highest total relaxin activity,
and highest specific activity. Therefore, this procedure (Doczi,
1963) was selected for extraction. Subsequent steps developed for
the isolation of porcine relaxin were adaptations of methods previously
used for the isolation of sheep pituitary gonadotropins (Sherwood
et al., 1970a,b). The acid-acetone extract was further purified
approximately 2.5-fold by gel filtration with Sephadex G-50 as
described in the legend to Figure 1.

Table 1.   *RECOVERY OF PROTEIN AND RELAXIN ACTIVITY FROM 1 kg OF*
FROZEN PORCINE OVARIES.

Extraction Method	Protein Yield g/kg	Total Biological Activity U/kg	Specific Activity U/mg
a) 40% ethanol - 0.15 M acetate (pH 5.5)	10.4[a]	190,000[b]	18
b) 0.2 M acetate (pH 5.0)	46.1	120,000	3
c) 70% acetone - 0.15N HCl	1.9	780,000	410

[a]Protein determined by biuret reaction (Gornall et al., 1949).

[b]Activity determined with mouse interpubic ligament bioassays
(Steinetz et al., 1969) employing Warner-Lambert Reference
Standard W1164, 48E2103a which contained 1,000 units (U) per mg.

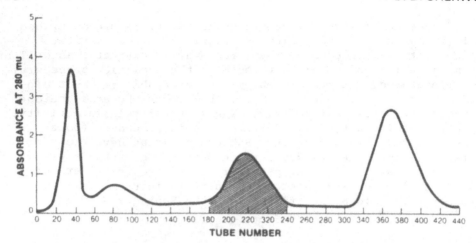

Figure 1.   Gel filtration of the acid-acetone extract (1.92 g
            protein) on a 9.4 x 115 cm column of Sephadex G-50 at
            4°C.   The column was equilibrated and run with 0.2 M
            CH₃COONH₄ buffer (pH 6.8).   The tubes containing nearly
            all of the relaxin activity (denoted by hatching) were
            pooled to form the Sephadex G-50 fraction (546 mg protein).
            (From Sherwood and O'Byrne, 1974).

Relaxin activity in the Sephadex G-50 fraction was further
purified and resolved into three highly purified porcine relaxin
preparations designated CMB, CMa, and CMa' by ion exchange
chromatography as described in the legend to Figure 2.   Table 2
summarizes the protein yields, relative potencies, confidence limits,
total relaxin activity, and ·percentage of relaxin activity recovered
in the principal porcine relaxin preparations obtained throughout
purification.   The yield of each of the highly purified relaxin
preparations CMB, CMa and CMa' was approximately 35 mg per Kg frozen
ovaries.   The relative potencies of these relaxin preparations were
2,500 to 3,000 U per mg, and they did not differ significantly
from one another. All relaxin activity is generally pooled for
biological studies.   When all relaxin activity is combined, the
total recovery of relaxin is 200-240 mg per Kg ovaries, and
approximately 70% of the relaxin activity present in the original
porcine relaxin extract is recovered.

Characterization of Porcine Relaxin

Molecular weights of the three relaxin preparations were
determined by means of sedimentation equilibrium analysis (Schachman,

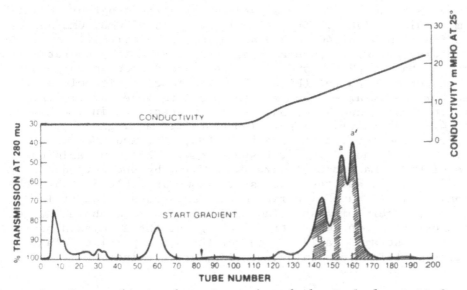

Figure 2. Ion exchange chromatography of the Sephadex G-50 fraction (546 mg) on a 2.5 x 27 cm column of CM-cellulose. The column was equilibrated and run with 0.08 M CH$_3$COOONH$_4$-CH$_3$COOH (pH 5.5) until unadsorbed protein was eluted. A linear gradient of equilibrating buffer plus NaCl was then applied to remove the three contiguous peaks which contained relaxin activity. The content of the tubes denoted by hatching were pooled to form the three relaxin preparations CMB, CMa, and CMa'. (From Sherwood and O'Byrne, 1974).

Table 2. RECOVERY OF PROTEIN AND RELAXIN ACTIVITY FROM 1 kg OF FROZEN PORCINE OVARIES.

Fraction	Yield of protein (mg)	Lower confidence limit	Relative potency	Upper confidence limit	Total units	Recovery %
Acid-acetone extract (17)[a]	1920 ± 140 (13)[b]	367	406	449	779,500	100
Sephadex G-50 (18)	546 ± 24 (10)	995	1063	1147	580,400	75
CMB (3)	38 ± 4 (4)	2010	2440	2960	92,720	12
CMa (3)	34 ± 3 (4)	2560	3070	3690	104,380	13
CMa' (3)	36 ± 2 (4)	2060	2530	3100	91,080	12

[a] Number of mouse interpubic ligament bioassays (Steinetz et al. 1960). Warner-Lambert References Standard W1164, 48E2103a (1,000 U/mg) employed as standard.

[b] Mean protein recoveries and their standard errors, determined from number of experiments in parenthesis.

1963). An estimated partial specific volume based on amino acid
composition (Schachman, 1957) was used to calculate apparent weight-
average molecular weights. The molecular weights of CMB, CMa and
CMa' were found to be 6,340, 6,370 and 6,180, respectively. Analytical
acrylamide disc gel electrophoresis of porcine relaxin preparations
CMB, CMa and CMa' at pH 4.3 showed a single broad protein component
near the center of each gel (Figure 3). The isoelectric points of
the three porcine relaxin preparations were determined by electrofocusing (Vesterberg and Svensson, 1966), as described in the legend
to Figure 4. Each relaxin preparation contained a single major
protein peak. The isoelectric points of CMB, CMa, and CMa' were
pH 10.55, pH 10.72 and pH 10.77, respectively. The amino acid compositions of CMB, CMa and CMa' were determined by the method of
Moore *et al.* (1958); and the results are shown in Table 3. When the
phenylalanine within each preparation was assigned a value of 1
residue, the recovery of most amino acids approached a whole integer;
moreover close agreement was obtained among the three relaxin preparations for most amino acids. None of the three porcine relaxin
preparations contained histidine, proline, or tyrosine.

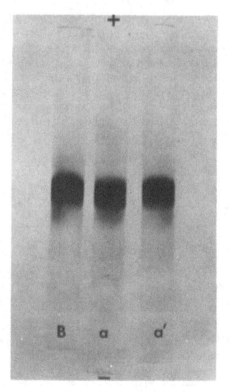

*Figure 3.   Analaytical acrylamide disc gel electrophoresis performed
              at pH 4.3 (Reisfeld et al., 1962) at 6mA per gel for 60
              min.   (From Sherwood and O'Byrne, 1974).*

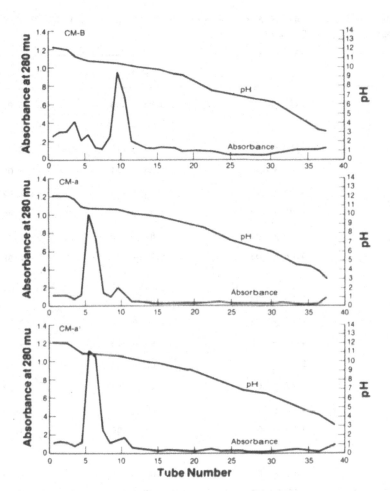

Figure 4. *Electrofocusing of 5 mg of CMB, CMa, and CMa' was conducted at 4°C in a 2% ampholyte solution at 650 V for 44 hr. At the termination of the run 3-ml fractions were collected and the pH and absorbance of each fraction was determined. (From Sherwood and O'Byrne, 1974).*

Table 3.   AMINO ACID ANALYSIS OF PURIFIED PORCINE RELAXIN PREPARATIONS
           CMB, CMa, AND CMa'.

Amino acid	CMB	CMa	CMa'
Lysine	3.20 ± .03[b]	3.05 + .04	3.08 ± .08
Histidine	-[c]	-	-
Ammonia	2.89 ± .01	3.89 ± .29	3.28 ± .01
Arginine	4.51 ± .05	5.25 ± .11	5.09 ± .06
Aspartic acid	2.86 ± .02	2.84 ± .05	2.72 ± .05
Threonine	1.85 ± .03	2.34 ± .06	1.72 ± .03
Serine	2.75 ± .03	2.81 ± .05	2.78 ± .08
Glutamic acid	4.66 ± .03	4.71 ± .11	4.58 ± .04
Proline	-	-	-
Glycine	3.20 ± .02	3.62 ± .08	3.31 ± .04
Alanine	2.28 ± .04	2.68 ± .04	2.13 ± .05
Half-cystine	4.84 ± .07	4.92 ± .15	4.95 ± .02
Valine	3.47 ± .04	3.65 ± .03	3.54 ± .05
Methionine	0.83 ± .03	0.83 ± .03	0.82 ± .05
Isoleucine	3.16 ± .02	3.26 ± .07	3.28 ± .04
Leucine	3.75 ± .04	3.93 ± .06	3.68 ± .06
Tyrosine	-	-	-
Phenylalanine[a]	1.00 ± .00	1.00 ± .00	1.00 ± .00

[a] The μmoles of phenylalanine obtained with each run were assigned one residue.

[b] The mean amino acid residues and their standard errors were calculated from four
analyses and were not corrected for destruction during hydrolysis.

[c] Histidine, proline, and tyrosine were either absent or present in trace amounts too
low to permit calculation.

Since no major contaminants were perceived with analytical acrylamide disc gel electrophoresis, electrofocusing, or amino acid analysis, it was concluded that the three preparations of porcine relaxin were sufficiently homogenous to allow further characterization studies. At that time, it was clear that relaxin was approximately the same size as insulin and, like insulin, required intact disulfide bonds for biological activity (Cohen, 1963; Frieden and Hisaw, 1953). Therefore, the disulfide bonds in relaxin were cleaved in order to determine whether relaxin, like insulin, consists of two chains linked by disulfide bonds. The three highly purified porcine relaxin preparations CMB, CMa, and CMa' were reduced with 2-mercaptoethanol and alkylated with iodoacetic acid (Crestfield *et al.*, 1963) and then separated from urea and other reagents by means of gel filtration, as described in the legend to Figure 5. Nearly all of the protein eluted in an asymmetrical peak designated 2. The shape of this peak suggested it contained two components of similar size. The elution profile of reduced CMa (peak 2) was compared to unreduced CMa by gel filtration on a long column of Sephadex G-50 in the presence of

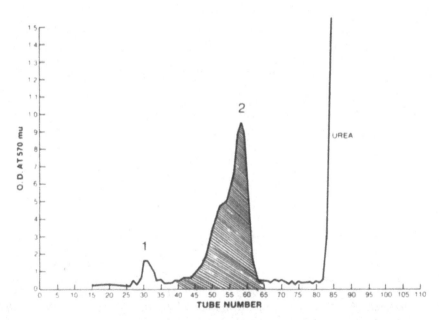

Figure 5. Gel filtration of reduced CMa (25 mg) on a 4 x 40 cm column of Sephadex G-50 which was equilibrated and run with 50% acetic acid. Protein was determined by means of ninhydrin determinations (Moore et al., 1958). The assymetrical peak 2 (denoted by hatching) was pooled and lyophilized for subsequent analysis. (From Sherwood and O'Byrne, 1974).

guanidine hydrochloride, as described in the legend to Figure 6. When reduced CMa was passed through the long column of Sephadex G-50, two major components were detected when the absorbance was read at 230 nm. When unreduced relaxin preparation CMa was passed through the Sephadex G-50 column, it eluted as a single symmetrical peak with an elution volume smaller than the two components of reduced CMa. It was concluded that porcine relaxin preparation CMa consists of two components which we originally designated α and β subunits but here acknowledge the preferred designations of A and B chains. Reduced and carboxymethylated A and B chains of porcine insulin were used as molecular weight markers and passed through the same Sephadex G-50 column. The molecular weights of the A and B chains of porcine relaxin were found to be 3,170 and 3,650, respectively when calculated according to the method of Bryce and Crichton (1971). Reduction, alkylation, and gel filtration of porcine relaxin preparations CMB and CMa' demonstrated that they also consist of two chains of a similar size.

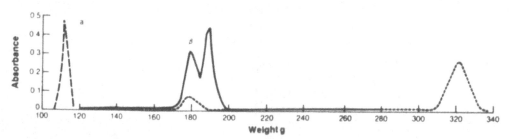

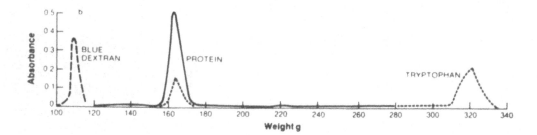

Figure 6. *Gel filtration of: (a) reduced CMa obtained, as described in the legend to Figure 5, and (b) unreduced CMa. The column (1.7 x 100 cm) contained Sephadex G-50 (Superfine) and was buffered with 0.01 M CH_3COONa-CH_3COOH, pH 5.0, containing 6 m guanidine hydrochloride. Each relaxin sample (3 mg) was charged in a volume of 0.2 ml equilibrating buffer containing 2 mg of Blue Dextran and 0.1 mg tryptophan. Blue Dextran was located by reading the absorbance at 630 mm (— —). Protein was located by reading the absorbance at 230 nm (—) and 280 nm (- - -). (From Sherwood and O'Byrne, 1974).*

The A and B chains of porcine relaxin preparation CMa were resolved by gel filtration on a long (2.7 x 200 cm) column of Sephadex G-50, and their amino acid compositions were determined (see Table 4). The A chain contained 22 amino acids; whereas, the B chain contained 28 to 31 amino acid residues. In addition to histidine, proline, and tyrosine, which were absent from the intact molecule, the A chain contained neither tryptophan nor phenylalanine; and the B chain contained no methionine.

To recapitulate, a simple procedure was developed for the preparation of high yields of three highly purified preparations of porcine relaxin. The relaxin preparations, designated CMB, CMa, and CMa', contained 2500 to 3000 U per mg biological activity when measured by the mouse interpubic ligament bioassay. Physicochemical analyses indicate the three purified relaxin preparations have molecular weights of approximately 6,300; isoelectric points ranging from pH 10.55 to pH 10.77; and contain no histidine, proline, or tyrosine. Porcine relaxin consists of two chains of similar size designated A and B. Amino acid analyses of the chains obtained from relaxin preparation CMa shows that it contains 22 amino acids in the A chain and 28 to 31 amino acids in the B chain.

RAT RELAXIN

Isolation of Rat Relaxin

We isolated rat relaxin in order to overcome limitations associated with the use of the porcine relaxin radioimmunoassay for the measurement of relaxin levels in the blood of rats (see Chapter 11). It was our objective to isolate sufficient relaxin to enable the development of a homologous radioimmunoassay for rat relaxin. Our initial effort was to determine the day of pregnancy when the relaxin content within the ovaries is highest. Anderson *et al.* (1973) earlier reported that levels of biological activity remained low through day 12 of pregnancy and increased between days 14 to 20 to peak values by day 20 of pregnancy. We confirmed these observations by determining relaxin immunoactivity levels within extracts of rat ovaries obtained throughout pregnancy. Sperm positive Sprague-Dawley derived rats were obtained from the Holtzman Co., Madison, Wisconsin; and the concentration of relaxin immunoactivity within ovarian extracts was determined with a porcine relaxin radioimmuno-assay. Consistent with Anderson *et al.* (1973), relaxin immunoactivity levels in ovarian extracts were detectable on day 10 and were maximal on day 20 of pregnancy (Figure 7).

Ovaries collected from 25 rats on day 20 of pregnancy (approximately 2.5 g) were finely ground at 4°C with a glass homogenizer in an extraction solvent consisting of 0.14 M sodium chloride and

Table 4. *AMINO ACID ANALYSIS OF RELAXIN A AND B. CHAINS OBTAINED FROM PORCINE RELAXIN PREPARATION CMa.*

Amino Acid	Chain A			Chain B		
	24 hr	72 hr	Residue	24 hr	72 hr	Residue
Lysine	2.0	1.9	2	1.1	1.1	1
Histidine	None	None		None	None	
Ammonia	1.8	1.8		3.2	3.0	
Arginine	2.9	2.8	3	2.8	2.8	3
Cm Cysteine	3.9	3.9	4	1.5	1.5	1 or 2
Aspartic acid	1.0	1.0	1	2.1	2.0	2
Threonine	0.9	0.8	1	1.6	1.4	1 or 2
Serine	0.9	0.7	1	2.7	2.0	3
Glutamic acid	2.0[a]	2.0	2	3.0	3.0	3
Proline	None	None		None	None	
Glycine	1.0	1.0	1	3.1	3.0	3
Alanine	1.0	1.0	1	1.5	1.4	1 or 2
Valine	1.0	1.0	1	2.7	2.9	3
Methionine	0.9	0.9	1	None	None	
Isoleucine	1.9	1.9	2	1.8	1.8	2
Leucine	2.0	2.0	2	2.0	2.1	2
Tyrosine	None	None		None	None	
Phenylalanine	None	None		1.0	1.0	1
Tryptophan						2[b]

Hydrolysis was conducted in 5.7 N double glass-distilled HCl under vacuum for 24 and 72 hr.

[a] All residues expressed relative to glutamic acid which was assigned two residues in the A chain and three residues in the B chain.

[b] Tryptophan determined spectrophotometrically by the method of Bencze and Schmid (1957).

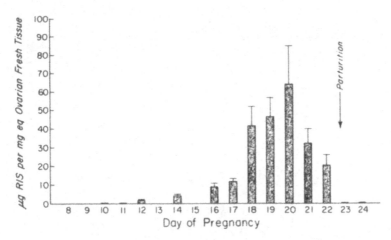

Figure 7. *Ovaries collected from two rats on each day of pregnancy*
indicated above were extracted with a solvent consisting of
0.14 M sodium chloride and 0.01 M sodium phosphate, pH 7.0.
Relaxin immunoactivity levels were determined with the
porcine relaxin radioimmunoassay (Sherwood et al., 1975).
Mean relaxin immunoactivity levels and their standard
errors are expressed relative to a relaxin immunoactivity
standard (RIS) which was an extract of rat ovaries obtained
on day 19 of pregnancy.

0.01 M sodium phosphate, pH 7.0. The relaxin extract was separated
from tissue residue by centrifugation at 45,000 rpm for 1 hr at
$4^{\circ}C$, dialyzed against 0.025% sodium chloride at $4^{\circ}C$, and lyophilized.
The rat relaxin was then purified approximately 10-fold by gel
filtration with Sephadex G-50 as described in the legend to Figure 8.
A small amount of relaxin activity was found in the first peak
eluted from the column (tubes 22-31). The contents of tubes containing nearly all of the relaxin activity were pooled to form
the Sephadex G-50 fraction.

Relaxin activity within the Sephadex G-50 fraction was further
concentrated about 10-fold and resolved into two highly purified
preparations designated CM1 and CM2 by ion exchange chromatography,
as described in the legend to Figure 9. Table 5 summarizes the
protein yields recovered in the relaxin fractions obtained throughout
the isolation procedure. The mean total yield of rat relaxin in
CM1 plus CM2 was 0.28 mg per g equivalent of ovarian tissue.

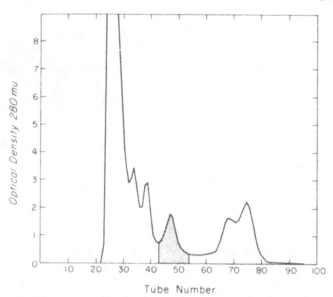

Figure 8. *Gel filtration of rat relaxin extract (70 mg protein) on*
a 2 x 90 cm column of Sephadex G-50 at 4°C. The column
was equilbrated and run with 0.01 M CH₃COONH₄-CH₃COOH (pH
5.0). The contents of tubes containing nearly all of the
relaxin activity (denoted by hatching) were pooled to form
the Sephadex G-50 fraction (5 mg protein). (From Sherwood,
1979).

Characterization of Rat Relaxin

The molecular weights of CM1 and CM2 were determined by means of
sedimentation equilibrium analysis employing the same experimental
conditions used for porcine relaxin. The molecular weights of CM1
and CM2 were 5,950 and 6,015, respectively.

Analytical acrylamide disc gel electrophoresis of CM1 and CM2
at pH 4.3 showed a single protein band near the center of each
gel. CM2 migrated slightly faster than CM1 but not as fast as
porcine relaxin (Figure 10).

The isoelectric points of CM1 and CM2 were determined by
electrofocusing (Vesterberg and Svensson, 1966), as described in
the legend to Figure 11. Electrofocusing resulted in the concentration of relaxin biological activity in CM1 and CM2 at pH 7.6 and
pH 9.4, respectively. The amino acid compositions of the two preparations of rat relaxin were determined by the method of Moore
et al. (1958). An additional sample of each was hydrolyzed in 6N
HCl containing dimethyl sulfoxide for half-cystine determinations

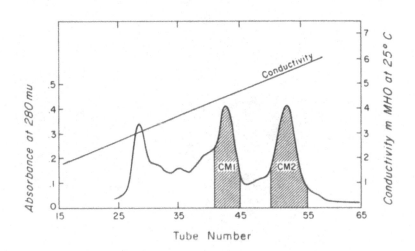

Figure 9.   *Ion exchange chromatography of the Sephadex G-50 fraction*
              (5 mg) on a 1.2 x 5.5 cm column of carboxymethyl cellulose.
              The column was equilibrated and run with 0.01 M CH₃CHOONH₄-
              CH₂COOH (pH 5.0) until unadsorbed protein was eluted.   A
              linear gradient of equilibrating buffer plus NaCl was then
              applied to remove adsorbed protein.   The contents of tubes
              containing relaxin activity (denoted by hatching) were
              pooled to form the two relaxin preparations, CM1 and CM2
              (0.35 mg protein each).   (From Sherwood, 1979).

Table 5.   RECOVERY OF PROTEIN PER GRAM OF FROZEN RAT OVARIAN TISSUE.

Fraction	Protein yield (mg/g) [a]
Rat relaxin extract	28.56 ± 1.26 (16)
Sephadex G-50	2.25 ± 0.15 (14)
CM1	0.14 ± 0.01 (9)
CM2	0.14 ± 0.01 (9)

[a] Mean protein recoveries and their standard errors were
determined from the number of experiments in parentheses.
Protein was determined by the method of Lowry et al. (1951).

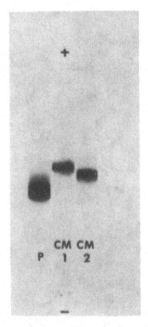

Figure 10.   Analytical acrylamide disc gel electrophoresis of porcine
*   relaxin (P), CM1, and CM2 was performed at pH 4.3*
*   (Reisfeld et al., 1962) employing 6 mA per gel for 45 min.*
*   (From Sherwood, 1979).*

(Spencer and Wold, 1969). The results are presented in Table 6.
When the assignment of residues was done as described in the legend,
the recovery of most amino acids approached a whole integer. The
amino acid compositions of CM1 and CM2 were similar but not identical--
the estimated numbers of residues for ten of the amino acids were the
same, and the estimated number of residues for the remaining seven
amino acids differed by only one residue.

      Slab gel analytical disc gel electrophoresis of reduced and
unreduced rat relaxin was conducted at pH 8.3 in Tris-HCl buffer
containing sodium dodecyl sulfate according to a modification
(Sherwood, 1979) of the procedure of Laemmli (1970). Reduction of
relaxin was conducted by placing 10-20 μg protein in sample buffer
containing 5% 2-mercaptoethanol, followed by heating at 90°C for
10 min. Figure 12 shows that unreduced CM1 and CM2 migrated with
unreduced porcine relaxin. After reduction, CM1, CM2 and porcine
relaxin migrated faster than the unreduced relaxin preparations.
Reduction did not influence the migration of cytochrome C which
does not consist of multiple chains linked by disulfide bonds.
From this experiment it was concluded that rat relaxin, like

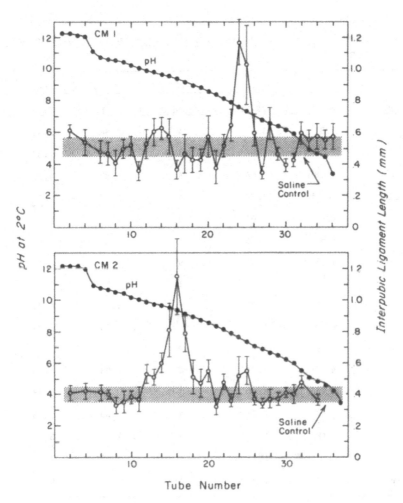

Figure 11. *Electrofocusing of 150 μg of CM1 and CM2 was conducted*
at 4°C in a 2% ampholyte solution at 650 V for 44 hr. At
the termination of the run, 3-ml fractions were collected
and the pH of each fraction was determined at 4°C. The
relaxin activity in each fraction was determined with the
mouse interpubic ligament bioassay (Steinetz et al., 1960).
Seven mice were used per fraction. The means and their
standard errors are shown in the figure above.
(From Sherwood, 1979),

Table 6. *AMINO ACID ANALYSIS OF RAT RELAXIN PREPARATIONS OF CM1 AND CM2.*

Amino acid	CM1			CM2		
	24 hr	72 hr	Residue	24 hr	72 hr	Residue
Lysine-	3.87	3.84	4	2.86	2.91	3 (3)[a]
Histidine-	1.37	1.36	1	1.24	1.33	1 (0)
Arginine-	4.08	4.04	4	4.82	4.71	5 (6)
Aspartic acid	3.55	3.89	4	2.72	2.50	3 (3)
Threonine	2.38	2.07	3	1.71	1.42	2 (3)
Serine	3.69	2.75	4	3.88	2.68	4 (4)
Glutamic acid-	8.78	8.65	9	8.12	8.12	8 (5)
Proline	-[b]	-[b]	1	-[b]	0.93	1 (0)
Glycine-	5.09	5.07	5	5.79	5.75	6 (4)
Alanine	4.45	4.35	4	4.96	5.07	5 (2)
Half-cystine	3.56[c]	-	4	4.10[c]	-	4 (6)
Valine-	3.51	3.81	4	4.08	4.05	4 (4)
Methionine-	0.86	0.90	1	0.84	0.78	1 (1)
Isoleucine	3.62	3.75	4	3.50	3.48	4 (4)
Leucine-	4.18	4.16	4	4.01	3.98	4 (4)
Tyrosine-	1.01	1.11	1	1.08	1.10	1 (0)
Phenylalanine-	0.98	1.08	1	0.78	0.85	1 (1)

The mean micromoles per residue were determined by setting the amino acids designated with a dash to the whole integers shown above. The tryptophan contents of CM1 and CM2 were not determined.

[a] The numbers of amino acid residues in porcine relaxin preparation CMa (Sherwood and O'Byrne 1974) are in parentheses.

[b] Proline peaks were too low to permit accurate measurement.

[c] Hydrolysis solution contained dimethylsulfoxide.

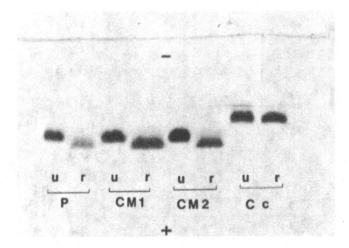

Figure 12. Slab gel analytical acrylamide disc gel electrophoresis of unreduced (U) porcine relaxin (P), CM1, CM2, cyto-chrome c (Cc), and reduced (r) porcine relaxin (P), CM1, CM2, and cytochrome c (Cc). (From Sherwood, 1979).

porcine relaxin, apparently consists of two chains of similar size which are linked by disulfide bonds.

No difference in biological potency between CM1 and CM2 was found (Figure 13). It appears that porcine relaxin is not a suitable standard for determining the relative potency of rat relaxin preparations with the mouse interpubic ligament bioassay. Larkin (1974) reported that the slope of the dose-response curve obtained with rat ovarian extract was significantly lower than the slope of the dose-response curve obtained with sow ovarian extract. We found that the response obtained with rat relaxin was less than that obtained with porcine relaxin (Figure 14). Why highly purified rat relaxin is less active than porcine relaxin in the mouse interpubic ligament bioassay is not clear. Rat relaxin may (a) be cleared from the blood more rapidly than porcine relaxin, (b) have its biological activity potentiated to a lesser degree than porcine relaxin by the repository vehicle 1% benzopurpurine 4B employed with the bioassay, (c) have been partially inactivated during the isolation procedure, or (d) interact with target tissue receptors less effectively than porcine relaxin.

To recapitulate, a procedure has been developed for the preparation of two highly purified forms of rat relaxin designated CM1 and CM2. CM1 and CM2 have molecular weights of approximately 6,000. CM1 has an isoelectric point of pH 7.6, and CM2 has an

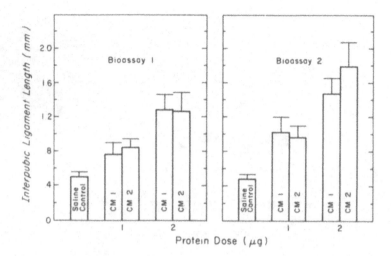

Figure 13. Bioassays of CM1 and CM2 were conducted with the mouse
interpubic ligament bioassay (Steinetz et al., 1969)
employing 10 mice per dose. The means and their standard
errors are shown above (From Sherwood, 1979).

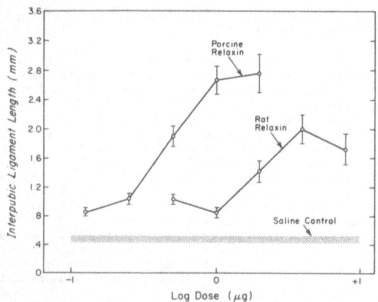

Figure 14. Comparison of biological responses obtained with multiple
doses of highly purified rat and porcine relaxin. The
bioassay (Steinetz et al., 1960) employed 20 mice per
dose. The means and their standard errors are presented
above (From Sherwood, 1979).

isoelectric point of pH 9.4. The amino acid compositions of CM1
and CM2 are similar but not identical. Rat relaxin apparently
consists of chains linked by disulfide bonds since reduced preparations
of CM1, CM2, and porcine relaxin migrate faster than unreduced
preparations when subjected to analytical acrylamide disc gel
electrophoresis in sodium dodecyl sulphate.

SUMMARY

Techniques have been developed for the isolation of porcine and
rat relaxin, and characterization studies have been conducted
with both highly purified hormone preparations. The total yield
or porcine relaxin ranged from 0.2 to 0.24 mg per gram equivalent
ovarian fresh tissue, and this yield was similar to the total yield
rat relaxin preparations CM1 plus CM2 which was 0.28 mg per gram
equivalent ovarian tissue. The characterization studies indicate
that rat relaxin is similar, but not identical, to porcine relaxin.
Rat relaxin, like porcine relaxin, apparently consists of two
chains linked by disulfide bonds since reduced preparations of
relaxin from both species migrate faster than unreduced preparations.
Moreover, the migration of reduced rat relaxin as one apparent
band seems to show that the chains of rat relaxin, like those of
porcine relaxin, are of similar size (Figure 12). No clear differences
in the sizes of porcine and rat relaxin were found when determined
by sedimentation equilibrium analyses (approximately 6,000). The
comparison of rat relaxin preparations CM1 and CM2 to porcine relaxin
preparation CMa on the basis of their estimated compositions of
the amino acid residues shown in Table 6 indicates that the rat
relaxin preparations may contain a few more residues than porcine
relaxin preparation CMa (Sherwood, 1979). The amino acid composition
of rat relaxin is similar, but not identical, to that of porcine
relaxin. The estimated numbers of residues for seven amino acids
within CM1 and eight amino acids within CM2 are identical to those
within porcine relaxin preparation CMa (Table 6). Perhaps the
most noteworthy differences between the amino acid contents of rat
relaxin and porcine relaxin are 1) the presence of histidine,
proline, and tyrosine in rat relaxin and 2) the relatively high
content of glutamic acid plus glutamine in rat relaxin.

In addition to their amino acid compositions, there are other
differences between porcine and rat relaxin. The isoelectric
points of rat relaxin preparations CM1 (pH 7.6) and CM2 (pH 9.4)
are lower than the isoelectric points of the three porcine relaxin
preparations, which range from pH 10.55 to pH 10.77. The electrophoretic mobilities of porcine relaxin and the rat relaxin preparations
CM2 and CM1 which are shown in Figure 10 differ but are consistent
with the differences in their isoelectric points. Porcine relaxin,
which has the highest isoelectric point, migrates fastest; and rat
relaxin preparation CM1, which has the lowest isoelectric point,

migrates slowest toward the cathode at pH 4.3. The biological
response obtained with rat relaxin also appears to be less than
that obtained with porcine relaxin (Figure 14).

Rat relaxin, like porcine relaxin, consists of multiple forms
which contain biological activity. The polymorphism of relaxin
may be attributed to genetic differences in amino acid sequences,
differences in amide content, or deletion of amino acids from the
N- or C-terminal.

The highly purified relaxin preparations described in this
chapter have been used for recent physiological and structural
studies. Both porcine and rat relaxin have been employed for the
development of relaxin radioimmunoassays. The development of those
radioimmunoassays and their utilization for physiological studies is
described in Chapter 11. Porcine relaxin, isolated by the
technique described in this chapter, has also been used for concurrent
amino acid sequence studies by two research groups (James *et al.*,
1977; Schwabe *et al.*, 1976, 1977); and these studies are described
in Chapters 4 and 5.

REFERENCES

Anderson, L. L., Bast, J. D. and Melampy, R. M. (1973). Relaxin in
     ovarian tissue during different reproductive stages in the
     rat. J. Endocr. 59:371.
Bencze, W. L.and Schmid, K . (1957). Determination of tyrosine and
     tryptophan in proteins. Anal. Chem. 29:1193.
Bryce, C. F. A. and Crichton, R. R. (1971). Gel filtration of
     proteins and peptides in the presence of 6 M guanidine
     hydrochloride. J. Chromatogr. 63:267.
Cohen, H. (1963). Relaxin: Studies dealing with isolation,
     purification and characterization. Trans. NY Acad. Sci.
     25:313.
Crestfield, A. M., Moore, S. and Stein, W. H. (1963). The
     preparation and enzymatic hydrolysis of reduced and S-carboxy-
     methylated proteins. J. Biol. Chem. 238:622.
Doczi, J. (1963). Process for the extraction and purification
     of relaxin. U. S. Pat 3,096,246.
Fevold, H. L., Hisaw, F. L., and Meyer, R. L. (193). The relaxative
     hormone of the corpus luteum. Its purification and concentration.
     J. Am. Chem. Soc. 52:3340.
Freiden, E. H. (1963). Purification and electrophoretic properties
     of relaxin preparations. Trans. NY Acad. Sci. 25:331.
Frieden, E. H. and Hisaw, F. L. (1953). The biochemistry of relaxin.
     Rec. Prog. Horm. Res. 8:333.

Frieden, E. H., Stone, N. R. and Layman, N. W. (1960). Nonsteroid
    ovarian hormones. III. The properties of relaxin preparations
    purified by counter-current distribution. J. Biol. Chem.
    235:2267.
Griss, G., Keck, J., Engelhorn, R. and Tuppy, H. (1967). The
    isolation and purification of an ovarian polypeptide with
    uterine-relaxin activity. Biochim. Biophys. Acta. 140:45.
Hisaw, F.L. (1926). Experimental relaxation of the pubic ligament
    of the guinea pig. Proc. Soc. Exp. Biol. Med. 23:661.
Gornall, A. G., Bardawill, C. J. and Davis, M. M. (1949). Determin-
    ation of serum proteins by means of the biuret reaction. J.
    Biol. Chem. 177:751.
James, R., Niall, H., Kwok, S., Bryant-Greenwood, G. (1977).
    Primary structure of porcine relaxin: homology with insulin
    and related growth factors. Nature (London) 267:544.
Koenig, V. L. and King, E. (1950). Extraction studies of sheep
    pituitary gonadotropic and lactogenic hormones in alcoholic
    acetate buffers. Arch Biochem. 26:219.
Laemmli, U. K. (1970). Cleavage of structural proteins during the
    assembly of the head of bacteriophage T_4. Nature (London)
    227:680.
Larkin, L. H. (1974). Bioassay of rat metrial gland extracts for
    relaxin using the mouse interpubic ligament technique.
    Endocrinology 94:567.
Lowry, O. H., Rosebrough, N. J., Farr, A. L. and Randall, R. J.,
    (1951). Protein measurement with the Folin phenol reagent.
    J. Biol. Chem. 193:265.
Moore, S., Spackman, D. H. and Stein, W. H. (1958). Chromatography
    of amino acids on sulfonated polystyrene resins. Anal. Chem.
    30:1185.
Reisfeld, R. A., Lewis, U. J. and Williams, D. E. (1962). Disk
    electrophoresis of basic proteins and peptides on polyacrylamide
    gels. Nature (London) 195:281.
Schachman, H. K. (1957). Ultracentrifugation, diffusion and
    viscometry. In: Methods in Enzymology. Colowick, S. P. and
    Kaplan, N. O., eds., Vol. 4, Academic Press, New York.
Schachman, H. K. (1963). The ultracentrifuge; problems and
    prospects. Biochemistry 2:887.
Schwabe, C., McDonald, J. K. and Steinetz, B. G. (1976). Primary
    structure of the A-chain of porcine relaxin. Biochem. Biophys.
    Res. Commun. 70:397.
Schwabe, C., McDonald, J. K. and Steinetz, B. G. (1977). Primary
    structure of the B-chain of porcine relaxin. Biochem. Biophys.
    Res. Commun. 75:503.
Sherwood, O. D. (1979). Purification and characterization of rat
    relaxin. Endocrinology 104:886.
Sherwood, O. D. and O'Byrne, E. M. (1974). Purification and
    characterization of porcine relaxin. Arch. Biochem. Biophys.
    160:185.

Sherwood, O. D. and Crnekovic, V. E. (1979). Development of a homologous radioimmunoassay for rat relaxin. Endocrinology 104:893.

Sherwood, O. D., Grimek, H. J. and McShan, W. H. (1970a). Purification and properties of follicle-stimulating hormone from sheep pituitary glands. J. Biol. Chem. 245:2328.

Sherwood, O. D., Grimek, H. J. and McShan, W. H. (1970b). Purification of luteinizing hormone from sheep pituitary glands and evidence for several physicochemically distinguishable active components. Biochim. Biophys. Acta   221:87.

Sherwood, O. D., Rosentreter, K. R., and Birkhimer, M. L. (1975). Development of a radioimmunoassay for porcine relaxin using ^{125}I-labeled polytyrosylrelaxin. Endocrinology 96:1106.

Spencer, R. L. and Wold, F. (1969). A new convenient method for estimation of total cysteine-cysteine proteins. Anal. Biochem. 32:185.

Steinetz, B. G., Beach, V. L., Kroc, R. L., Stasilli, N. R., Nussbaum, R. E., Nemith, P. J., and Dun, R. K. (1960). Bioassay of relaxin using a reference standard: A simple and reliable method utilizing direct measurement of interpubic ligament formation in mice. Endocrinology 67:102.

Steinetz, B. G., Beach, V. L. and Kroc, R. L. (1969). Bioassay of relaxin. In: Methods in Hormone Research. R. I. Dorfman, ed., Vol. 2A, 481, Academic Press, New York.

Vesterberg, O. and Svensson, H. (1966). Isoelectric fractionation, analysis and characterization of ampholytes in natural pH gradients. Acta Chem. Scand. 20:820.

DISCUSSION FOLLOWING DR. O. D. SHERWOOD'S PAPER

Dr. Bradshaw
     To me, the most interesting thing about rat and porcine relaxin
which you didn't even mention, is the apparent loss of one disulfide
bond. It is of course the disulfide structure of relaxin that makes
it so strikingly similar to insulin. This would seem to be a very
big change. Do you want to comment on that?

Dr. Sherwood
     There appear to be three possibilities. (1) Rat relaxin may have
one rather than two interchain disulfide linkages. (2) Rat relaxin
may lack the intrachain disulfide linkage in the A chain. (3) Our
estimate of 4 half-cystine residues may be incorrect. It should be
appreciated that the yields of rat relaxin are low and that our
estimate of the amino acid compositions of rat relaxin preparations
CM1 and CM2 are based on a single amino acid analysis. Rat relaxin
may have 6 half-cystine residues and 3 disulfide linkages as is the
case with porcine relaxin.

Dr. Frieden
     At various times, as I think I mentioned this morning, we have
also looked at the chemical composition of porcine relaxin using
the NIH-R-P1 preparations.

     We began our fractionation using Bio-Gel P-10 fractionation on
which relaxins are separated rather well from contaminants. Sephadex
G-50, as has already been indicated, will work perfectly well. When
we looked at the active fractions from Bio-Gel P-10 on gel electrophoresis at pH 8.8, two bands could be discerned; at lower pH (5.0)
four bands, migrating toward the cathode, can be seen.

     When we examined these by isoelectric focusing, we found two
major peaks of relaxin activity; one with an isoelectric point of
10.7; another at 9.7; and a third band of activity with considerably
lower isoelectric point. This indicated to us that we might be
successful in separating these samples by the use of column electrophoresis using the Porath technique.

     The first slide I think will show the separation we achieved
on a 60 centimeter column of G-25 operated at pH 9.0, with a cathode
at the bottom (Figure 1). The first peak that comes off is the most
rapidly moving peak and, therefore, the one with the highest isoelectric point.

     As you can see, you can get a reasonably decent separation on
this column of three distinct components.

     The pattern of the extreme right shows the original preparation,
after having been purified on Bio-Gel P-10.

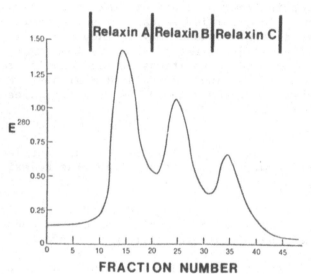

Figure 1. *Column electropherogram of 59 mg Bio-Gel--purified relaxin*
on a 1.8 x 63 cm column of Sephadex G-25. The buffer was
0.025 M NH$_4$OAc, pH 9.0. The experiment was continued for
36.5 hours at a current of 27 m.a., with the cathode at
the bottom of the column. Gel electropherograms of material
recovered from each of the three pools are superimposed.
An electropherogram of the original sample is shown at
the far right.

The next slide shows again the original preparation, and then each of the three active fractions which have been repurified by rerunning them each on the electrophoresis column and each one appears to be reasonably homogenous (Figure 2).

Now, with respect to biological activity, each of the fractions labeled A,B, and C here are active. We used the guinea pig palpation assay. Gel pattern b, which actually we call Fraction A for other reasons, is active at about 2,200 guinea pig units per milligram. Fraction B (gel pattern c) is a little bit less active, although it is probably statistically not that much different, about 1,600. But fraction C (Gel fraction d) seems to be significantly less active, having an activity about half that of the most actively moving fraction.

Dr. Steinetz was kind enough to do some immunoreactivity studies for us. A and B were equally active in precipitating anti-relaxin

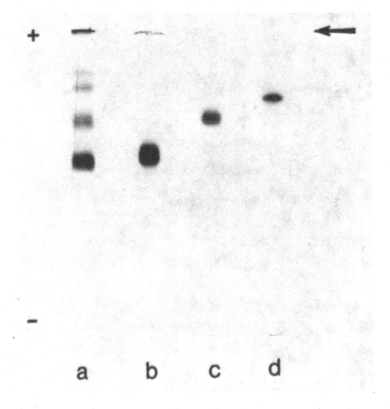

Figure 2.   Porcine relaxin fractions separated by electrophoresis.

antibody. But C had only about 35 percent of the activity of their
standard. The others actually were reported to have about 150
percent of the standard.

The next slide shows the comparison of these three fractions
with samples of CMa, CMa^1, and CMB, again kindly provided by Dr.
Steinetz. a, b, and c are CMa, CMa^1 and CMB (Figure 3).

Now, we verified the observation reported just now, that you
don't separate the three fractions, CMa, CMa^1, and CMB in the
Reisfeld gel electrophoresis procedure. But at pH 5.0, in an
ammonium acetate buffer they do, in fact, separate.

d, e, and f are our preparations--relaxin A, relaxin B, and
relaxin C--at the same pH and run under the same conditions. Although
there are slight differences, it looks like relaxin A and relaxin B
correspond pretty well to CMa and CMB, respectively. Relaxin C,
the last one over, is a little bit different.

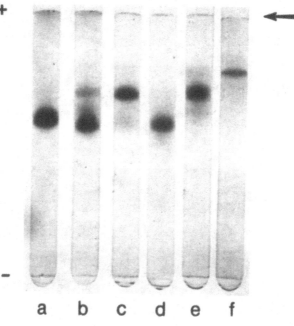

Figure 3. *Porcine relaxin fractions separated by electrophoresis at
pH 5 and compared to fractions CMa, CMa^1 and CMB, indicated
as a, b and c, respectively.*

The final slide shows the amino acid composition of our preparations, and these have been reported now on three different preparations of these materials. I'll call your attention primarily to two facts: One is that both relaxin A and relaxin C do, in fact, contain one residue of proline each. I am at a loss to explain that with respect to relaxin A, since it corresponds so nicely to CMa[1] (Table 1).

Relaxin C seems to be a different varient.

Relaxin B does, in fact, correspond very well to the material that Schwabe and McDonald have sequenced.

The small amounts of tyrosine and histidine in relaxin C may or may not be the result of heterogeneity; they may also indicate the presence of a contaminant.

Dr. Sherwood
If the two relaxin preparations described by Dr. Frieden (relaxin A and relaxin C) are devoid of contamination it would appear that we have at least two more forms of porcine relaxin to consider.

Dr. Frieden
Yes. I am still very much puzzled about our A and your A.

Dr. Sherwood
Have either Dr. Niall or Dr. Schwabe ever had reason to suspect that proline is present in either porcine relaxin preparation CMa or CMa[1]?

Dr. Bradshaw
Since Dr. Schwabe and Dr. Niall will be presenting the next two papers, it might be better to hold the discussion of this point until after they are finished.

Dr. Schwabe
I have a question. First, I think that was a nice piece of work. It certainly has spawned a regular relaxin explosion and it was a very necessary step.

I have two or three questions, however, one of which has been touched upon by the Chairman of this in suggestions already pertaining to the cystine. The others are the graph that you have published by the separation of the two chains. You recall it? The first chain that comes out is the larger one. It's the B chain. It has more peptide bonds. It has all the aromatic residues, yet in your graph, it has the lesser optical density. It has a small peak.

Assuming that there is one B chain for every A you should have had, first a large peak and then a small peak for the a chains coming out. Would you agree?

TABLE 1. *AMINO ACID ANALYSIS OF RELAXIN PEPTIDES.*

Amino Acid	Relaxin A (moles/mole Phe)	Relaxin B	Relaxin C	CM-a[2]	Cm-B	Schwabe and McDonald	James et al.
Alanine	2.5	2.6	3.1	2.7	2.3	2	2
Arginine	5.6	5.0	3.9	5.3	4.5	5	6
Aspartic acid	2.9	2.9	3.0	2.8	2.9	3	3
Half-cystine	5.3	6.0	5.4	4.8[3]	4.9[3]	6	6
Glutamic Acid	4.8	4.8	4.7	4.7	4.7	5	5
Glycine	3.75	3.6	3.4	3.6	3.2	3	4
Histidine	0	0	0.4	--	--	0	0
Isoleucine	3.6	3.4	2.8	3.3	3.2	4	4
Leucine	4.1	4.1	3.9	3.9	3.75	4	4
Lysine	3.3	3.05	3.3	3.05	3.2	3	3
Methionine	0.85	0.77	0.74	0.83	0.83	1	1
Phenylalanine	1.00	1.00	1.00	1.00	1.00	1	1
Proline	1.15	0	0.96	--	--	0	0
Serine	3.2	3.4	2.8	2.8[4]	2.75[4]	3	4
Threonine	2.1	2.1	1.7	2.3[4]	1.85[4]	2	2
Tryptophan	1.6	1.4	1.0	--	--	2	2
Tyrosine	0	0	0.2	--	--	0	0
Valine	3.7	3.6	3.2	3.65	3.5	4	4

[1] Phenylalanine was assigned one residue
[3] These samples were not oxidized
[2] From Sherwood and O'Byrne (1974)
[4] Uncorrected for destruction during hydrolysis

Dr. Sherwood
    Shall we look at that slide? Are you talking about the reduced--

Dr. Schwabe
    Yes. Porcine relaxin.

Dr. Sherwood
    Can we look at that slide?

Dr. Schwabe
    Yes.

Dr. Sherwood
    Projectionist, I would say about 43 or 44, and that could be
off plus or minus 10.

Dr. Schwabe
    Bingo! The first coming out on the left is designated Beta there,
which is a larger chain, which has, therefore, more peptide bond
absorption and the aromatic contribute significantly in the 230
range. It should have been a much larger peak.

Dr. Sherwood
    Your point is well taken.

Dr. Schwabe
    Thank you.

Dr. Sherwood
    The porcine relaxin was reduced, alkylated, and then dried
by lyophilization. As you know the reduced and alkylated B chain of
porcine relaxin is difficult to work with as it is relatively
unsoluble and tends to form aggregates. My interpretation is that the
relatively low optical density associated with the B chain is a
reflection of a low yield of the B chain relative to that of the A
chain.

Dr. Schwabe
    Secondly, I am puzzled by your ability to determine molecular
weights by autocentrifugation in the range of 6,000 to an accuracy
of 6,154 versus 6,003. I understand we have difficulties with 6,000
molecular weight molecules.

Dr. Sherwood
    It is my perception that molecular weight determination by means
of sedimentation equilibrium analysis will generally provide a value
which is within 10% of the correct value when an accurate partial
specific volume in employed for the calculation of the molecular
weight. In my presentation I indicated that the three porcine

relaxin preparations have molecular weights of approximately 6,000 and presented the precise values which were obtained (CMB = 6,340, CMa = 6,370, CMa' = 6,180) merely to document that point. The correct molecular weight of porcine relaxin could differ by approximately 600 from these values.

Dr. Schwabe

Pardon me for one more question. What have you done to determine the cystine content of rat relaxin? Obviously this is a very important point. The analysis alone can really be misleading.

Dr. Sherwood

We have conducted only the single amino acid analysis. It is possible that there may be more half-cystine in the molecule.

Dr. Boime

Dave, in one of your slides it looked like CM-1 did not have proline either. Did I misread that? Is it sure that there is proline both in CM-1 and CM-2?

Dr. Sherwood

As you know the absorbance obtained with proline during amino acid analysis is low relative to that of other amino acids. With rat relaxin preparation CM1 there was insufficient absorbance to permit an accurate determination of the quantity of proline. Nevertheless, proline was prsent in quantities sufficient to permit the suggestion that one residue of proline is present per molecule of rat relaxin preparation CM1.

Dr. Boime

In the rat, did you confirm the presence of two chains by isoelectric focusing under reduced conditions?

Dr. Sherwood

No, we did not. Following complete reduction of all disulfide linkages the biological activity of rat relaxin, like that of porcine relaxin, would likely be destroyed. It would be extremely expensive and difficult to obtain sufficient rat relaxin to conduct an isoelectric focusing experiment in which the reduced chains are located on the basis of their optical density.

Dr. Greenwood

I think it is a general question for anybody who isolates, so it is not directed specifically at David's paper. I am interested in how you distinguish between polymorphism, which is genetic and intrinsic, and proteolysis, which is an extrinsic factor?

I think that we need to be able to show the existence of these multiple relaxins in the gland or to show that they are reduced

or increased by using protease inhibitors before we can jump the
next step to say there are many relaxins and these are genetic
polymorphic forms. And I'm hoping somebody has got some data in the
next couple of days to show whether this is so.

Dr. Bradshaw
     I think that Dr. Niall and perhaps Dr. Schwabe will address
this point in their talks.

ON THE STRUCTURE AND FUNCTION OF RELAXIN

Christian Schwabe, J. Ken McDonald and
Bernard G. Steinetz

Department of Biochemistry, Medical University
of South Carolina, Charleston, S.C. 29403
CIBA-GEIGY Corporation, Ardsley, NY 10502

INTRODUCTION

The endocrinological events leading to parturition are poorly
understood. There are obvious species differences and no generali-
zations are possible at this time. In 1926 Hisaw called attention
to the fact that in some mammals an ovarian factor is produced that
leads to an enlargement of the birth canal in preparation for parturition. Subsequent work showed that this factor suppressed uterine contractions that might be harmful to the fetus. Hisaw and his
coworkers also demonstrated that this ovarian factor was not a
steroid but a protein susceptible to proteolytic action. He determined some physical properties of his new factor, relaxin, and
compared them in an almost visionary fashion with the properties of
insulin. Importantly, the involvement in parturition of a distinct
hormone was demonstrated for the first time. The next thirty years
of relaxin research was dominated by studies concerning the physiology of relaxin. The investigation of the biochemistry of relaxin
suffered from the absence of an accurate and convenient bioassay.
In 1930 Fevold *et al.* introduced the guinea pig assay which was
rather elaborate and not sufficiently objective. The introduction
of the mouse assay system by Steinetz *et al.* (1959) and the discovery of Kliman and Greep (1958) that the activity of relaxin in
mice could be enhanced more than 100-fold by simultaneous injection
of an adjuvant provided a better basis for the purification of relaxin. In the 1960's highly purified relaxin preparations were
obtained by Frieden (1963); Cohen (1963); Doczi (1963); and Griss
et al. (1967). In fact the preparations by Doczi and Griss yielded
3000 guinea pig units per milligram of relaxin, i.e., were virtually pure by present standards. Sherwood and O'Byrne (1974)

published a paper describing the large-scale preparation of relaxin. This procedure opened the way for the primary structure determination of relaxin (Schwabe *et al.*, 1976; 1977a,b,c). This structure was confirmed by James *et al.* (1977) within one year (for the A chain) and three months (for the B chain) with some variance in C-terminal residues of the B chain. Evidence for the insulin-like crosslinking (Schwabe and McDonald, 1977) has not yet been published by other laboratories.

ISOLATION AND CHEMISTRY

Utilizing the isolation method and the chromatographic step on CM cellulose described by Sherwood and O'Byrne (1974), we isolated the pure relaxin from both NIH-R-P1 preparation as well as from fresh pregnant sow ovaries. A very useful additional step proved to be chromatography on Sephadex G-75 superfine in 6 M guanidine·HCl. The relaxin did not chromatograph as a single species on ion exchange columns suggesting that charge differences existed between the various forms of relaxin. All the relaxin material obtained under these conditions had the same specific activity both in the symphysis pubis assay as well as the uterine motility inhibition assay. The amino acid composition of the various fractions occasionally differed by a serine and arginine residue suggesting that the difference between the various subspecies of relaxin might indeed be due to a less rigidly defined activation system for a putative prorelaxin compared to the well defined system that activates proinsulin.

The final obstacle to be removed from sequencing could commence was the separation of the two chains, named A and B chains by analogy to insulin. Fortuitously the first reduction and alkylation experiment was performed using radioactive iodoacetic acid. In order to obtain complete reduction and alkylation the reaction was allowed to proceed in 6 M guanidine·HCl. During dilution of the reaction mixture and preparation for dialysis, a precipitate was discovered which proved to be the B chain. The A chain remained in solution as shown by the distribution of radioactivity. This was confirmed by spectral analysis of the precipitate and the supernatant solution (Figure 1).

The sequence studies were performed using enzymes, namely dipeptidyl aminopeptidase I, carboxypeptidase A, lysosomal carboxypeptidase B, as well as the automated chemical sequence analysis in a Beckman 890C protein sequencer. In order to obtain a preliminary sequence with dipeptidyl aminopeptidase, a tyrosylated relaxin was used. This was necessary because the otherwise nonspecific DAP I does not act if arginine is at the N-terminal position of the peptide. The cyanogen-bromide-treated A chain, following treatment with DAP 1, gave rise to a set of overlapping dipeptides and thus interpretable sequence information (Figure 2). These data were in

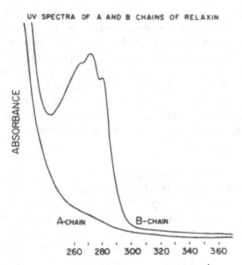

Figure 1. *Ultraviolet spectra of equal amounts of the A and B chain of relaxin.*

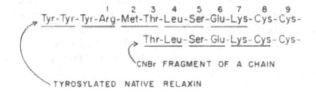

Figure 2. *Example of the use of DAP I for sequence analysis. The sequence of the A chain of relaxin begins at the #1. The tyrosine has been polymerized onto the molecule prior to digestion. The second line shows the CNBr-treated A chain. Note overlapping dipeptides produced by this procedure. The peptides were isolated by thin-layer chromatography on cellulose plates in butanol:formic acid:water (70:15:15).*

complete agreement with those obtained from the automatic protein sequencer.

The B chain sequence was inaccessible to either enzymatic or chemical approaches. Digestion of the B chain with trypsin yielded four peptides, two of which contained arginine, one containing lysine, and one lacking a basic amino acid. The lysine peptide did not contain a free amino group and was therefore tested with pyrrolidonecarboxyl peptidase (PCA peptidase). The existence of a pyro-

glutamate residue was demonstrated by thin-layer chromatography and
the PCA recovered for hydrolysis and amino acid analysis. The
tryptic peptides were then isolated in larger amounts by high
pressure liquid chromatography and each subjected to chemical
sequence analysis. It remained to place the peptides into the proper
sequence within the B chain. This was achieved by masking the lysine
residue with succinic anhydride and thus preventing the action of
trypsin between the lysine containing peptide and the neighboring
tetrapeptide. With one of the two tetrapeptides fixed the remainder
of the chain could be deduced.

In order to locate the disulfide crosslinks, the total molecule
was subjected to tryptic hydrolysis and the peptides isolated as
shown in Figure 3. Crosslink peptide 2 was expected to give a PTH
alanine and one crosslinked peptide after one cycle of Edman degradation if the crosslinking was identical to that in insulin. This
was in fact observed. The crosslinking between relaxin A-22 and
B-22 had earlier been established by digestion of intact relaxin
with lysosomal carboxypeptidase. Thus cysteines A-8 and A-13 had
to be an intra-chain disulfide bond just as in insulin.

Although the remaining amino acids were only 40% homologous with
insulin it seemed justifiable to ask whether the relaxin sequence
could be fitted to a three-dimensional insulin structure. This
question was answered affirmatively through the work of Dr. Blundell
(Birkbeck College, London, England). He built the model seen in
Figure 4 and noted that the sequence of relaxin fits the insulin
coordinates without stress or strain. This was further confirmed by

PORCINE RELAXIN

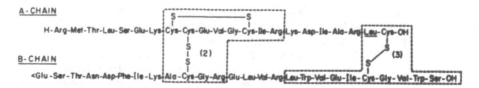

PORCINE INSULIN

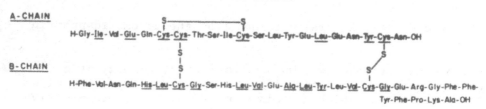

Figure 3.   The primary sequence of relaxin and insulin. The cross-
            linked peptides isolated after tryptic digestion are
            enclosed by broken lines.

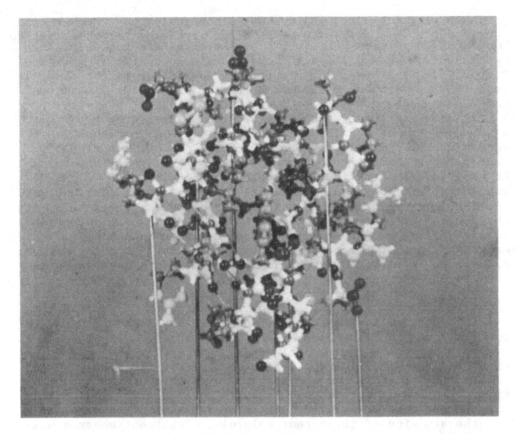

*Figure 4.   The three-dimensional model of relaxin built on the
insulin coordinates. The critical tryptophan residue is
seen edge-on in the center and the Arg-Met N terminus of
the A chain in the lower right hand corner (Bedarkar et
al., 1977).*

the similarity of the circular dichroism spectra of relaxin and insulin
in solution. The final answer to this question of course, will be
obtained when we are able to grow sufficiently large crystals of
relaxin to perform an X-ray analysis.

STRUCTURE-FUNCTION RELATIONSHIPS

The structure-function relation studies for relaxin are at about
the stage at which corresponding studies concerning insulin were ten
years ago. Today, literally hundreds of insulin-derivatives exist.
Through chemical modification it has been shown conclusively that
the glycine residue at the N terminus of the A chain, the asparagine
at the C terminus of the A chain and the C-terminal octapeptide of

the B chain of insulin are indispensable for activity. The N-terminal residue of the B chain can be modified with very large derivatives
without loss of insulin activity. These studies are not only aimed
at better understanding the action of insulin, but also at the production of slow-release insulin that might better serve the diabetic
patient. By comparison, modification of relaxin at the C terminus
of the B chain does not seem to modify the biological activity.
With histidine and tyrosine absent from the molecule the two tryptophan residues can be oxidized with N-bromosuccinimide without interference with the remainder of the structure. To our surprise, 50%
(i.e., one equivalent of tryptophan) could be oxidized without
inhibiting relaxin activity. When the second equivalent of tryptophan began to oxidize, biological activity was lost proportionately
to the loss of tryptophan. We interpret these data to mean that the
tryptophan readily accessible to water (position 25 of the B chain)
is oxidized first and the change of the indole to an oxindole,
a change which might force the C-terminal tail into an abnormal position, does not interfere with biological activity. The tryptophan
located in the hydrophobic pocket is oxidized last and concomitantly
with its disappearance the activity of relaxin disappears. This
observation suggests that the surface from which the edge of tryptophan B-18 protrudes is also the surface that interacts with the receptor. As seen in Figure 4 the N-terminal end of the A chain is
wrapped around this putative active site, particularly the two
terminal residues arginine and methionine. These two residues can
be removed very readily and specifically by cleavage with cyanogen
bromide. We have performed this cleavage under controlled conditions
and determined that des-arginylmethionine relaxin has only 20% to
30% of the activity of the parent molecule. Treatment under conditions of the CNBr cleavage, but without CNBr, leaves a fully-active
hormone. We are thus slowly beginning to obtain an outline of what
might constitute the active site of relaxin and are beginning at the
same time to learn how the insulin predecessor had to change through
millions of years to arrive at the activity that is unrelated to the
parent molecule and very specific for only the female of the species
and for one specific function during a very short period of her life
cycle (Figure 5).

EVOLUTION OF THE HORMONE

     The close relationship of relaxin to insulin and to the insulin-
like growth factor poses the question of how this diversity of
structure and function might have come about from a common ancestral
gene. In this context it seemed interesting to find out whether
sharks possess relaxin activity and whether they use a similar type
of molecule to exert the relaxin effect. Ovaries from pregnant sand
tiger sharks, when treated by the methods used for pregnant sow
ovaries, yielded a molecule similar in chemical properties to relaxin
that possessed relaxin activity in guinea pigs but not in mice.

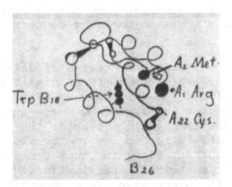

*Figure 5. Schematic drawing of the hypothetical receptor interaction
site of relaxin. The tryptophan and the Arg-Met dipeptide,
shown as solid dots, have been identified as being important
for biological activity.*

The amino acid analysis of this relaxin revealed that it is more
closely related to insulin than "modern" porcine relaxin (Table 1).
Thus, the gene duplication theory seemed to be verified when one
considers that sharks are an ancient form of life that already

*Table 1.   AMINO ACID COMPOSITION OF HOG, SHARK AND RAT RELAXINS
AND RELAXIN-LIKE PEPTIDES FROM SOW OVARIES.*

RESIDUES	SHARK	52-2	53-2	RAT	SOW
ASP	5	11	9	4	3
THR	2	4	4	3	2
SER	6	4	6	4	3
GLU	6	16	15	9	5
PRO	2	4	4	1	0
GLY	5	6	5	5	3
ALA	5	6	5	4	2
1/2 CYS	4	4	4	4	6
VAL	2	7	5	4	4
MET	1	6	2	1	1
ILE	5	5	5	4	4
LEU	4	7	10	4	4
TYR	1	2	1	1	0
PHE	2	2	3	1	1
HIS	1	2	2	2	0
LYS	5	5	7	4	3
TRP*	1	1	1	3	2
ARG	3	3	6	4	5
FACTOR*	0.203	0.400	0.351		.200
DALTONS	6,352.2	10,201.6	10,122.0	5950.0	5,480

*DETERMINED BY UV SPECTROSCOPY.

existed in the late Cambrian period (About five hundred million
years ago). The immediate questions arising concern the role of
relaxin in the shark.

At about this time we reexamined a series of marginally-active
peptides obtained from large-scale purification of hog ovarian relaxin. These fractions (52-2, 53-2) were very difficult to purify
but eventually we reached the point where we were sure that the
molecules at hand were not the relaxin of which the structure had
been published. Importantly, the peptide in fraction 53-2 was somewhat larger, contained proline, histidine, and tyrosine and possessed
only about 5% of the porcine relaxin activity in mice and about 32%
of the porcine activity in guinea pigs. The second peptide (52-2)
had less relaxin activity and contained six methionine residues
instead of the usual one. Shark relaxin is very similar to these
peptides as regards the histidine, tyrosine and proline contents.
All four preparations (shark relaxin, hog relaxin and ovarian
fractions 52-2 and 53-2) appear to contain only four residues of
cysteine. Recently Sherwood (1979) reported that rat relaxin also
has four cysteine residues and contains proline, histidine and
tyrosine.

This finding casts a shadow of doubt on the idea that diversity
has come about by specific duplication followed by slowly divergent
development of the two copies until different functions have evolved.
Instead, it is conceivable that gene duplication has been a major
preoccupation of perhaps single cellular organisms during early
evolutionary stages and that a large mass of potential DNA has been
accumulated which could be considered the genetic destiny of a cell
line. The larger this pool, the more potential for development might
exist in a specific line of single cellular organisms. According
to this hypothesis insulin and relaxin have started out at the same
time from a normal distribution of genetic material that would give
rise to related peptides. Several of these related peptides might
have acquired a function that imparted advantages to an organism.
Under evolutionary pressure, the requirement for certain functions
would become more specific causing single copies of the gene pool
to be selected from the normal distribution of relaxin or insulin-
like peptides to fulfill a more and more restricted function.
Finally, the result would be one major hormone and a number of
"runners-up" that did not quite fit this specific need of a particular species. The consequence of this model would be that every
hormone should have a few parahormones less active or barely recognizable and that different species could favor a different copy of
the normal distribution of suitable genes. Thus pregnant sows are
using the molecule that has been isolated and analyzed and sharks
may be using the molecule (for whatever reason) that looks somewhat
more like insulin but also seems closely related to rat relaxin.
In sow ovaries we find secondary relaxin molecules that have shark
relaxin-like features and might be the "losers" in the internal

competition for function. It will be exceedingly interesting to see
which copy of the relaxin gene pool humans are using and we hope
to be able to provide the answer in the near future.

REFERENCES

Bedarkar, S., Turnell, W. G., Blundell, T. L. and Schwabe, C. (1977).
    Relaxin has conformational homology with insulin. Nature
    270:449.
Cohen, H., (1963). Relaxin: studies dealing with isolation,
    purification, and characterization. Trans. N.Y. Acad. Sci.
    25:313.
Doczi, J. (1963). Process for extraction and purification of
    relaxin. U. S. Patent 3,096,246.
Fevold, H., Hisaw, F. L., and Meyer, R. K. (1930). The relaxative
    hormone of the corpus lutuem. Its purification and concentra-
    tion. J. Am. Chem. Soc. 53:3340.
Frieden, E. H. (1963). Purification and electrophoretic properties
    of relaxin preparations. Trans. N. Y. Acad. Sci. 25:331.
Griss, G., Keck, J., Engelhorn, R. and Tuppy, H. (1967). The
    isolation and purification of an ovarian polypeptide with uterine
    relaxin activity. Biochim. Biophys. Acta 140:45.
Hisaw, F. L. (1926). Experimental relaxation of the pubic ligament
    of the guinea pig. Proc. Soc. Exp. Biol. Med. 23:661.
James, R., Niall, H., Kwok, S. and Bryant-Greenwood, G. (1977).
    Primary structure of porcine relaxin: homology with insulin
    and related growth factors. Nature 267:544.
Kliman, B. and Greep, R. O. (1958). The enhancement of relaxin-
    induced growth of the pubic ligament in mice. Endocrinology
    63:586.
Schwabe, C. and Braddon, S. (1976). Evidence for one essential
    tryptophan residue at the active site of relaxin. Biochem.
    Biophys. Res. Commun. 68:1126.
Schwabe, C. and McDonald, J. K. (1977). Relaxin: a disulfide
    homolog of insulin. Science 197:914.
Schwabe, C., McDonald, J. K. and Steinetz, B. (1976). Primary
    structure of the A chain of porcine relaxin. Biochem. Biophys.
    Res. Commun. 70:397.
Schwabe, C., McDonald, J. K. and Steinetz, B. (1977). Primary
    structure of the B chain of porcine relaxin. Biochem. Biophys.
    Res. Commun. 75:503.
Sherwood, O. D. and O'Byrne, E. M. (1974). Purification and charac-
    terization of porcine relaxin. Arch. Biochem. Biophys. 160:185.
Sherwood, O. D. (1979). Purification and characterization of rat
    relaxin. Endocrinology 104:886.
Steinetz, B., Beach, V. L. and Kroc, R. L. (1959). The physiology
    of relaxin in laboratory animals, in: "Recent Progress in the
    Endocrinology of Reproduction", C. H. Lloyd, ed., Academic
    Press, New York.

DISCUSSION FOLLOWING DR. C. SCHWABE'S PAPER

Dr. Jeffrey
       (Washington University, St. Louis, Missouri): I assume that
there is no insulin with less than three disulfides that has been so
far identified. How about shark insulin?

Dr. Schwabe
       Correct. I haven't seen any insulin that has less than the
prerequesite disulfide bonds.

Dr. Niall
       One point I can perhaps add to that. Katsoyannis has made a
synthetic insulin which has no intrachain disulfide bond in the A
chain. He finds low, but nevertheless, detectable activity, in this
insulin analogue with two half cystines replaced by alanines. Though,
I think this is a situation, which you would agree, is far from
being sorted out, it is at least theoretically possible to have
insulin like activity with only two disulfide bridges in the molecule.

Dr. Schwabe
       That is a very good point. Disulfide bonds are, of course,
not a directing force in structure formation.

Dr. Bylander
       (Kent State University): I noticed on the last slide you showed
there is a nerve growth factor shown on the slide. I would like
to hear your comments on how it fits in with the insulin and proinsulin evolutionary scheme.

Dr. Schwabe
       Well, you would have to ask that, wouldn't you? Now, this is
a personal bias, you will understand, and at the risk of losing a
few important parts of myself, I feel nerve growth factor does not
fit.   The x-ray crystallographers argued about the nerve growth
factor (NGF) during the Insulin Symposium in Aachen, West Germany.
When Dr. Dodds presented NGF data in the context of insulin and
relaxin, Blundell strongly disagreed and felt that some of the
criteria that they all had agreed upon are not met by nerve
growth factor, i.e., the backbone structure and the hydrophobic core
are not preserved. Now, I think we have to leave it at that. I
personally feel that perhaps there is a bit too much in terms of
modification and assumptions necessary in order to suggest a gene
duplication process beginning with insulin and ending with NGF.

Dr. Bylander
       I had noticed, by comparing sequences that this nerve growth
factor between residues 89 through 110 by the usual numbering shceme,
that there are 8 to 20 absolute homologies between the A chain and the

more basic chain of relaxin, which are not the regions that are most
homologous when you compare relaxin and insulin.

Dr. Schwabe
    Well, it might be totally correct; I'm not sure. I can only
give a hunch at this point, and I want it to be registered as such.

    The other think I would like to say, in terms of relaxin is
often included as a growth factor. I personally don't think relaxin
is a growth factor. I have looked at the result of relaxin action
on the synthesis during a recent one-month stay in Munich. Dr. Timpl
and I used an immunofluorescent technique which distinguished between
the various procollagens and collagens produced in the symphysis
pubis. Ever since, I have the impression that relaxin should not
be classified as a growth factor. Besides that, of course, the effect
on the uterus, as far as the uterine motility suppression is
concerned, doesn't fit. The only thing that could possibly fit is
some classical work that has been done on the glycogen content of
the uterus which supposedly increases under the influence of relaxin.
Relaxin might be a quasi insulin for uterine structures.

Dr. Greenwood
    Dr. Schwabe, could you clarify in my mind for me the definition
of a parahormone? Is that a hormone that has lost out, as you put
it so dramatically, or has it acquired another function?

Dr. Schwabe
    No. Para means next to like paramour; you know that. So a
little bit illegal. The choice of word doesn't have any specific
meaning. In my scheme, of course, it is one of the runners-up that
lost the internal competition for function in a particular species.
You know, I could call it an isohormone.

Dr. Greenwood
    It is quite interesting to us, of course, because what you have
shown is a tyrosine containing relaxin-related peptide in sows'
ovaries which, of course, would iodinate with anything. That means
it raises the possibility that when you iodinate that with an
antiserum, your measuring changes, in a parahormone in, for example,
human plasma.

Dr. Schwabe
    Yes, that is a possibility. Now, we would have to specify the
antigenic potency of that hormone to recognize the regular relaxin
antibodies, and we do not know very much about that. Of course,
it could lead to erroneous results. There is a distinct possibility
that your early RIA has detected this pararelaxin. In fact in honor
of yourself, we have lovingly adopted the term Hawaiian Relaxin to
designate the tyrosine relaxin.

Dr. L. L. Anderson
     This is a little bit of a sideline, but do you know anything about the histology of the shark ovary and the kinds of cells that produce relaxin and about what might be a production rate of the hormone?

Dr. Schwabe
     No, absolutely nothing. I have, in fact, talked to Dr. Callard not long ago, who is the Chairman of Biology at Boston University. He had quite a keen interest in this subject. When I asked him an opinion similarly formulated to yours, he said, "Well, you known, I can't tell you anything for sure, but I can see many reasons why a shark would have relaxin".

     First of all, you know, of course, that sharks have made their own attempt at mammalian-type reproduction. There is a wide variety of subspecies. You go from very primitive, almost egg-laying animals to something that is very close to a regular placental animal. Of course, we would like to get a good sample of every one of the stages of complexity and see whether the relaxin changes. I haven't the faintest idea about the relaxin location within the shark ovaries, but perhaps you could take a look at it. We would be happy to send you a sample.

Dr. Bradshaw
     I feel I should comment on the nerve growth factor question since we introduced the relationship of NGF and insulin originally. Clearly, I must take issue with Dr. Schwabe's response, which, in fact, surprises me, because it turns out the nerve growth factor is more similar to relaxin than either are to insulin. In the comparison of relaxin to insulin, if you take away the disulfide bonds, you find you are left with very little homology, which you noted in an early paper on the subject. Further, you have told us today that now you can even take away one of the disulfides. Thus while the relationship with insulin seems to be fading, the relationship to nerve growth factor is not. As was pointed out the region surrounding the B20 (insulin) half-cystine is similar in NGF and relaxin but unlike the IGF's or insulin. Furthermore, it is certainly very interesting that nerve growth factor and relaxin are both made as precursors of at least 22,000 molecular weight. Thus, both come from much larger molecules which we know nothing about. Therefore, it hardly seems appropriate to cite an unpublished structure as proof that nerve growth factor did not evolve from the same precursor that produced relaxin, the IGF's and insulin. I think that would be rather premature.

Dr. Schwabe
     I would like to make a response. I would like to tell the audience that we do find some of this stuff. Having done so, I

would like to say that my response was rather guarded in that
respect. I think that the processing that you're referring to, you
seem to feel that it is a rather established thing, that you could
use this as an argument. I feel that the large precursor processing
is far from being proved in the relationship of relaxin and insulin
or any of these factors. So I don't think that it is necessarily
a positive argument one way or the other.

Dr. Bradshaw
    I will let Dr. Gast deal with that in his talk.

CHEMICAL STUDIES ON RELAXIN

H. D. Niall, R. James, M. John, J. Walsh,
S. Kwok, G. D. Bryant-Greenwood, G. W. Treager
and R. A. Bradshaw

Howard Florey Institute, University of Melbourne
Parkville, Australia 3052, Department of Anatomy
and Reproductive Biology, University of Hawaii
at Manoa, Hololulu, Hawaii 96822, Department of
Biological Chemistry, Washington University
St. Louis, MO 63110

INTRODUCTION

Relaxin is a low molecular weight peptide hormone (6000 daltons)
with multiple biological effects during pregnancy in mammals. It
relaxes the pubic symphysis, causes inhibition of uterine contractions, softens the cervix and stimulates mammary gland development.
While it has been identified in several non-mammalian species, its
physiological role in these is unclear.

Relaxin from pregnant sow and rat ovaries has been purified and
characterized to the point of amino acid analysis (Sherwood and
O'Byrne, 1974; Sherwood, 1979). Porcine relaxin was found by
Sherwood and O'Byrne to separate on carboxymethyl cellulose columns
in three components, designated CM-B, CM-a and CM-a', in the order
of their elution (Sherwood and O'Byrne, 1974). The two groups (our
own, and that of Schwabe and coworkers) have reported on the amino
acid sequence of porcine relaxin (James et al., 1977; Schwabe et al.,
1976; Schwabe et al., 1977). Discrepancies between the two proposals
for the structure, and the need to establish the differences between
the three forms of pig relaxin led us to undertake further chemical
studies. These were aimed at finding the basis for the observed
molecular heterogeneity by sequence analysis of CM-B, CM-a and CM-a'.

163

Isolation

        Proteolysis during isolation procedures could cause or contribute
to the appearance of multiple molecular forms of porcine relaxin.
Using the basic procedure of Sherwood and O'Byrne (1974), we carried
out multiple small side purifications of relaxin from ovaries collected at various stages of pregnancy. Ovaries were pooled in
batches of 70-80 g, carefully matched according to the fetal crown-
rump lengths, and frozen at once in liquid nitrogen to minimize
proteolysis. Batches corresponding to early, middle and late
pregnancy were worked up with and without the addition of 2 mM
phenylmethylsulfonyl fluoride, 10 mM disodium EDTA and 0.02% sodium
azide to solutions used for purification. Peaks equivalent to CM-B,
CM-a and CM-a' were obtained. It was found that the yields of
relaxin purified in the presence of these reagents were 2-4 fold
higher than in their absence (Kwok *et al.*, 1980). This provides
evidence that proteolytic destruction of relaxin takes place to a
significant degree during the Sherwood-O'Byrne isolation procedure.
However, the relative proportions of CM-B, CM-a and CM-a' did not
change appreciably. This suggests either that they are endogenous
components present in the corpora lutea *in vivo*, or that they are
generated by proteases which are not adequately inhibited by the
above agents. Further studies are in progress to establish which
of these alternatives is correct.

Sequence Analysis

        Our earlier sequence studies were carried out on fraction
CM-a' as defined by Sherwood and O'Byrne. In order to define better
the origin of the microheterogeneity of the relaxin components, small
pools were taken, across the CM-a and CM-a' peaks, and subjected
to N- and C-terminal analysis. N-terminal analysis revealed no
significant heterogeneity in any component--i.e. the A chain amino-
terminal sequence $arg^1-met^2-thr^3$...was the only one identified.
However, digestion with carboxypeptidases A, B and Y revealed clear
differences between pools. Relaxin obtained from the descending
portion of the CM-a' region (Pool IV, Figure 1) released arginine,
glycine and tryptophan, in that order, on timed digestions with
carboxypeptidase Y. No amino acids were released from this pool on
carboxypeptidase A digestion. Carboxypeptidase B digestion released
arginine only. Thus the C-terminal sequence of this component of
relaxin was - trp - gly - arg. Larger amounts of relaxin pooled
from this region of the elution profile were subjected to total
sequence analysis using procedures similar to those earlier
described (James *et al.*, 1977). However, in the present experiments
it was possible to carry out a complete automated sequence analysis of
the C-terminal tryptic peptide from the B chain. The sequence
leu^{17}-trp-val - glu - ile - cys - gly - ser - val - ser - trp - gly -
arg^{29} was obtained in two independent experiments in a Beckman 890C

sequentor using polybrene as a carrier and ^{35}S-phenylisothiocyanate
as the coupling agent. This sequence is identical to that earlier
reported by us except for the absence of the threonine residue
previously attributed to position 27. The remainder of the B-
chain sequence and the A chain sequence confirmed our earlier work
(James *et al.*, 1977).

Digestion of aliquots from earlier eluting regions of the CM-a
and CM-a' peaks revealed that pool III had carboxyl-terminal
threonine, and pool II carboxyl terminal thr-ala. In addition to
these residues small amounts of carboxyl-terminal leucine were
released from pool I. When digestion with carboxypeptidase A was
followed by digestion of the same samples with carboxypeptidase Y,
arginine, glycine and tryptophan were released in addition. This
allowed us to propose that the C terminal sequences of relaxin
fractions from the CM-a and CM-a' regions of the elution profile
were as illustrated in Figure 1. No other differences were found
between the relaxin fractions by a series of experiments involving
complete sequence analysis of the A chain by Edman degradation and
N-terminal sequence analysis of the B chains by Edman degradation
after removal of the pyrrolidone carboxylic acid residue at B1 by
enzymatic treatment. Confirmatory data was obtained by tryptic
digestion of intact relaxin pools and isolated chains followed by
fingerprinting by two dimensional chromatography-electrophoresis
on cellulose thin layer plates. Peptides were located by light
spraying with ninhydrin or fluorescamine, eluted, and subjected to
amino acid analysis and Edman degradation. The detailed results will
be reported elsewhere. Particularly valuable in establishing the
differences between the major components of CM-A and CM-a' were
experiments in which aliquots of pools II and IV were digested with
chymotrypsin for short time intervals. Cleavage-carboxyl-terminal
to trp^{27} gave rise to short peptides (gly - arg from pool IV, and
gly - arg - thr - ala from pool II) which were isolated on cellulose
thin layer plates and sequenced as described above. This established
beyond reasonable doubt the differences between the multiple molecular
forms of relaxin in CM-a and CM-a'.

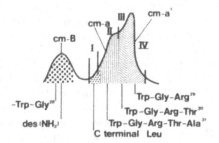

*Figure 1.   C terminal sequences of porcine relaxin fractions from
CM-a and CM-a' regions of the elution profile.*

Similar experiments were carried out on CM-B. These were less
conclusive in that this peak contains small amounts of a non-relaxin
peptide containing tyrosine and histidine. However, the major component of CM-B was found to be a variant of relaxin lacking the
arginine residue at B^{29}. Also present was a form of relaxin with
C-terminal - trp - gly - arg. A plausible explanation for the early
elution of this peptide from the column is that it has suffered
deamidation during isolation, possibly at position A10 (Glutamine).

DISCUSSION

The heterogeneity of porcine relaxin as purified by the Sherwood
and O'Byrne procedure can be put on a structural basis by the above
experiments. Quantitatively there are three major components dif-
fering only in the length of the B chain through the presence or
absence of residues at its carboxy terminus. Thus, the major
component of CM-B has a B chain of 28 amino acids (ending in B^{28}
glycine). The major component of CM-a has 31 residues, with the
C terminal sequence - gly^{28} - arg^{29} - thr^{30} - ala^{31}. The major
component of CM-a' has carboxyl terminal gly^{28} - arg^{29}. Minor
relaxin components are also present. The form ending in B^{30} thr
elutes between the B^{29} and B^{31} forms. Its presence presumably
explains the difficulty in resolving CM-a and CM-a' as distinct
peaks. An additional minor component found in CM-B is probably a
deamidated form of the B^{29} form of relaxin. The status of a putative
B^{32} leucine form of relaxin (from pool I) is uncertain, since we
could no isolate enough of this material for definitive sequence
analysis. It is possible that the C-terminal leucine in this pool
derives from a non-relaxin contaminant present in low concentration.
This point should be definitively settled when the nucleic acid
sequence of the relaxin-specific messenger RNA is determined.

The results of the present study indicate that our earlier
reported sequence (James *et al.*, 1977) for porcine relaxin (CM-a')
was incorrect in one respect. The threonine residue we thought was
present at position B^{27} was not found in our more detailed studies.
Moreover, the reason for our misinterpretation of earlier data now
becomes clear. In the earlier work we sequenced up to residue B^{26}
(serine) by Edman degradation and placed the last four residues as
thr^{27} - trp^{28} - gly^{29} - arg^{30} on the basis of timed digestions with
carboxypeptidase Y. This enzyme in short incubations (5-30')
clearly released arg, gly and trp in that order. On more prolonged
digestions (2-6 hrs) appreciable amounts of threonine and serine were
released, the threonine appearing first. We concluded that the
threonine preceded trp^{28} in the sequence, and that the serine
released by the enzyme was in fact serine B^{26}. Our present studies,
on carefully pooled aliquots from the CM-a region show that this
conclusion was incorrect, since complete Edman degradation, twice
repeated, showed a continuous sequence...val^{25} - ser^{26} - trp^{27} -

gly^{28} - arg^{29}. However, the finding of a form of relaxin with the additional residue (thr^{30}) explains the earlier observations. In the carboxypeptidase Y digestions we were working in fact on a mixture of B^{29} (arg) and B^{30} (thr) relaxins. The enzyme removes the threonine only very slowly--thus its late appearance in the digest, subsequent to the release of arg, gly and trp. In the present work, with more selective pooling of the CM-a' peak, we were able to obtain separately the B^{29} and B^{30} forms of relaxin.

These studies do not completely resolve the differences between the sequence proposals for porcine relaxin put forward by Schwabe *et al.* (1977) and by our own group (Figure 2). In the two proposals for the A chain, the only difference is at position 10 where we find glutamine (James *et al.*, 1977) and Schwabe *et al.* (1976) have glutamic acid. This difference is readily explained by deamidation of their relaxin during isolation. Our finding that CM-B may contain a desamido form of relaxin lends some support to this suggestion. The differences between the B chain sequences, however, are less easy to explain. Schwabe *et al.* report a 26 amino acid B-chain ending in the carboxyl-terminal sequence-- cys - gly - val - trp - ser. Our sequence for the predominant form is--cys - gly - ser - val - ser - trp - gly - arg and the form with the shortest B chain (the major compnent of CM-B) still has 28 amino acids, with C-terminal glycine. These differences are clearly not explicable on the basis of proteolytic shortening of the B chain of the relaxin sequenced by Schwable *et al.* since in comparison with our B chain sequence one serine residue is missing internally from their structure and the last two residues are inverted in order (Schwabe *et al.*, 1977). It seems unlikely that this is due to genetic differences in the relaxins, since we have obtained the same sequence in relaxin isolated from both Australian and United States pig ovaries. At present we feel that technical problems in sequencing will prove to be the explanation for the disparity in the sequences of the two groups.

The origin of the heterogeneity of porcine relaxin is still unclear. However, all of the 3 major and 2-3 minor forms we have characterized are consistent with an oriding from a single gene product with a unique amino acid sequence. Thus, it is not necessary to postulate allelic forms or genetic variations. The variants which differ in the length of the B chain could arise by enzyme cleavage, at slightly different sites of a single chain prorelaxin. Alternatively, as noted above, we have not yet excluded proteolytic degradation during isolation. Although Sherwood and O'Byrne found no significant difference in the activities of CM-a, CM-a' and CM-B in a mouse pubic symphysis assay (Sherwood and O'Byrne, 1974) these forms could differ in their specific activities on other relaxin target tissues. For this reason, it seems desirable, if not essential, that a single molecular form of relaxin be used as the reference standard for those working in the field.

A further consideration is the need for a new nomenclature. The terms CM-B, CM-a, and CM-a' may still be convenient for the moment to describe the relaxin preparations commonly used for clinical or biological experiments. However, they ought really be specified in terms of their chemical structures (e.g. relaxin B^{29}) now that these are known.

	Present work and James *et al.* (1977)	Schwabe *et al.* (1976, 1977)
A chain	Gln^{10}	Glu^{10}
B chain	Ser^{24} Val Ser Trp Gly Arg^{29}	Val^{24} Trp Ser^{26}
	Ser Val Ser Trp Gly Arg Thr^{30}	
	Ser Val Ser Trp Gly Arg Thr Ala^{31}	

Figure 2. Amino acid sequence proposals for porcine relaxin.

Synthesis

In other studies of relaxin chemistry we are currently attempting the synthesis of relaxin by the solid phase procedure. Progress to date (Tregear *et al.*, 1979), which is encouraging, has been recently reviewed and will not be discussed in detail here. The structural homology between insulin and relaxin allows the use for relaxin synthesis of strategies earlier shown to be effective for insulin. Dr. Tregear, working as a guest scientist at the Shanghai Institute of Biochemistry, has recently succeeded in several chain combination experiments. This is the key problem in the synthesis of relaxin since incorrect disulfide pairing readily occurs when the isolated synthetic A and B chains are combined. Dr. Treagear working in collaboration with Dr. Du Yu-cang of the Shanghai Institute has recombined successfully the separated chains from native porcine relaxin, with restoration of about 25% of the biological activity of the native hormone in a uterine contractility bioassay.

Native and synthetic chains have also been combined, again to give a product with significant (10-20%) biological activity. This positive result led to the successful combination of chains from insulin and relaxin to form hybrid molecules: relaxin A + insulin B ("relaxulin") and insul A + relaxin B (insulaxin"). In preliminary experiments these hybrids were biologically inactive in both insulin (mouse convulsion) and relaxin (uterine contractility) bioassays. However, they should prove fascinating models for studies of the structural requirements for antigenicity and receptor binding of these hormones.

ACKNOWLEDGEMENTS

We thank Dr. J. W. Jacobs for carrying out one of the sequenator experiments on the relaxin B chain. This work was supported by grants from the National Institutes of Health to Dr. H. D. Niall and G. D. Bryant-Greenwood. R. A. Bradshaw participated in this work while a Josiah Macy Jr. Foundation Faculty Scholar at the Howard Florey Institute, University of Melbourne. S. Kwok was supported during these studies by a Lalor Foundation Fellowship at the Howard Florey Institute.

REFERENCES

James, R. H., Niall, H. D., Kwok, S. and Bryant-Greenwood, G. (1977). Primary structure of porcine relaxin: homology with insulin and related growth factors. Nature 267:544.

Kwok, S., Bryant-Greenwood, G. D., and Niall, H. D. (1980). Evidence for proteolysis during purification of relaxin from pregnant sow ovaries. Endocr. Res. Commun. 7:1.

Schwabe, C., McDonald, J. K. and Steinetz, B. G. (1976). Primary structure of the A-chain of porcine relaxin. Biochem. Biophys. Res. Commun. 70:397.

Schwabe, C., McDonald, J. K. and Steinetz, B. G. (1977). Primary structure of the A-chain of porcine relaxin. Biochem. Biophys. Res. Commun. 70:397.

Schwabe, C., McDonald, J. K. and Steinetz, B. G. (1977). Primary structure of the B-chain of porcine relaxin. Biochem. Biophys. Res. Commun. 75:303.

Sherwood, O. D. and O'Byrne, E. M. (1974). Purification and characterization of porcine relaxin. Arch. Biochem. Biophys. 160:185.

Sherwood, O. D. (1979). Purification and characterization of rat relaxin. Endocrinology 104:886.

Tregear, G. W., Kemp, B., Borjesson, B., Thompson, A., Scanlon, D., Collier, M., John, M., Niall, H. and Bryant-Greenwood, G. (1979). In: Peptides. Proc. Sixth American Peptide Symposium. Pierce Publ., Illinois, USA (In Press).

DISCUSSION FOLLOWING DR. H. D. NIALL's PAPER

Dr. Frieden
    If I understand you correctly, the work at Shanghai was not with
the synthetic hypothetical procompound, but actually, a recombination
of separated oxydized chains. Is that correct?

Dr. Niall
    Yes, that's correct, it has been with separate chains.

Dr. Frieden
    Very similar to the work done with synthetic insulin?

Dr. Niall
    Right. That was why we initiated this interaction.

Dr. Schwabe
    This interesting work on the combination of insulin A and relaxin
B chains proves another point in evolution, that man's mind isn't so
different. We always reach the same point at almost the same time.
I'm very excited to hear that you have been successful with things
that we have obviously tried and are still trying.

    Can you tell how much combination you got between the insulin
A chain and the B chain of relaxin? And secondly, if the yield was
significant to any degree, I would like to remind you that this might
be a further confirmation of the compatability of the two structures,
the insulin structure as well as the hypothetical model of relaxin.

Dr. Niall
    Yes. The formation of the hybrid was essentially quantitative
in terms of the chain, which was not in excess. And I don't know
quite how the people in China did it, but presumably they had one
chain in excess and were able to bring it to one hundred percent
based on that.

    In the case of native, this gave about 25 percent activity, and
presumably this means that virtually all of it has joined up in some
way or another, but only about a quarter of the molecules have joined
in the confirmation required to give activity.

    As regards to your second point, I couldn't agree more. Even
though neither of these molecule hybrids turned out to have any
activity, I think the very fact that they can be formed illustrates
the conservation of the core part of the molecule where the chains
interlink. Clearly this may very strongly serve evolutionarily.

Dr. Bradshaw

But that assumes that the disulfide formed the right way, which you don't know.

Dr. Niall

We don't know the disulfide formed the right way, though we do know that the product is biologically active.

Dr. Bradshaw

I'm sure it's going to come out that way, but without activity, you would have to do a chemical measurement.

Dr. Greenwood

It's a very mundane question on the heterogeneity of CMB. On your data, there's a 28 relaxin in there and there's a deamidated material. I recall that Gill Bryant, some years ago, showed that you could actually radioiodinate CMB with chloramine T and bind with antibody. Hence there is a tyrosine-containing peptide in CMB, as there is in "purified" NIH-RXN, which will iodinate with chloramine T. The implication is that there are tyrosine-containing peptides in RXN. Have you seen this in CMB?

Dr. Niall

Yes. Let me qualify that by saying, yes--in many batches of purification, whereas the CMa and CMa' appeared to have no histidine, tyrosine, or proline at all. If any one of the components has traces of what we regard as impurities, 5 or 10 percent, very small ratios of other amino acids, it would be the CMB. However, we have obtained preparations of CMB with virtually no tyrosine at all. But I'm not surprised to hear that occasionally it occurs in CMB.

Dr. Rawitch

(University of Kansas): I think it might be appropriate to comment on some calculations that we did, since several people have alluded to the fact that, if you compare sequences, that you can make argument for differences between relaxin and insulin, just looking at the amino acids. Benefitting from the sequence work, the very nice work that has been reported here today, we took the sequences of insulin and relaxin and did some simple calculations which predict secondary structure, specifically (Maxfield, Scheraga and Chou-Fasman) predictions for helix and beta structures.

You can construct a number of profiles and make a very convincing case just based on the helix preference of the residues that both the A and B chains of insulin will overlie their counterparts in relaxin in such profile with good qualitative correspondence. So that is another piece of evidence which suggests that they are homologous in terms of secondary structure, quite apart from CD measurements.

Dr. Schwabe

The protease inhibitor stuff is surprising to me, as I noted by your hesistant way of presenting it, that you too have questions. First of all, the peaks disappeared uniformly, whereas you stated there was no inhibition of the possible conversion of one form to the other. Secondly, you used PMSF, and what do you hope to inhibit with PMSF? Don't you use acid pH immediately, as you extract hormone?

Dr. Niall

Yes. We used a procedure which is identical to the one which you describe.

Dr. Schwabe

You think of a serine protease usually as neutral protease?

Dr. Niall

Yes.

Dr. Schwabe

I do not understand why you did not use the pepstatin as an inhibitor for acid proteases?

Dr. Niall

These are the initial ones we looked at, and I think the results speak for themselves. One can come up with various arguments as to what we might use. But then Dr. Kwok could perhaps comment further. We saw a very dramatic effect of PMSF, ADT'I, and so on.

Dr. Bradshaw

I think it is important to distinguish just when the proteolysis goes on. It may well go on from the point of sacrifice until you disrupt the tissue.

Dr. Schwabe

Then you don't get the inhibitor there either.

Dr. Bradshaw

But then you disrupt the tissue before you do the acid precipitation. There are examples of serum protease that can survive identical treatment and are carried through onto the first gel filtration column. However, I think your point is an excellent one and that probably the acid protease inhibitors ought to be looked at.

Dr. Greenwood

What was the data for the quote on the important amino acids in relaxin for receptor binding?

Dr. Niall
    If you look at the receptor, what is thought to be the
receptor binding of insulin, and see which residues are there and see
what their substituted for in relaxin, there is no homology at all.
So it is very, very unlikely that relaxin will have any insulin
activity.

Dr. Bradshaw
    There may or may not be. It would have something to do with
the active site of relaxin. It might be the same and then it might
be different.

THE TOPOGRAPHY OF PORCINE RELAXIN:

LOCATION OF THE TRYPTOPHAN RESIDUES

R. James[+], H. D. Niall* and R. A. Bradshaw[+]

Howard Florey Institute, University of Melbourne,
Parkville, Victoria, Australia*
Department of Biological Chemistry, Washington
University School of Medicine
St. Louis, MO[+]

The amino acid sequence of porcine relaxin is distinctly similar
to that of insulin, particularly in regard to the placement of the
cystine residues, suggesting the likelihood of three-dimensional
homology as well. Two computer-modeling studies have produced
structures consistent with this possibility. While the overall
correctness of these predictions can only be adequately tested by
x-ray crystallographic analyses, solution methods can determine if
the placement of certain side chains is compatible. By use of charge
transfer titrations, the solvent availability of the two tryptophan
residues located in the B chain has been examined. N-Methylnicotin-
amide chloride forms weak complexes with indole moieties that are
readily detected by visible absorption measurements. Such reactions
occur in proteins if the tryptophan residues are fully exposed which
was found to be the case in relaxin. Furthermore, Trp B-18 was also
fully available, by this criterion, when the Trp-Gly-Arg sequence
was removed from the carboxyl terminus of the B chain by carboxypeptidase Y. These results clearly favor only one of the predicted
orientations of Trp B-18 and suggest an altered position of the
carboxyl terminal region of the B chain than that previously proposed. (RAB was a Josiah Macy Jr. Foundation Faculty Scholar at
the HFI during the tenure of these studies).

DISCUSSION FOLLOWING DR. R. A. BRASHAW'S PAPER

Dr. Niall
     Thanks, Ralph, for that presentation. Any questions on the
study? Dr. Schwabe.

Dr. Schwabe
     A technical question, Ralph, about the chain. The backbone of
the two models is almost superimposable, as you showed, right? That
means the difference is in the C -C bond. You can rotate that
tryptophan: right? What is the energy between one or the other
position of tryptophan?

Dr. Bradshaw
     That would be hard to predict. The two models, suggested by
Neil Isaacs and Guy Dodson, differ only in the rotation around the
alpha-beta bond. Thus, the plane of the ring just swings through
180°.

Dr. Schwabe
     Is there any energy barrier between one or the other position?

Dr. Bradshaw
     I'm sure there is but I don't know what the order of magnitude
it is. Are you suggesting that it could sit in more than one position?

Dr. Schwabe
     Well, what I'm saying is that it is actually an interesting
possibility, but it's trivial, if there is no energy barrier to hold
the tryptophan in one versus the other position.

Dr. Bradshaw
     I would guess that there would be an energy barrier, but there
is no way I can predict it. Hydrophobic interactions can provide
a fair amount of energy. Alternatively, steric considerations could
be equally important in determining whether the ring can pass back
and forth between the two orientations. I should mention that the
charge transfer data really aren't consistent with tryptophan ring
movement. Rather they indicate that the tryptophan is available
at least a majority of the time.

Dr. Rawitch
     Having two tryptophans and no tyrosine, it is tempting to con-
sider the possibility of looking at the intrinsic fluorescence, which
might give you some information with respect to environment. I
wonder, are there any intrinsic fluorescent measurements or quenching
studies?

Dr. Bradshaw

We haven't made such measurements, but I think this would be an ideal molecule to do such studies on.

Dr. Schwabe

The tryptophans are severely quenched. I haven't quantified it, but the fluorescent yields for the tryptophan components in the molecule come nowhere near what they should be.

Dr. Bradshaw

Yes. I'm certain that the internal one, despite the fact that we think it is relatively available to solvent, would probably be quenched.

I don't know about the other one. It is a bit harder to guess what it may be doing. I don't think that any of the predicted models were very comfortable with the C terminal region of the beta chain and with good reason. There is a lot of flexibility there. As I pointed out, we think it should be moved over a bit, but that is only a guess. It is one part of the molecule that really requires the crystallographers to tell us what is going on.

Dr. Niall

Perhaps I could before turning over the microphone, Ralph, just comment, in regard to tryptophan accessibility, that we found that in the course of sequence studies, that that particular buried or apparently buried tryptophan (B18) is in fact, very accessible to chymotryptic digestion at brief time intervals with low concentrations of enzyme. Of course, other bonds are split at the same time, but the enzyme is able to get very rapidly at that particular bond joining tryptophan[18] to valine[19]. So it is not buried from that particular point of view.

MESSENGER RNA DEPENDENT SYNTHESIS OF A PROTEIN

CONTAINING RELAXIN RELATED SEQUENCES

Michael J. Gast, Hugh D. Niall and Irving Boime

Department of Pharmacology
School of Medicine
Washington University, St. Louis, MO

INTRODUCTION

Serum relaxin levels in pregnant rats, sows, and guinea pigs are very low during most of gestation (Sherwood *et al.*, 1975); mean relaxin concentrations in the sow range between 0.1 and 2.0 ng/ml throughout the first 100 days of pregnancy. During this period small electron dense cytoplasmic granules begin to appear in luteal cells. This granule population continued to increase in late gestation, reaching a maximum several days before parturition. About 24-48 hours before delivery a rapid disintegration of the cyto-plasmic granules occurs. Serum levels of relaxin rise rapidly and then drop precipitously during parturition and lactation (Belt *et al.*, 1971). Studies in rat ovarian homogenates also suggest a steady, gradual rise in relaxin production throughout pregnancy (Sherwood and Crnekovic, 1979). The stimuli for the initial production of the hormone, the factors controlling its secretion and storage during pregnancy, and the reasons for its explosive release at term remain obscure. Relaxin has traditionally been assigned to the class of pregnancy-related hormones, but at least one study suggests that in humans the protein is also present in non-pregnant sera (Bryant-Greenwood *et al.*, 1977).

Because of our interest in follicular and luteal maturation we examined relaxin biosynthesis as a model for ovarian gene expression during the menstrual cycle and pregnancy. We show here that ovarian mRNA directs the synthesis of a high molecular weight protein con-taining relaxin related sequences (RCP). RCP mRNA is first detectable in the corpus luteum of the cycle and eventually represents increasingly larger proportion of total ovarian RNA as gestation advances.

MATERIALS AND METHODS

Ovaries were obtained fresh from Hunter Packing Co., E. St.
Louis, Ill. Corpora lutea or follicles were excised (Figure 1) and
placed in homogenizing buffer containing 50 mM Tris-HCl pH 7.8, 0.88 M
sucrose, 25 mM KCl, 5 mM $MgCL_2$, 7 mM βMe, and 0.5 mM EDTA. Whole
corpora lutea were homogenized in a motor driven glass homogenizer and
then spun at 10,000 x g for 10 min to remove nuclei and cell debris.
RNA was extracted as previously described (Szczesna and Boime, 1976).
Yields of total luteal RNA ranged from 0.5 to 1.0 mg per gram of
luteal tissue.

Protein synthesis in the presence of 0.3 μM $[^{35}S]$ cysteine
(specific activity 500 Ci/mmol) was assayed in cell-free lysates of
wheat germ or in reconstituted ascites lysates following the procedure of Szczesna and Boime (1976). Following incubation, deoxy-
cholate (DOC) and Triton-X-100 (TX) were added to scaled-up reaction
mixtures to a final concentration of 1% for each detergent, and then
centrifuged at 100,000 x g for 45 minutes to remove ribosomes. The
supernate was then mixed with phosphate buffered saline (PBS) and
an appropriate antiserum. Detergent concentrations were readjusted
to 1%. During competitive binding experiments, 20 μl of unlabelled
protein (6 mg/ml) was added prior to the addition of antiserum.

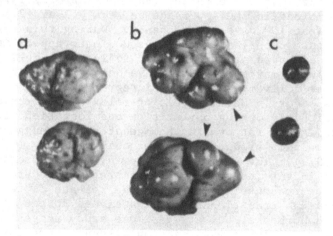

*Figure 1.   Ovarian tissue used in the preparation of RNAs for the study
of relaxin biosynthesis and luteal maturation.   Ovaries
were obtained fresh from a local slaughterhouse.   They were
characterized as either follicular (A) or luteal (B).   If
sows were pregnant, duration of gestation was assessed by
fetal size (see Methods).   The corpora lutea (C), which
are the large, dark spherical projects in the ovaries at
center (arrows) were obtained by carefully excising the
ovarian capsule and dissecting away all non-luteal tissues.*

The final volume of the immunoprecipitation mixture was 400 μl.
Mixtures were incubated at 4°C for 16 hours, and 25 μl of sheep anti-
rabbit antiserum was then added. Incubation was continued for an
additional three hours at room temperature.

The immunoprecipitates were centrifuged at 9,000 x g for two min
and the pellets were washed three times with PBS, resuspended in a
buffer containing 1% SDS and then analyzed on 15% acrylamide gels
(300:1 acrylamide:bis) Laemmli, 1970). Gels were stained and destained
and labelled proteins were detected by fluorography (Laskey and
Mills, 1975) or impregnation with 1M salicylate (J. Chamberlain,
personal communication).

For pregnancy time course experiments, the gestational period
was determined on the basis of fetal crown-rump length. Collections
were made in the 1-3 cm (embryonic), 5-12 cm (early fetal stages)
and greater than 22 cm (late fetal stage) size ranges. RNA was
isolated from these ovaries as well as from follicular and luteinized
ovaries of non-pregnant animals.

Authentic relaxin was isolated according to Sherwood and O'Bryne
(1974). A highly purified fraction of relaxin corresponding to peak
CMa' was used for this work. Relaxin antisera were prepared by
emulsifying purified porcine relaxin in sterile water and complete
Freund's adjuvant. Adult male New Zealand White rabbits were initially
immunized by footpad injection of 1 mg and were re-injected with 0.1 mg
of relaxin at bi-weekly intervals. The animals were bled from a
lateral ear vein one week after each injection. Antiserum was stored
at -20°C until used in an immunoassay. HCG-α antiserum was a gift
of Drs. Steven Birken and Robert Canfield.

Ten-40% sucrose gradients (12 ml) of total ovarian RNA were prepared as described previously (Daniels-McQueen *et al.*, 1978).
Gradients were subjected to centrifugation at 150,000 x g for 18 hours
at 5°C. Fractions (0.3 ml) were collected, pooled, and RNA precipitated by addition 1/9 of a volume of 20% KAc and two volumes of
ethanol (prechilled to 20°). Translation and immunoprecipitation
were carried out as described above.

RESULTS

Based on its structural similarities with insulin (James *et al.*,
1977), we expected an mRNA coding for relaxin would direct the
synthesis of a protein having a molecular weight of 12,00 daltons
("preprorelaxin") or perhaps 9,000 daltons ("prorelaxin") in the
ascites system (James *et al.*, 1977). When reaction mixtures were
incubated with luteal RNA, relaxin anti-serum immunoprecipitated a
major product with an apparent molecular weight fo 23,000 daltons
(RCP) (Figure 2, lane 2). Analysis of reaction mixtures incubated

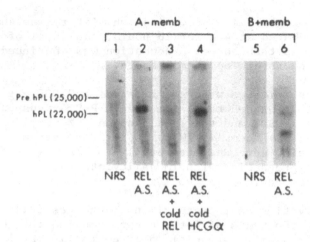

Figure 2.   *Fluorograph of a NaDODSO₄/polyacrylamide gel electrophoreto-*
gram of [³⁵S] cystein labelled proteins isolated by immuno-
precipitation.   Reconstituted S-100-ribosome extracts
derived from ascites tumor cells were incubated in the
presence (lanes 5 and 6) and absence (lanes 1-4) of micro-
somal membranes.   The ribosomes were removed by centri-
fugation and aliquots from the supernatant fraction were
treated with relaxin antiserum.   The immunoprecipitates
were dissolved in SDS buffer and applied to gels
(approximately 5,000 cpm/lane).   HPL and pre-hPL were
labelled with [³⁵S] methionine and served as markers.
Lanes 1 and 5, normal rabbit serum was substituted for
relaxin antiserum; Lane 2, 20 µl of undiluted relaxin
antiserum was used in the immunoprecipitation reaction;
Lane 3 and Lane 4, 120 µg of unlabelled relaxin and hCG-α,
respectively were added prior to addition of relaxin anti-
serum.

in the absence of RNA or in the presence of RNA from term placenta
did not reveal this protein.   In addition, when reaction mixtures
containing luteal RNA were precipitated with normal rabbit serum, RCP
was not observed (Figure 2, lane 1).

    To further verify the presence of relaxin sequences within the
23,00 MW product we attempted to inhibit RCP binding to relaxin antiserum by the prior addition of a large excess of unlabelled relaxin to
the reaction mixture.   It is clear that RCP was not precipitated when
unlabelled relaxin was added.   An identical concentration of hCG-α
did not compete with RCP in the immunoprecipitation reaction (Figure
2, Lanes 3 and 4).   Bovine serum albumin and β-HCG also failed to
inhibit this binding (data not shown).

Because relaxin is a secretory protein we anticipated that RCP would contain a signal sequence. Indeed, in lysates containing ascites microsomal membranes luteal RNA directed the synthesis of a 20,000 molecular weight protein (Figure 2, Lane 6). Synthesis of this protein was not observed in identical reaction mixtures containing no RNA. Binding of the 20 K protein to relaxin antiserum was completely inhibited by the addition of purified relaxin (data not shown). These results suggest that TCP contains a 3000 dalton signal peptide.

Using RCP production as a marker of ovarian function, we examined protein synthesis in both the non-pregnant and pregnant state. There was no detectable RCP in immunoprecipitates from reaction mixtures containing RNA from an early follicular ovary preparation (Figure 3, Lane 1). However, a significant amount of RCP synthesis was seen using RNA derived from non-pregnant, luteinized ovaries (Figure 3, Lane 2). The binding of this protein to relaxin anti-serum was completely inhibited by unlabelled relaxin (data not shown).

In translation mixtures containing luteal RNA from pregnant sows, the levels of RCP seem to increase from early to mid and late gestation (Figure 3, Lanes 3-5).

To further enrich and characterize the mRNA encoding RCP, crude ovarian RNA was subjected to sucrose gradient centrifugation. Measurement of absorbance across the gradient revealed characteristic peaks of tRNA (4S) and rRNA (18S and 28S (Figure 4A). RNAs isolated from fractions collected between the 4S and 18S regions of the gradient were translated in ascites lysates. The peak of RCP mRNA activity was found in gradient fraction 3 (Figure 4B). The mRNA encoding preplacental lactogen (12S) sedimented in the region corresponding to fraction 4 when a parallel gradient of crude RNA from term placenta was analyzed. From these data we estimate that RCP mRNA sediments at 11S.

DISCUSSION

Data presented here strongly suggest that relaxin is synthesized as a part of a large 23,000 dalton ovarian polypeptide. We have shown that this relaxin-containing protein contains a signal sequence (characteristic of many secretory proteins) of 2 to 3 thousand daltons. Further characterization of RCP mRNA in sucrose density gradients reveals an mRNA of molecular weight 375-400,000 daltons-- which is sufficient to encode a protein molecular weight of 20-25,000 daltons.

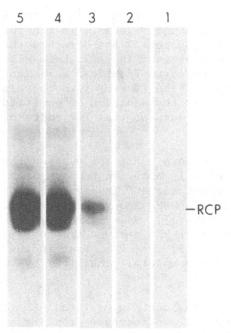

Figure 3. *Fluorograph of NaDODSO$_4$/polyacrylamide gel electrophoretogram or proteins synthesized in the presence of 2 µgm. RNA isolated from tissue at various stages in the ovarian maturational cycle. Proteins were translated in the re-constituted ascites lysate system containing [^{35}S] cysteine and immunoprecipitated with relaxin antiserum. Equal counts were applied to each lane. Lane 1, RNA from follicular ovaries of immature animals. Lane 2, RNA from corpora lutea of nonpregnant sows. Lane 3, RNA from corpora of early gestation (CR length 1-3 cm). Lane 4, RNA from luteal tissue of mid gestation (5-1/2 cm CR length). Lane 5, RNA from ovaries of sows near parturition (CR length > 22 cm).*

RCP is much larger than relaxin (molecular weight 6,000) and its presumed "pre- Pro-" (molecular weight 12,000) and "Pro" (molecular weight 9,000) forms. Mains and Eipper (1978) and Roberts *et al.*, (1978) working with the precursor to ACTH/β lipotropin have shown that proteins containing different biological activities may be derived from post-translational processing of common precursor

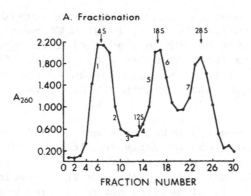

A. Fractionation

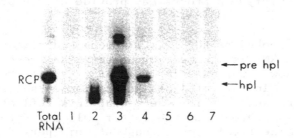

B. Immunoprecipitation

Figure 4.   Sucrose gradient analysis of total ovarian RNA. Approximately 2.8 mg of RNA was fractionated on a 10 to 40% sucrose gradient (upper panel). Fractions 1 to 7 were collected and equivalent amounts of RNA were translated in ascites lysate. 12S (arrow) represents the location of the mRNA encoding pre-placental lactogen in a parallel gradient of crude placental RNA. Translation mixtures containing ovarian RNA from gradient fractions 1-7 were then immunoprecipitated with relaxin antiserum. Lanes 1-7 (bottom panel) represent a fluorograph showing the distribution of immunoprecipitated proteins labelled with [^{35}S] cysteine.

molecule. The existence of an extra protein portion in RCP suggests that relaxin is derived through a cascade of post-translational processing step analogous to the ACTH/βLPH model. In future work we hope to examine more closely the nature of this extra protein segment in RCP and the conversion of the RCP molecule to authentic relaxin.

For several years, ovarian relaxin production outside of pregnancy has been controversial (O'Byrne *et al.*, 1978). We have demonstrated small, but definite amounts of RCP in translation mixtures containing RNA isolated from corpora lutea of non-pregnant sows. Thus, RCP mRNA is present within the total RNA population of the cycling ovary. These data strongly suggest that relaxin synthesis is occurring in the non-pregnant state.

We are unable to demonstrate the presence of RCP messenger among RNA's derived from preparations of early follicular ovary. This implies that relaxin is not a product of these small, pre-ovulatory follicles. We cannot exclude the possibility that levels of RCP produced in these translational assays, however, were undetectable using our immunoprecipitation techniques. Survey of these crude RNAs with complementary DNA probes may provide a more precise answer to this question.

We have also looked at RCP mRNA production during pregnancy. It is clear that RCP mRNA is the most prevalent mRNA present during gestation in the sow. Our data imply an increase in the proportion of RCP mRNA present in the total RNA population of sow corpus luteum as pregnancy progresses. It is likely that this reflects an increase in relaxin synthesis throughout the latter half of gestation. Serum levels of the hormone remain low throughout this period, rising significantly only during the last two weeks of pregnancy in the sow. The increase which we observe in mRNA levels appear to more closely parallel rising levels of relaxin in luteal tissue and correspond to growth in the population of electron dense granules in ctyoplasm. In addition, while our translational assays provide an indication of steady state RNA concentrations in a given RNA preparation, such data must be interpreted with caution, since *in vitro* systems do not always accurately reflect *in vivo* cellular events. Again, direct measurement of RCP mRNA levels with a homogenous complementary DNA probe is essential to confirm these results.

The question of the stimuli for onset and maintenance of relaxin synthesis remains unanswered. Our data suggest that luteinization, rather than pregnancy, induces synthesis of RCP and mRNA. This model implies that early control of relaxin synthesis in the sow is not a function of any agent elaborated by the placenta, but does not exclude involvement of pituitary hormones. Elucidation of the factors responsible for relaxin induction should provide crucial information about the control of ovarian gene expression during the menstrual cycle and pregnancy.

REFERENCES

Belt, W. D., Anderson, L. L., Cavazos, L. F. and Melampy, R. M.
    (1971). Cytoplasmic granules and relaxin levels in porcine
    corpora lutea. Endocrinology. 89:1.
Bryant-Greenwood, G.D., Greenwood, F.C., Hale, R.W. and Morislige,
    W. K. (1977). Hormonal evaluation of the intrauterine pro-
    gesterone contraceptive system. J. Clin. Endocrinol. Metab.
    44:721.
Chan, S. J., Keim, P. and Steiner, D. F. (1976). Cell-free synthesis
    of rat preproinsulins: characterization and partial amino acid
    sequence determination. Proc. Natl. Acad. Sci. 73:1964.
Daniels-McQueen, S., McWilliams, D., Birken, S., Canfield,R., Landefeld,
    T. and Boime, I. (1978). Identification of mRNAs encoding the
    α and β subunits of human choriogondotropin. J. Biol. Chem.
    253:7109.
James, R., Niall, H., Kwok, S., and Bryant-Greenwood, G. (1977).
    Primary structure of porcine relaxin: homology with insulin
    and related growth factors. Nature 267:544.
Laemmli, U. K. (1970). Cleavage of structural proteins during the
    assembly of the heat of bacteriophate T_4. Nature 227:680.
Laskey, R. A. and Mills, A. D. (1975). Quantitative film detection
    of ^3H and ^{14}C in polyacrylamide gels by fluorography. Eur. J.
    Biochem. 56:335.
Mains, R. E. and Eipper, B. A. (1978). Coordinate synthesis of
    corticotropins and endorphins by mouse pituitary tumor cells.
    J. Biol. Chem. 253:651.
O'Byrne, E. M., Carriere, B. T., Sorenson, L., Segaloff, A., Schwabe,
    C. and Steinetz, B. G. (1978). Plasma immunoreactive relaxin
    levels in pregnant and non-pregnant women. J. Clin. Endocrinol.
    Metab. 47:1106.
Roberts, J. L., Phillips, M., Rosa, P. A. and Herbert, E. (1978).
    Steps involved in the processing of common precursor forms of
    adrenocorticotropin and endorphin in cultures of mouse pituitary
    cells. Biochemistry. 17:3609.
Sherwood, O. D., Chang, C. C., Bevier, G. W. and Dziuk, P. J. (1975).
    Radioimmunoassay of plasma relaxin levels throughout pregnancy
    and at parturition in the pig. Endocrinology 97:834.
Sherwood, O. D. and Crnekovic, V. E. (1979). Development of a homo-
    logous radioimmunoassay for rat relaxin. Endocrinology 104:893.
Sherwood, O. D. and O'Bryne, E. M. (1974). Purification and
    characterization of porcine relaxin. Arch. Biochem. Biophys.
    160:185.
Szczesna, E and Boime, I. (1976). mRNA-dependent synthesis of
    authentic precursor to human placental lactogen: conversion to
    its mature hormone form in ascites cell-free extracts. Proc.
    Nat. Acad. Sci. 73:1179.

DISCUSSION FOLLOWING DR. M. GAST'S PAPER

Dr. *Soloff*

(Medical College of Ohio): What percentage of the total mRNA present in late gestation would you estimate that relaxin mRNA is?

Dr. *Gast*

That's an excellent question and requires precise quantitation with complementary DNA probes, I think. I would guess that it's a relatively high percentage, of the order of five percent; but that's a guess, that's not a hard answer.

Dr. *Soloff*

Could you get some estimate by comparing the amount of radioactive peptide precipitated with relaxin antibody with the total amount of radioactivity precipitated with trichloroacetic acid?

Dr. *Gast*

I think that that's a difficult way to handle that question. I'm not sure it is an entirely appropriate measure in our systems. The problem is, we do a lot of operations to products following immunoprecipitation. We measure the counts directly, bring them up in a blue mix and dilute them out in a gel buffer, and so on.

Dr. *Jeffrey*

Mike, would you be prepared to say anything about further transformations of the presumptive pro-relaxin at this time? It is a very large pro-molecule as such. Have you looked at conversion from the twenty-one thousand to the six?

Dr. *Gast*

John, we haven't looked at that directly. In some of our work, we have seen, with the membrane systems, other molecular weight forms of RCP that are of lower molecular weight than 20,000 to 21,000 molecules, minus the signal sequence. We haven't investigated those thoroughly yet, although we have in our laboratory looked at a variety of other types of processing steps involving glycosylation for example. Through various instrumentations, we may be able to examine this phenomenon *in vitro*.

Dr. *Diehl*

(Tuskeegee Institute): Have you looked at mRNA production around day 14 compared to other days of pregnancy?

Dr. *Gast*

Are you talking about in a porcine model?

Dr. *Diehl*

Yes.

Dr. Gast
The cuts that we took from pregnancy were rather arbitrary.
What I looked at in my earliest pregnant animals was fetuses of
approximately one to two centimeters in crown-rump length. This is,
I think, a relatively embryonic stage, just based on the maturation
and development- of the limb buds, and so on. But since we got our
animals from the slaughterhouse, we are not in a position to quantify the number of days of pregnancy, and so on. Perhaps one day
somebody like Dr. Sherwood can help us in that regard.

I must point out that if you look at the continuum, and recall
the slide that we used, there was RCP present in the non-pregnant
corpus luteum already. I think you have to carefully consider how
fine a gradation you're going to make in checking how the messenger
RNA levels increase over the period of earliest gestation.

Dr. Rawitch
I just wondered what your evidence was for lack of glycosylation.

Dr. Gast
That is an excellent question. First of all, we translated
RCP in the wheat germ system. There is good evidence that wheat
germ lysates do not participate in asparagine linked glycosylation
in vitro.

Next, as a check and balance for that, we looked at the ability
of tunicamycin treated membranes, which prevent core glycosylation
at asparagine residues, and found a 21,000 molecular weight product
identical to RCP.

The third thing, of course, is in the information we presented
on the sucrose density gradient, and that is that the messenger
RNA is of a size sufficient to produce a purely protein product of
20,000 to 25,000 molecular weight. I think those three points
decrease the possibility of glycosylation.

Dr. Sherwood
It has been suggested that insulin and relaxin may have a
common ancestral origin (Schwabe *et al.*, *Recent Progress in Hormone
Research* 34:123, 1978). How does the relaxin containing precursor
form which you have described relate to that which is known about
the precursor for insulin?

Dr. Gast
Dave, I wish I could. In fact, the only homology that we know
of between the two is that they both contain a pre-sequence. This
is, again, characteristic of many secretory proteins. We are in
the process of doing other work to define these things, but at this
time we have no direct evidence for a proportion of the molecules
such as the C peptide type of a portion of the molecule, nor do we

have an idea of what the extra protein portions of this molecule
represent.

Dr. Frieden

I reviewed a paper recently on the synthesis of insulin in
hagfish and in sea raven pancreas. It turns out that the signal
peptide for pre-proinsulin in both tissue peptides brings the
molecular weight of the first product up to about 11,000 to 13,000.
So it's a 26-amino acid sequence. Thus, there is a pro pre-proinsulin
sequence and then a proinsulin sequence.

CHEMISTRY OF BOVINE RELAXIN

Michael J. Fields, Phillip A. Fields and Lynn H. Larkin

Department of Animal Science
Institute of Food and Agricultural Sciences
Department of Anatomy, College of Medicine
University of Florida, Gainesville, FL

The physiological role of relaxin (relaxation of pelvic ligaments and cervical softening) demonstrated in other species makes the potential use of this hormone appealing to the cattle industry.

There are several problem areas in cattle production where relaxin might be useful. The first is embryo recovery and transfer. Relaxin administered to the diethylstilbestrol primed cow (Graham, 1952; Graham and Dracy, 1953; Eggee and Dracy, 1966) and ovariectomized heifer (Zarrow *et al.*, 1954) dilated the cervix. Dilatation of the cervix would facilitate embryo recovery via the cervix and eliminate the need for complicated surgery. Harper *et al.* (1961) reported that the mechanical stimulation of the cervix and myometrium during nonsurgical embryo transfer resulted in expulsion of the embryo. Relaxin has been shown to inhibit the myometrial contractions of other species, however, its effect on myometrial contractions of the cow uterus has not been tested.

A second potential use for relaxin in the cow would be to increase cervical dilation and relaxation of pelvic ligaments at parturition, particularly in the heifer. The use of sires with increased propensity to pass on a greater growth potential has inadvertently increased calf birth weight. This, in combination with the practice of breeding heifers at one year of age before they have reached their full growth potential, has resulted in increased calving difficulties.

Although Donker (1956) was unable to show that relaxin effected milk ejection in the cow, there is the potential effect of relaxin on lactation (Schwabe *et al.*, 1978).

191

Before attempting to show a physiological role and clinical application for relaxin in the cow, the initial approach was to demonstrate the presence of relaxin in the cow, its tissue source, and, subsequently, the chemistry of this isolate. Previous studies indicate the ovary would be the major source of the hormone in the cow.

Relaxin has been characterized in the ovary of the rat (Sherwood, 1979; Fields and Larkin, 1979) and pig (Sherwood and O'Bryne, 1974). These two species require the ovary for maintenance of pregnancy. Although individual variation does exist (some cows continue pregnancy, give birth to viable offspring, but will have a retained placenta), the essentiality of the corpus luteum by the cow during the third trimester of pregnancy has been shown by McDonald *et al.* (1954), Tanabe (1966), Estergreen *et al.* (1967) and Erb *et al.* (1968). In addition to the ovary, tissues such as blood, placenta and allantoic fluid were evaluated for relaxin activity.

ISOLATION

Blood, extracted according to Albert and Money (1946), from third trimester pregnant cows yielded and extract that promoted a linear (P < .01) increase in growth of the interpubic ligament of the mouse (Steinetz *et al.*, 1960). The biological activity was less than 1 unit/ml of serum.

Crude extracts of third trimester placenta, allantoic fluid or eluates from gel filtration (Sephadex G-50) of the placenta contained no demonstrable bioactivity when tested in the mouse uterus bioassay. Although extraction (Griss *et al.*, 1967) of the ovary from the pregnant cow resulted in less than 1 unit/mg crude extract (Table 1), this indicated that the corpus luteum was the tissue with the highest concentration of relaxin. Emphasis was thus shifted to the CL of late pregnancy. Laboratory technique was monitored by extraction of third trimester pregnant sow ovaries.

When the crude extracts from the third trimester pregnant cow and sow were prepared according to the procedure of Griss *et al.*, (1967) and Fields *et al.* (1980) and chromatographed on Bio-Gel P-10, dissimilar protein elution profiles were seen (Figure 1).

BIOLOGICAL ASSAYS

Bio-Gel P-10 eluates within each peak were combined, freeze dried, filtered and tested in the mouse uterine motility assay (Kroc *et al.*, 1959). The cow and sow crude extracts yielded a relaxin rich fraction that eluted in the 6,000 molecular weight (MW) range. Bovine relaxin biological activity of 71 units/mg protein was lower

*Table 1. TISSUES AND FLUIDS FROM THE THIRD TRIMESTER PREGNANT
COW EXAMINED FOR RELAXIN.*

Source	Quantity Extracted		Biological Activity[a] Units/mg Crude Extract
Plasma	3	1	< 1.0[b]
Placenta (Crude Extract)	1	kg	N.D.[c]
Chromatographed	157	mg	N.D.
Allantoic Fluid	3	1	N.D.
Ovary + CL	1.13	kg	< 1.0
CL	546	gm	1.9
Sow Ovary + CL	200	gm	200.0[d]

[a]Bioactivity was calculated in terms of relative potency of the NIH
standard (NIH-R_P1 460 units/mg) as determined with the mouse uterine
motility inhibition assay as described by Kroc *et al.* (1959).

[b]1 ml blood yields 5.6 mg crude extract.

[c]N.D.--Nondetectable

[d]units mg/protein

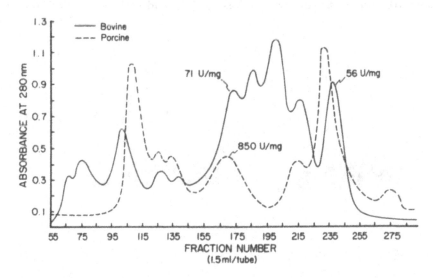

*Figure 1. Column chromatography of the crude CL extracts from the
third trimester pregnant cow (250 mg) and sow (150 mg)
on a Bio-Gel P-10 column (2.6 x 70 cm) with .2 M ammonium
acetate buffer (pH 5.0) at a flow rate of 18 ml/h. (With
permission from Fields et al., Endocrinology, 1980,
107:869).*

than the 850 units eluted for the sow. Unexpectedly, a fraction with
relaxin activity was detected from the bovine eluates that eluted
after the 1,400 MW standard bacitracin, that was not seen with the
porcine eluates (Figure 2). Biological activity was similar between
these two fractions, however, protein yield was much lower for the
later eluting material. Gel filtration of the sow extract did not
demonstrate a later eluting fraction having biological activity.

In addition to inhibiting the myometrial contractions of the
mouse uterus, the 6,000 MW bovine relaxin promoted growth of the mouse
interpubic ligament (Figure 3). Analysis by least squares regression
showed a linear regression (P < .01) of interpubic ligament growth on
log dose of 6,000 MW bovine relaxin, no divergence from parallelism
with porcine WL 150 standard and no quadratic regression component.
Precision of the assay (λ = SE/slope) of less than 0.4 indicated a
sensitive assay with a minimum of variability. The control mice injected with estradiol and relaxin vehicle, 1% benzopurpurine 4B, did
not show an interpubic ligament response.

The low levels of relaxin detected in the cow reported by Wada
and Yuhara (1960 a,b,; 1961) and Fields *et al.* (1980) help to explain
the recent unsuccessful attempts to detect relaxin in serum from the
pregnant cow (Sherwood *et al.*, 1975; Lesmeister, 1975). In addition,
our earlier attempts to detect relaxin in crude extracts of bovine CL

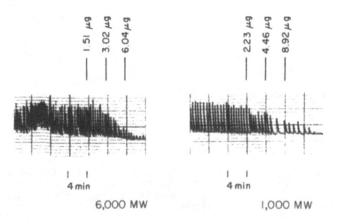

*Figure 2.   Representative example of effect of relaxin isolated from
corpora lutea of the third trimester cow on spontaneous
uterine contractions. Bioactivity was calculated in terms
of relative potency of the NIH porcine standard (NIH-R-P1
460 units/mg) simultaneously tested in the contralateral
uterine horn to which the unknown was tested. Units expressed in terms of μg protein added to bath.*

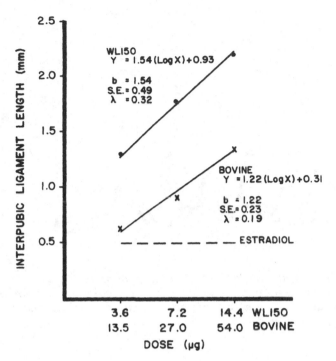

Figure 3. Mouse interpubic ligament bioassay (Steinetz et al., 1960) of Bio-Gel P-10 6,000 MW relaxin and the WL 150 porcine standard (150 units/mg). Potency of bovine relaxin calculated at 13 units/mg protein. (With permission from Fields et al., Endocrinology, 1980, 107:869).

were hampered by a factor that caused myometrial contractions masking relaxin bioactivity. This uterine contracting factor was isolated by chromatography on Bio-Gel P-10 (Fraction 180-211, Figure 1). The factor elicites a sudden tetanic contraction following a return to normality (Figure 4). Although a similar factor was isolated from the sow ovary it caused no difficulty in the assay because of the high biological activity of porcine relaxin.

Bioactivity of the factor was not destroyed and in many cases enhanced when incubated at 100 C for 15 min or exposed to trypsin digestion for 14 h (Figure 4). The factor seemed to be specific for the smooth muscle of the uterus since the stimulatory response was not observed when tested with the isolated mouse ilium. Nor did the isolated eluate containing contracting factor promote growth of the interpubic ligament.

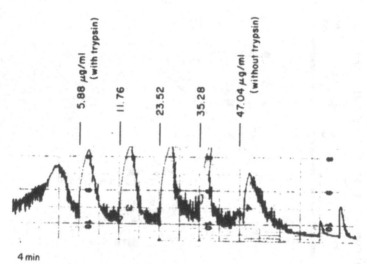

Figure 4.   Presence of a factor from the bovine CL that causes
            tetanic contractions of the spontaneous contracting mouse
            uterus.   CL crude extract incubated with and without 1%
            trypsin for 14 h.

        This factor remains undefined and its biological significance is
unknown.   Isolation of this factor does help to point out the caveats
of using the uterine motility bioassay for screening crude extracts
for relaxin activity in species containing low levels of relaxin.

ISOELECTRIFOCUSING

        Isoelectricfocusing (Fields et al., 1980) of the 6,000 MW
bovine relaxin isolated by Bio-Gel P-10 column chromatography
yielded three peaks with uterine motility inhibitory activity
(Figure 5).   These fractions with biological activity had high
isoelectric points as had been deomonstrated for isofocused porcine
relaxin (Table 2).   However, the bovine fractions were less active
biologically than the porcine isofocused relaxin.

        This observation of lower specific activity for bovine relaxin
has consistently been shown at each step of this study.

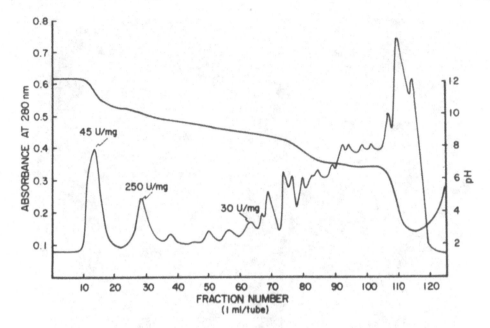

*Figure 5.   Isoelectricfocusing of Bio-Gel P-10 6,000 MW bovine relaxin.
Biological activity is indicated for the peak tube from
each protein peak. (With permission from Fields et al.,
Endocrinology, 1980, 107:869.*

Table 2.   COMPARISON OF ISOFOCUSED BOVINE AND PORCINE RELAXIN[a]

Isolate No.	Isofocused pH		Bioactivity[b] Units/mg Protein	
	Cow	Sow	Cow	Sow
15	11.5	11.4	45	2,500
30	10.1	10.2	250	2,760
65	8.8	8.9	30	400

[a]Isoelectricfocusing of the Bio-Gel P-10 6,000 MW isolated relaxin
according to the method of Karlsson and Ohman (1972).

[b]Bioactivity determined by uterine motility inhibition assay (Kroc
et al., 1959).

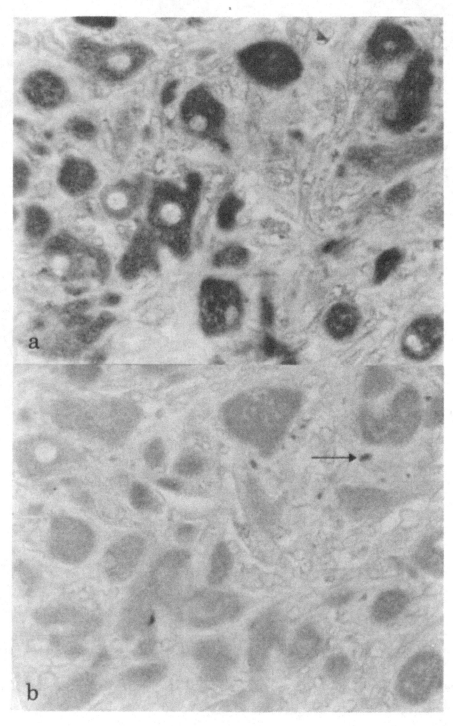

Figure 7.   *Sectional micrograph (x 1,000) of corpora lutea from the
pregnant cow prepared with the immunoperoxidase bridge
technique as described by Mason et al. (1969).   a) Section
treated with an antiserum (#R 19) to relaxin produced
against electrophoretically purified C2 relaxin (Larkin
et al., 1977) and used at a 1:50 dilution.   Stained cells
had irregular outlines with a clear nuclear profile
indicating lack of staining in the nucleus.   b) Control
in which the immunoperoxidase stain was applied exactly
as in a) except that serum from a rabbit not immunized
against relaxin was substituted for the relaxin antiserum
in the intitial phase of the procedure.   Although cellular
outlines are evident, density of stain was greatly
reduced.   Arrow indicates areas of red blood cells containing endogenous peroxidase that served as a positive
control.*

IMMUNOREACTIVITY

Using the immunodiffusion technique (Ouchterlony, 1953) bovine 6,000 MW relaxin was shown to crossreact with a rabbit antiserum prepared against electrophoretically purified porcine relaxin (Larkin *et al.*, 1977; Larkin *et al.*, 1979). With this antiserum in the center well, a continuous precipitin line with no spurring was seen between porcine (NIH-R-P1) and bovine relaxin (Figure 6). The reaction of identity between bovine and porcine relaxin preparations indicates a high degree of similarity between the three molecules detected.

Additional simmilarity of the immunodeterminants of bovine and porcine relaxin was shown with immunohistochemical localization of relaxin in the luteal cell of mid-to late pregnant cows, according to the immunoperoxidate procedure of Mason *et al.* (1969). The dark brown reactive product was localized in the cytoplasm with no staining within the nucleus and interstitial stromal spaces (Figure 7). Little or no specific staining was seen in the luteal cell from the cycling or early pregnant cow. No staining resulted when normal rabbit serum was substituted for the antiporcine relaxin antiserum or when the antiserum was absorbed with a purified porcine relaxin preparation.

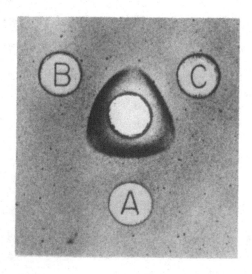

Figure 6.   Immunodiffusion assay showing immunological crossreaction of porcine relaxin antiserum to (A) NIH-R-P1 porcine standard; (B) Bio-Gel P-10 bovine 6,000 MW: and (C) "1,000 MW" relaxin.

SUMMARY

Two small polypeptides with uterine and pubic symphysis relaxin activity were detected in extracts from the CL of third trimester pregnant cows. Fractions having relaxin activity eluted in the 6,000 and 1,000 MW range when chromatographed on Bio-Gel P-10. The 6,000 and "1,000" MW fractions were shown to inhibit spontaneous contractions of the mouse uterus and the 6,000 MW fraction promoted formation of the mouse interpubic ligament that paralleled that of porcine relaxin. Agar diffusion studies with an antiserum to highly purified porcine relaxin showed a continuous precipitin line with no spurring between the two bovine relaxin fractions and NIH-R-P1 porcine relaxin standard. Electrofocusing of the 6,000 MW fraction demonstrated three fractions which were capable of inhibiting contractions of the mouse uterus. Relaxin isolated from porcine ovaries treated in exactly the same manner as that of the cow also had three high pH fractions with bioactivity. Treatment of the three isoelectrifocused bovine fractions and the "1,000 MW" fraction from Bio-Gel P-10 with the reducing agent dithiothrietol eliminated biological activity. Although bovine and porcine relaxin had similar biochemical characteristics, the bovine relaxin preparations had lower biological activity. In addition, the relaxin activity detected in the later eluting bovine fraction was absent from chromatographs of porcine relaxin. Relaxin was shown with immuno-histochemical staining to reside in the cytoplasm of the luteal cell of the pregnant cow.

REFERENCES

Abramowitz, A. A., Money, A. L., Zarrow, M. X., Talmage. R. V. N., Kleinholz, L. H., and Hisaw, F. L. (1944). Preparation, bio-assay and properties of relaxin. Endocrinology 34:103.

Albert, A., and Money, W. L. (1946). Methods of concentration of relaxin from blood serum and urine. Endocrinology 38:56.

Donker, J. D. (1956). Lactation studies. I. Effects upon milk ejection in the bovine of various injection treatments using oxytocin and relaxin. J. Dairy Sci. 39:537.

Eggee, C. J., and Dracy, A. E. (1966). Histological study of effects of relaxin on the bovine cervix. J. Dairy Sci. 49:1053.

Erb, R. R., Gomes, W. R., Randell, R. D., Estergreen, V. L., Jr., and Frost, O. L. (1968). Effect of ovariectomy on concentra-tion of progesterone in blood plasma and urinary estrogen excretion rate in the pregnant bovine. J. Dairy Sci. 51:420.

Estergreen, V. L., Jr., Frost, O. L., Gomes, W. R., Erb, R. E., and Bullard, J. F. (1967). The effect of ovariectomy on pregnancy maintenance and parturition in dairy cows. J. Dairy Sci. 50:1293.

Fields, M. J., Fields, P. A., Castro-Hernandez, A., and Larkin, L. H. (1980). Evidence for relaxin in corpora lutea of late pregnant cows. Endocrinology 107:869.

Fields, P. A. and Larkin, L. H. (1979). Isolation of rat relaxin. Anat. Rec. 193:537.

Graham, E. F. (1952). Some mechanical and hormonal methods of dilating the bovine cervix. Thesis. South Dakota State University, Brookings.

Graham, E. F., and Dracy, A. E. (1953). The effect of relaxin in mechanical dilation of the bovine cervix. J. Dairy Sci. 36:772.

Griss, G., Keck, J., Engelhorn, R. and Tuppy, H. (1967). The isolation and purification of an ovarian polypeptide with uterine relaxin activity. Biochem. Biophys. Acta 140:45.

Harper, M. J., Bennett, J. P., and Rowson, L. E. A. (1961). A possible explanation for the failure of nonsurgical ovum transfer in the cow. Nature 190:788.

Karlsson, C., and Ohman, J. (1972). Electrofocusing in the pH-range 9-11 separation of cytochrome C., LKB Application Note 16 MLB/an-32.

Kroc, R. L., Steinetz, B. G., and Beach, V. L. (1959). The effects of estrogens, progestogens, and relaxin in pregnant and non-pregnant laboratory rodents. Ann. NY Acad. Sci. 75:942.

Larkin, L. H., Fields, P. A. and Oliver, R. M. (1977). Production of antisera against electrophoretically separated relaxin and immunofluorescent localization of relaxin in the porcine corpus luteum. Endocrinology 101:679.

Larkin, L. H., Suarez-Quian, C. A. and Fields, P. A. (1979). In vitro analysis of antisera to relaxin. Acta Endocrinologica 92:568.

Lesmeister, J. L. (1975). Hormonal effects of pelvic development and calving difficulty in beef cattle. Ph.D. Thesis, University of Nebraska, Lincoln.

Mason, T., Pfifer, R., Spicer, S., Swallow R., and Dreskin, R. (1969). An immunoglobulin-enzyme bridge method for localizing tissue antigen. J. Histochem. Cytochem. 17:563.

McDonald, L. E., McNutt, S. H., and Nichols, R. E. (1954). Retained placenta; experimental production and prevention. Amer. J. Vet. Res. 15:22.

Ouchterlony, O. (1953). Antigen-antibody reactions in gels. Acta Path. Microb. Scand. 32:231.

Schwabe, C., Steinetz, B., Weiss, G., Segaloff, A., McDonald, J. K., O'Byrne, E., Hochman, J., Carribre, B. and Goldsmith, L. (1978). Relaxin. Rec. Prog. Horm. Res. 34:123.

Sherwood, O. D., and O'Byrne, E. M. (1974). Purification and characterization of relaxin. Arch. Biochem. Biophys. 160:185.

Sherwood, O. D. (1979). Purification and characterization of rat relaxin. Endocrinology 104:887.

Steinetz, B. G., Beach, V. L., Kroc, R. L., Stasilli, N. R., Nirssbaum, R. E., Nemith, P. J., and Dun, R. K. (1960). Bioassay of relaxin using a reference standard: A simple and reliable method utilizing direct measurement of interpubic ligament formation in mice. Endocrinology 67:102.

Tanabe, T. Y. (1970). The role of progesterone during pregnancy in dairy cows. Penn. Agri. Expt. Sta. Bull. 774.

Wada, H. and Yuhara, M. (1960a). Extraction of relaxin from sow ovary and cow tissues. Jap. J. Zootech. Sci. 31:241.

Wada, H. and Yuhara, M. (1960b). Amino acids in acid hydrolyzate of relaxin extract. Jap. J. Zootech. Sci. 31:243.

Wada, H. and Yuhara, M. (1961). Concentration of relaxin in the blood serum of pregnant cow and cow with ovarian cyst. Proc. Silver Jubilee, Kyoto University.

Zarrow, M. X., Sikes, D., and Nehen, G. M. (1954). Effects of relaxin on the uterine cervix and vulva of young, castrated sows and heifers. Amer. J. Physiol. 178:687.

DISCUSSION FOLLOWING DR. M. J. FIELD'S PAPER

Dr. Bradshaw
    In the gel filtration data you presented you have two fractions
of 6,000 and 1,000 molecular weight. However, in your isoelectric
focusing experiments, you showed three fractions. How do the
latter ones compare to the 6,000 to 1,000 MW fractions.

Dr. Fields
    Only the 6,000 molecular weight fraction has been isoelectric-
focused at this time. The isoelectricfocused 6,000 molecular weight
bovine and porcine relaxin has three bioactive peaks with similar
isoelectric points. I would expect the 1,000 molecular weight
fraction to be quite different.

Dr. Soloff
    Are the cows lactating when you look at the ovaries?

Dr. Fields
    No. Relaxin activity was only demonstrated in corpora lutea
of late pregnant cows very near giving birth to the calf. These
are difficult animals to acquire.

Dr. Gast
    Mike, I enjoyed your localization studies, and I thought you had
excellent controls. I've one other question, though, based on some
of the other things we've talked about. Did you take a look at histochemical localization in any other tissues of these animals near
term, for example, placental tissue?

Dr. Fields
    No, Mike. In view of the report on a relaxin prohormone and
the similar structures between relaxin and insulin it would be
interesting to look at the pancreas.

Dr. Greenwood
    This is almost the same type of question. I think Dr. Anderson
showed a slide this morning of bovine relaxin levels five days into
parturition. Am I right that the CL in the cow, like the pig, just
goes by the end of pregnancy?

Dr. Fields
    Yes. There is a rapid regression of the corpora lutea at the
time of parturition.

Dr. Greenwood
    So then you wouldn't expect any ovarian relaxin early in
pregnancy or lactation?

Dr. Fields

No, at least I wouldn't expect it to be of corpora lutea origin since the cow does not have a CL for up to 40 days post-parturition. But we have noticed in steroids that you can have sequestering of these hormones and then release later on. We have no evidence that relaxin is doing that but, if so, it certainly isn't coming from a CL.

Dr. Bradshaw

Let me ask you one other question, Dr. Fields. The 1,000 molecular weight relaxin is obviously intriguing. By average residue molecular weights we're talking.... if we accept that molecular weight, about nine to ten residues. And if at least one of those is disulfide or two of them are in half cystine, it sounds like oxytocin. Therefore, I begin to suspect--particularly with your own data, namely immunological data--that really what you've got is perhaps some kind of modified form of relaxin to think about, namely 6,000, that is somehow making it be retarded.

My question is--have you every had any other independent molecular weight data on that fraction?

Dr. Fields

We have been working on this now for, I guess, close to five years, and we have just decided to go to publication. With the same extraction and gel filtration technique we do not find a comparable low molecular weight fraction in the sow or rat corpora lutea. The 1,000 MW relaxin induces growth of the interpubic ligament of the mouse, but interpubic ligament growth is not parallel to that induced by porcine relaxin. This infers a difference between 6,000 and 1,000 MW bovine relaxin since porcine and 6,000 MW bovine relaxin induces interpubic ligament growth in a parallel fashion.

Another interesting aspect is that 1,000 MW relaxin runs to the end (cathode) of a 7.5% polyacrylamide gel (pH 8.5) in contrast to a lower Rf value for the 6,000 MW relaxin.

The question has been raised as to whether this 1,000 MW relaxin could be a 6,000 MW relaxin with a high carbohydrate content, i.e., sialic acid. Although a carbohydrate association with protein has been shown to result in a longer retention time on Sephadex, this has not been shown to be the case with Bio-gel. In addition, that problem was reported with low ionic strength buffers whereas we are working with .2 M ammonium acetate. It is, however, an interesting project that the low levels of relaxin found in the cow might be associated with a relaxin of longer half life.

Although verification of the molecular weight of the supposedly low molecular weight relaxin still awaits us, there does appear to be a distinct difference between the 6,000 and 1,000 MW isolate.

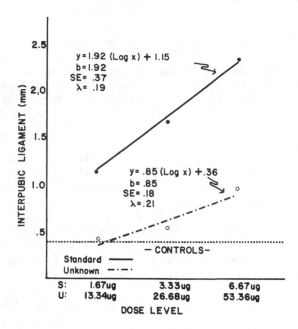

Figure 1. *Interpubic ligament bioassay of Sephadex G50 late eluting*
fraction rechromatographed on Sephadex G25 and the standard
WL 150 porcine relaxin. Analysis showed a linear
regression (P < .01) of interpubic ligament growth on
log dose of "1,000" MW bovine relaxin, divergence from
parallelism (P < .05) with the porcine relaxin and no
quadratic regression component.

Dr. Frieden

You have no data on the effect of that low molecular weight
material in the guinea pig....the guinea pig symphysis?

Dr. Fields

I would have to go back to Al Castro's dissertation on that,
actually to the raw data. Initially, all our bioassay work was with
the GP--however, we have no data on the low molecular weight material.
Repeatability was such a problem for us we have since turned to
Steinetz's mouse interpubic ligament bioassay.

Dr. Sherwood

Mike, do you have a feeling for how clean these three fractions
are that you get after isoelectricfocusing? Have you analyzed them
for homogeneity? Are you getting close enough and are the yields
high enough that one could begin immunoassay analysis and things of
that nature?

Dr. Fields

We are getting close to homogeneity. When we run the Bio-Gel P-10 relaxin towards the cathode (pH 8.5) on the polyacrylamide gels, we see approximately five bands. When we isofocus each polyacrylamide band, we see only one peak. Although this could simply reflect the amount of material that is applied to the gel we feel comfortable we are dealing with a fairly homogenous protein but we do have more work to do on this.

Dr. Bradshaw

The resolution of that question is going to be very, very interesting.

ISOLATION AND CHARACTERIZATION OF HIGH MOLECULAR WEIGHT FORMS OF RELAXIN

Simon C. M. Kwok* and Sandra Y. Yamamoto

Department of Anatomy and Reproductive
Biology
University of Hawaii at Manoa
Honolulu, Hawaii 96822

The striking structural homology with insulin suggests that relaxin may also be derived from a 9,000 dalton single peptide chain precursor. Therefore, in the past few years, we have been searching for a precursor of relaxin using two different approaches, namely, a) isolation of the precursor from pregnant sow ovaries and b) demonstration of the precursor in *in vitro* biosynthetic studies.

From a by-product fraction of relaxin production, we have isolated three forms of relaxin with apparent molecular weights of 19,000, 13,000 and 10,000 daltons (Kwok *et al.*, 1978). Both the 19,000 and 13,000 dalton components retained their high molecular weights after treatment with 8M urea, whereas 40% of the 10,000 dalton component was dissociated into 6,000 dalton relaxin. This was probably due to contamination by relaxin because of their close molecular weights. The 19,000 dalton component could be readily converted to 6,000 dalton relaxin by limited digestion with TPCK-trypsin, while the other two seemed to be sensitive to trypsin. All three high molecule weight forms were biologically active in the *in vitro* bioassay using rat uterine segments.

Since the 19,000 dalton component seemed to be the most promising candidate for the precursor of relaxin, we attempted to purify it further by ion-exchange chromatography. We found that most of the materials were not absorbed on CM-cellulose under the

*Present address: Department of Biochemistry, The University of
 Chicago, Chicago, IL   60637

conditions where relaxin would be tightly bound on the column
(Sherwood and O'Byrne, 1974). Therefore, we used it as a first step
to remove any relaxin contamination before further purification on a
DEAE-cellulose column using a linear gradient of 0-0.2M NaCl in 10 mM
Tris-HCl buffer, pH 8.1. Although precautions had been taken to
minimize proteolysis by using protease inhibitors during isolation
(Kwok *et al.*, 1980), the 19,000 dalton component was found to be
very heterogeneous when it was chromatographed on a DEAE-cellulose
column. Thus, we used a buffer containing 7M urea to minimize
protein-protein interactions. Under these denaturing conditions, the
19,000 dalton component was resolved into a number of peaks. Only
the first six peaks were immunoreactive, and two of them were predominant. When these two predominant forms were rechromatographed on
a Sephadex G-75 column in the presence of 6M guanidine HCl, they
produced single immunoreactive peaks with molecular weights of 11,000
and 14,300 daltons, respectively. The molecular weight of 19,000
daltons determined previously under non-denaturing conditions (1) may
be an over-estimate due to protein-protein interaction. Further
purification and characterization of these two major components are
in progress.

In our studies in relaxin biosynthesis, corpora luteal slices
from late pregnant sow ovaries were incubated with ^{3}H-leucine and
19 other unlabeled amino acids in a balanced salt solution at 37°C
for up to six hours. In some experiments, the tissue slices were
pulse-labeled for 30 min. and then chased for up to six hours.
Longer incubation time was not attempted because of cell death after
prolonged incubation. After incubation, the corpora luteal slices
were extracted with 1M acetic acid, and the extract was then
chromatographed on a Sephadex G-50 (fine) column. In all experiments,
a major radioactive peak (peak I) was detected at the void volume
followed by two small ones (peaks II and III) when the biosynthetic
product was analyzed on a Sephadex G-50 column (Figure 1). No
peak corresponding to the elution volume of relaxin was detected
even after six hours of incubation. There was no conversion of peak
I to the size of relaxin either in continuous labeling or in pulse-
chase experiments for up to six hours, probably due to the abnormally
slow conversion rate of relaxin. When the three peaks were pooled
and immunoprecipitated with antiserum raised against purified relaxin,
only peak I gave significant immunoprecipitable radioactivity. The
immunoprecipitate of peak I was then analyzed on a Sephadex G-75
column in the presence of 6M guanidine HCl. A single peak with a
molecular weight of 13,000 daltons was observed. The peak was
completely annihilated when the immunoprecipitation was carried out
in the presence of excess unlabeled relaxin.

In summary, we have isolated two major forms of relaxin with
molecular weights of 11,000 and 14,300 daltons. We have also
detected a biosynthetically radiolabeled, immunoreactive peptide

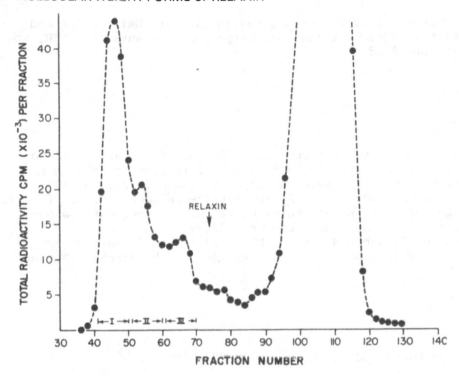

Figure 1.   Chromatography of an extract of corpora luteal slices
after incubation with ^{3}H-leucine for 3 hours on a 1.6 x
90 cm column of Sephadex G-50 (fine). The column was
eluted with 1M acetic acid containing 0.02% bovine serum
albumin at a flow rate of 18 ml/hour. Fractions of 1.5 ml
were collected. Aliquots from alternate fractions were
taken for measurement of total radioactivity. The arrow
marks the elution volume of relaxin.

with a molecular weight of 13,000 daltons. Whether these high
molecular weight forms of relaxin represent true precursors or
conversion intermediates of relaxin, remains to be determined. In
any event, relaxin seems to have a different biosynthetic pathway
from that of insulin despite structural similarities between these
two hormones.

ACKNOWLEDGEMENTS

     We wish to thank Drs. F. C. Greenwood and G. D. Bryant-Greenwood
of the University of Hawaii, Honolulu, Hawaii and Dr. H. D. Niall

of the University of Melbourne, Australia, for their advice and
suggestions.   These studies were supported by grants from NIH, HD-
06633 and HD-11908.

REFERENCES

Kwok, S. C. M., Bryant-Greenwood, G. D. and Niall, H. D.   (1980).
    Evidence for proteolysis during purification of relaxin from
    pregnant sow ovaries. Endocr. Res. Commun. 7:1.
Kwok, S. C. M., Chamley, W. A. and Bryant-Greenwood, G. D. (1978).
    High molecular weight forms of relaxin in pregnant sow ovaries.
    Biochem. Biophys. Res. Commun. 82:997.
Sherwood, O. D. and O'Byrne, E. M. (1974). Purification and
    characterization of porcine relaxin. Arch. Biochem. Biophys.
    160:185.

DISCUSSION FOLLOWING DR. S. C. M. KWOK'S PAPER

Dr. Bradshaw
    Obviously, we are getting more support for the idea that relaxin
is made in a higher molecular weight form.

Dr. Frieden
    Using either trypsin or fibrolysin, can you convert this to a
6,000 Dalton product?

Dr. Kwok
    Which form?

Dr. Frieden
    Well, either of the precursor forms, particularly that last
very sharp peak you showed.

Dr. Kwok
    I haven't tried that. That is a metabolically labeled protein.

Dr. Gast
    You said that you produced a protein that is only seen at the
void volume of your column up until six hours of incubation. You
didn't say if you characterized the protein further than just coming
through with the void volume of the column. Also, did you see
conversion intermediates after that six-hour time period?

Dr. Kwok
   No. At first, it was chromatographed on the Sephadex G-50
column in the presence of one molecular aspartic acid. It is in the
high volume, so it has a molecular weight of over 30,000 daltons.

Dr. Gast
   Did you later see a molecular weight of over 30,000 daltons?

Dr. Kwok
   Yes, on Sephadex G-50. The upper limit of the precipitate is
only 13,000 daltons. Apparently, it may bind to some other protein.

Dr. Gast
   What label did you use? Just for curiosity.

Dr. Kwok
   Well, I have used different ones, but mostly lysine and leucine.

Dr. L. L. Anderson
   I have a question for Dr. Gast.

   In relation to non-pregnancy and pregnancy and detection of
this activity, it would be interesting to look at the transition
from a non-pregnant to a pregnant state, say, between days 11 and
20 to determine whether you can detect when recognition is occurring
in terms of your system. We cannot see this by peripheral blood
assays, but it may be of interest in terms of maintenance of the
corpus luteum versus its imminent regression in a cycling animal.

Dr. Gast
   Lloyd, if I could expand on that. We do see RCP mRNA, as we
pointed out in the corpus luteum of the non-pregnant ovary.

   There are two critical transition periods to be examined here.
The first is the transition from the follicular ovary to the corpus
luteum of the cycle. The second is the transition from the corpus
luteum of the cycle to the corpus luteum of pregnancy. And the
question to ask is the obvious one that you have asked.

   Our hope was, by studying the levels of RCP mRNA, that we might
be able to more closely examine both of these periods of time. Again,
I think it might be difficult to examine those on a day-by-day basis.
I'm not sure, based upon the results we got with our non-pregnant
corpus luteum that we would see the tremendous induction or the
saving phenomena that people have talked about in the past.
Apparently the corpus luteum of the non-pregnant animal has a
capacity for milking relaxin as it is actively transcribing RCP
messenger RNA already. So the question might be: is the follicular
portion of the cycle the important period of time to look at in
terms of generation of RCP messenger RNA?

NEED FOR HUMAN RELAXIN

F. C. Greenwood and G. D. Bryant-Greenwood
University of Hawaii
Honolulu, HI   96822

There are four variations on the porcine relaxin radioimmunoassay which could be used to look at relaxin in human plasma.   Each
radioimmunoassay has a different degree of heterogeniety with
respect to the labelled hormone and to the antiserum, although all are
derived from porcine material. The most heterogenous system is that
originally used by Bryant in 1972, a labelled hormone selected from
NIH-R-P1 relaxin and an antiserum generated to the crude material.
A number of other RIAs have been reported (Sherwood *et al.*, 1975;
O'Byrne and Steinetz, 1976; Loumaye *et al.*, 1978). A less heterogenous
radioimmunoassay is that using pooled relaxins, CM-a', CM-a, CM-B,
from a CMC column used as a label, and an antiserum to the product
of an earlier purification step, the G2 area of a Sephadex column
(O'Byrne and Steinetz, 1976). This assay is markedly more homogenous
with respect to the antigen used for labelling and to that used for
immunization. Finally, the most homogenous RIA would be one of
these relaxins, CM-a' and an antiserum to this material (Afele *et
al.*, 1979); a system unable to pick up immunoactivity in human plasmas
in our hand. In studying these RIAs to look at heterologous relaxins
in plasma we have arrived at the following conclusions (Bryant-
Greenwood and Greenwood, 1979): the higher the degree of heterogeniety, the more total inhibition can be detected; each RIA looks at
a spectrum of plasma immunoactivities related to relaxin but we do not
know the structure of the molecules inhibiting in any of the radioimmunoassays; we cannot utilize the physiology of relaxin to support
the specificity of heterologous radioimmunoassays. By this we mean
that changes in plasma immunoactivity obtained by a heterologous
system yield evidence for specificity where these can be attributed
physiologically, e. g. a rise before parturition. On the other hand,
a rise in plasma immunoactivity on suckling in the sheep as
demonstrated by a porcine/anti-porcine system gives no evidence for

specificity until verified in the pig. When one considers the spectra
of immunoactivities measured by variants of the porcine/anti-porcine
assay, one has to concede on Occam's principle that the spectrum
would be widest with the most heterogenous assay through to the most
homogenous assay (CM-a'/anti-CM-a' system). In addition there is a
problem of sensitivity in heterologous assays where a sample of the
homologous hormone is not available, as is the case of human relaxin.
Demonstrating parallelism between dilutions of human plasma and over
the entire range of the standard curve of purified porcine relaxins
merely allows the inhibition of the human plasma to be expressed in
terms of equivalence of porcine relaxin, with caveats that a particular
label and a particular antiserum is used. The specific immunological
activity cannot be known until authentic samples of human relaxin are
obtained; only then can the true sensitivity of the heterologous system be expressed in terms of the human hormone rather than the porcine
material.

Hence, we perceive a need for a fully homologous and sensitive
radioimmunoassay for human relaxin. To this end we have collected
placentas obtained at elective cesarean section, and with the addition
of protease inhibitors, extracted the material, chromatographed these
extracts on Sephadex and CMC columns, monitoring the columns by the
porcine/antiporcine RIA on the assumption that at high concentrations,
human relaxin would be detected by this system. A final fraction is
active, by definition, in the RIA but more importantly is active in a
radioreceptor assay at a level equivalent to 1:20 to 1:50 that of
porcine CM-a' relaxin. We have yet to demonstrate *production* of this
human relaxin in the basal plate nor have we excluded completely the
possibility that some of the immunoactivity and perhaps of the bioactivity might be related to NGF or represent authentic human relaxin
produced elsewhere but bound to receptors in the placenta and isolated therefrom. A full report of this work has been prepared
(Yamamoto *et al.*, 1981). In discussions subsequent to this meeting,
with Dr. L. H. Larkin, University of Florida and Dr. M. Bigazzi,
Poggiosecco Hospital, Florence, it is apparent that their groups have
similar data on the human placenta using bioassay and histochemistry.

A further indication of the need for a human relaxin is suggested
by the results of a preliminary clinical trial using porcine relaxin
on cervical ripening and on the initiation of labor in women. Relaxin
was administered intravaginally in 10 ml of water mixed with 700 mg
of tylose granules (Hoechst) to make a viscous gel. After initial
dose trials, a 2 mg dose was chosen for a randomized, double-blind
trial of 30 relaxin-treated patients and an equal number of controls.
The gels, given 15 hours prior to surgical induction of labor, caused
a significant number of patients to establish labor with a significant
improvement in ther cervical score. It was concluded that 2 mg of
intravaginal relaxin was essentially comparable to 25 to 50 mg of
intravaginal $PGF_2\alpha$. A full account of this trial has been published
(MacLennan *et al.*, 1980). Larger trials are now indicated in order

to pick up possible side effects at the 1% incidence level, and of
course, human relaxin would be more appropriate if available.
Further, although it is acceptable to treat pregnant women intravaginally with porcine relaxin, human material would be required for
any intravenous studies in pregnancy with a view to the abolition
of premature labor.

Finally, although the existence of the human relaxin in the human
corpus luteum of pregnancy has been well established by Dr. B. Weiss
and his collaborators in a series of publications, the identification
production of a relaxin in human placenta with no apparent effect
on blood levels suggests a local action for this material and raises
the interesting possibility that relaxin may be both a systemic and
a local hormone.

REFERENCES

Afele, S., Bryant-Greenwood, G. D., Chamley, W. A. and Dax, E. M.
    (1979). Plasma relaxin immunoactivity in the pig at parturition
    and during nuzzling and suckling. J. Reprod. Fert. 56:451-457.
Bryant, G. D. (1972). The detection of relaxin in porcine, ovine,
    and human plamsa by radioimmunoassay. Endocrinology 91:1113-
    1117.
Bryant-Greenwood, G. D. and Greenwood, F. C. (1979). Specificity of
    radioimmunoassays for relaxin. J. Endocrinol. 81:239-247.
Loumaye, E., Teuwissen, B. and Thomas, K. (1978). Characterization
    of relaxin radioimmunoassay using Bolton-Hunter reagent.
    Gynecol. Ostet. Invest. 9:262-267.
MacLennan, A. H., Green, R. C., Bryant-Greenwood, G. D., Greenwood,
    F. C. and Seamark, R. F. (1980). Ripening of the human cervix
    and induction of labour with purified porcine relaxin. Lancet
    1(8162):220-223.
O'Byrne, E. M. and Steinetz, B. G. (1976). Radioimmunoassay (RIA)
    of relaxin in sera of various species using an antiserum to
    porcine relaxin. Proc. Soc. Exp. Biol. Med. 152:272-276
Sherwood, O. D., Rosentreter, K. R. and Birkhimer, M. L. (1975).
    Development of a radioimmunoassay for porcine relaxin using
    ^{125}I-labeled polytyrosyl-relaxin. Endocrinology 96:1106-1113.
Yamamoto, S., Kwok, S. C. M., Greenwood, F. C. and Bryant-Greenwood,
    G. D. (1981). J. Clin. Endocrinol. Metab. (submitted).

DISCUSSION FOLLOWING DR. F. GREENWOOD'S PAPER

Dr. *Bradshaw*
     You said you used 25 to 50 milligrams of prostaglandin in these studies?

Dr. *Greenwood*
     Yes.

Dr. *Steinetz*
     With regard to the work setting up a heterologous radiommunoassay for human relaxin, actually, the rabbits were immunized first with the thousand-unit material and then annestically challenged for the next six months with purified CM relaxin.

     It's an amnestic response and is a perfectly legitimate immuno-logical procedure to develop a highly effective antibody where you have a weak antigen.

     Secondly, we have never claimed to measure human relaxin. We measure something which cross-reacts with our antiserum to porcine relaxin, which is obviously produced by the human corpus luteum, since we detect it in ovarian vein blood in much higher concentration than in peripheral blood. Also, the levels drop much faster fol-lowing leutectomy than they do following caesarian section.

     Finally, we have done parallel bioassays in the guinea pig and immunoassay in the heterologous porcine system of human corpora lutea extraction and there is reasonable agreement between the bioassay and the immunoassay. The biological activity can be inhibited by addition of the porcine antiserum. Whatever we are measuring in the human serum and in the human ovary seems to be a peptide that has at least some of the characteristics of porcine relaxin.

Dr. *Greenwood*
     Yes. The CL extracted material is definitely biologically active and it is inhibited by an antiserum to porcine relaxin. The step from that into plasma is a big leap into the unknown. I would agree with you in saying that these assays can be used to look at relaxin like immunoactivity in human plasma.

Dr. *Steinetz*
     In regard to your human placental extract, you said it had biological activity. Could you tell us how much?

Dr. *Greenwood*
     In a radioreceptor assay the specific activity would be equivalent to 1/20th to 1/50th of the activity of CMa.

Dr. Steinetz
   In a radioreceptor assay?

Dr. Greenwood
   In a radioreceptor assay. Yes. We have to do a bioassay on
it, but I'm really loath to do a bioassay on very valuable material.

Dr. Boime
   Have you even taken biopsy material of human liver or kidney,
made a comparable homogenate, passed it through a Sephadex column,
and tested it in your receptor assay as a negative control?

Dr. Greenwood
   No, but I'm thinking of the controls which Dr. Mercado-Simmen
has done with muscle, but that's the other side of the coin. That's
not making a pseudo-extract. That's making a pseudo-receptor; so
my answer is still no.

Dr. Bradshaw
   What is your tissue for the radioreceptor assay?

Dr. Greenwood
   That is a uterine membrane preparation from the estrogen-primed
rat.

RADIOIMMUNOASSAY OF RELAXIN

O. D. Sherwood*

School of Basic Medical Sciences
Department of Physiology and Biophysics
University of Illinois
Urbana, IL 61801

INTRODUCTION

Until recently rigorous studies concerning the physiology of
relaxin biosynthesis and secretion were impeded by limitations
associated with the available relaxin assays. Relaxin bioassays lack
the sensitivity required for accurate measurements of the relaxin
levels which exist in the peripheral blood of many species during
pregnancy. Even with the pig, a species in which substantial quantities of relaxin are released by the ovaries during late pregnancy,
determination of relaxin levels in ovarian venous blood by mouse
interpubic ligament bioassay necessitates the concentration of relatively large volumes of plasma in order to attain the limits of assay
sensitivity (Belt et al., 1971). The relative insensitivity of
bioassays makes it impossible to use them for the measurement of
relaxin levels in small samplings of blood taken at frequent intervals
from animals. The opportunity to develop more sensitive and precise
relaxin assays became available with the advent of the radioimmunoassay in the 1960's.

In 1972 Bryant reported the development of the first radioimmunoassay for relaxin. With that radioimmunoassay the impure porcine
relaxin preparation NIH-R-P1 (442 U per mg), which contains approximately 20% biologically active relaxin and 80% uncharacterized
proteins, was used for the generation of an antiserum. Radioactive
iodine was incorporated into NIH-R-P1 by means of the chloramine T
oxidation procedure described by Hunter and Greenwood (1962). A
radioactive fraction obtained following gel filtration of radiolabeled NIH-R-P1 on Sephadex G-50 was selected as radioligand.
*Work originating from the author's laboratory was supported by
 NIH Grant 08700.

221

Bryant and her collaborators have reported relaxin immunoactivity in
sheep and human beings under many physiological conditions (Bryant
and Chamley, 1976a,b; Bryant et al., 1975, 1976; Chamley et al.,
1975) when that radioimmunoassay is employed. More recent studies
(Sherwood and O'Byrne, 1974) conducted with highly purified porcine
relaxin have demonstrated that biologically active porcine relaxin,
which has a molecular weight of approximately 6,000, lacks the amino
acids tyrosine and histidine which incorporate radioactive iodine
when the chloramine T procedure is used for radioiodination. Therefore, the molecules radioiodinated by Bryant were not these biologically active relaxin molecules. Kwok, McMurtry, and Bryant
(1976) reported that the substances detected with the Bryant (1972)
radioimmunoassay are proteins in the impure relaxin preparation NIH-
R-P1 which are larger than the biologically active relaxin molecules
which have molecular weights of 6,000. The nature of the proteins
measured with the radioimmunoassay of Bryant (1972) have not been
clearly defined; and, therefore, the studies which have been conducted
with that radioimmunoassay will not be summarized in this chapter.

In 1974 (Sherwood and O'Byrne, 1974) and 1979 (Sherwood, 1979a),
we reported the isolation and characterization of high purified porcine
and rat relaxin, respectively (Chapter 3). We have employed these
highly purified relaxin preparations for the development of homologous
radioimmunoassays for porcine relaxin (Sherwood et al., 1975a) and
rat relaxin (Sherwood and Crnekovic, 1979). The development of
these radioimmunoassays and their subsequent utilization for
physiological studies are described in this chapter. In order to
permit the discussion of physiological studies which have been
conducted with these relaxin radioimmunoassays, some experimental
details found in the original reports describing their development
(Sherwood et al., 1975a; Sherwood and Crnekovic, 1979) will be omitted
from this chapter.

PORCINE RELAXIN RADIOIMMUNOASSAY

Development of the Porcine Relaxin Radioimmunoassay

Radioiodination of porcine relaxin

The three highly purified preparations of porcine relaxin designated CMB, CMa, and CMa' (Sherwood and O'Byrne, 1974) which
are described in Chapter 3, were used for the development of the
porcine relaxin radioimmunoassay; and they are collectively designated
native relaxin. Conventional techniques which employ chloramine T
(Hunter and Greenwood, 1962) or the enzyme lactoperoxidase
(Marchalonis, 1969) for radioiodination incorporate radioactive
iodine into residues of tyrosine and histidine (see Figure 1A).
Porcine relaxin lacks both of these amino acids (Sherwood and
O'Byrne, 1974); and, as expected, initial efforts to radioiodinate

native relaxin according to the commonly used procedure of Hunter and Greenwood (1962) were not successful (Figure 1B). In order to radioiodinate relaxin, tyrosine molecules were incorporated into the hormone. Tyrosine was covalently bound to amino groups of native relaxin by an amide bond employing the reagent N-carboxy-L-tyrosine anhydride according to a modification (Sherwood et $al.$, 1975a) of the procedure described by Becker and Stahmann (1953) for the preparation of poly-peptidyl proteins. When an 8:1 molar ratio of N-carboxy-L-tyrosine anhydride to native relaxin was used, native relaxin incorporated 1.67 moles of tyrosine per mole of native relaxin. Mouse interpubic ligament bioassays showed that the modified native relaxin, designated polytyrosyl-relaxin, was as biologically active as native relaxin.

Polytyrosyl-relaxin readily incorporated ^{125}I when the chloramine T procedure of Hunter and Greenwood (1962) was employed for radio-iodination. A typical elution pattern showing the separation of ^{125}I-polytyrosyl-relaxin from free ^{125}I by gel filtration is shown in Figure 1C. The two or three tubes of ^{125}I-polytyrosyl-relaxin containing the highest radioactivity are routinely employed as the radioligand for the radioimmunoassay. The specific radioactivity of ^{125}I-polytyrosyl-relaxin obtained by this procedure ranges from 80-100 μCi per μg. ^{125}I-polytyrosyl-relaxin is diluted and frozen in PBS (0.14 M sodium chloride, 0.01 M sodium phosphate, pH 7.0) containing 1% ovalbumin and routinely used for four to five weeks without repurification.

Preparation of rabbit anti-porcine relaxin sera

Porcine relaxin antigen was prepared by emulsifying 4.0 mg native relaxin in 2 ml 0.9% saline and 2 ml complete Freunds adjuvant. Four adult male New Zealand white rabbits were initially immunized with 1.0 mg native relaxin at biweekly intervals by intradermal injections into three or four sites in the medial aspect of each thigh. After two months, 1.0 mg native relaxin was administered intra-muscularly at biweekly intervals for an additional two months in 1.0 ml 0.9% saline. Seven days after the ninth injection of porcine relaxin, 50 ml blood was removed by cardiac puncture. The four rabbits produced antiporcine relaxin sera suitable for use in the relaxin radioimmunoassay at final dilutions ranging from 1:50,000 to 1:200,000 (Figure 2). Antiserum from rabbit 1082 is routinely employed for the porcine relaxin radioimmunoassay.

Porcine relaxin radioimmunoassay procedures

Double antibody relaxin radioimmunoassays are conducted in 12 x 75 mm disposable glass culture tubes. Quantities of standard native

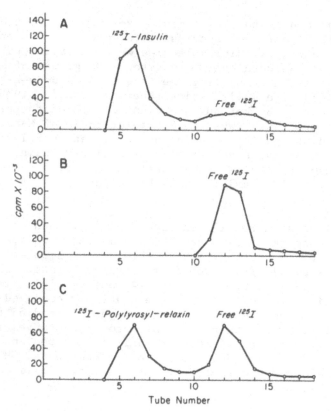

*Figure 1.   Radioactive ^{125}I elution profiles from Bio-Gel P-6 columns
            after the radioiodination procedure of Hunter and Greenwood
            (1962) was employed with (A) insulin, (B) native relaxin,
            and (C) polytyrosyl-relaxin.   (From Sherwood et al.,
            1975a).*

relaxin ranging from 8.0 to 2,000 pg or unknowns are placed in each
tube, and sufficient PBS-1% ovalbumin is added to bring the volume
to 500 µl.   Two hundred microliters of rabbit anti-porcine relaxin
serum 1082, diluted 1:20,000 in 0.05 M EDTA-PBS and containing 1:60
male rabbit serum, are added to each tube.   The contents are incubated
at 4°C for 24 hr.   One hundred microliters of ^{125}I-polytyrosyl-relaxin
(prepared by diluting the ^{125}I-polytyrosyl-relaxin obtained from
the BioGel P-6 column with PBS-1% ovalbumin so that on the day of
iodination 100 µl contains 55,000-58,000 cpm) are added to each tube,
and the contents are again incubated at 4°C for 24 hr.   Twenty-four
hours later 200 µl sheep anti-rabbit γ-globulin, at a dilution which
will enable maximum precipitation of bound ^{125}I-polytyrosyl-relaxin,

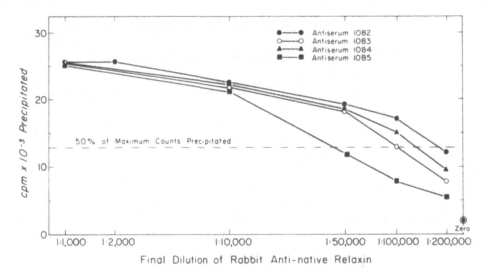

*Figure 2.   Titration curve of four rabbit anti-porcine relaxin sera
(From Sherwood, 1979b).*

are added to each tube. The contents are mixed and incubated at 4°C
for 72 hr. Three milliliters of cold PBS are then added to each
tube, and the tubes are centrifuged for 30 min at 1,000 x g at 4°C.
The supernatants are decanted and the precipitates are counted in an
automatic γ counter. Native relaxin standards and unknowns are
normally assayed in quadruplicate.

Characterization of the Porcine Relaxin Radioimmunoassay

Sensitivity

A typical standard curve obtained with the porcine relaxin
radioimmunoassay is shown in Figure 3. The "least-detectable dose"
(Feldman and Rodbard, 1971) which is consistently measured with
this radioimmunoassay is 32 pg of native relaxin. This is more than
1,000 times more sensitive then the mouse interpubic ligament bioassay which requires approximately 100 ng of porcine relaxin for
detection. When logit and log transformations are used, a linear
regression is obtained from 32 to 1,000 pg native relaxin. During
late pregnancy relaxin levels are normally determined with multiple
volumes of plasma or sera ranging from 1 to 20 μl.

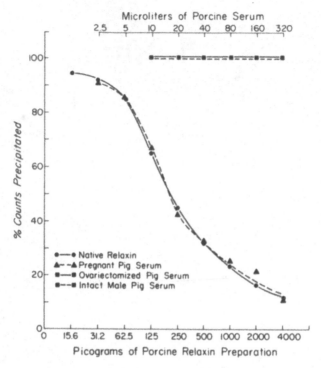

Figure 3.   Dose-response curves for porcine native relaxin, pregnant
            pig serum, ovariectomized female serum, and intact male
            pig serum in the porcine relaxin radioimmunoassay.
            (From Sherwood, 1979b).

Hormone specificity

All experiments which have been conducted indicate that the
radioimmunoassay is specific for relaxin. First, the slope of the
dose·response curve obtained with multiple volumes of late pregnancy
pig serum does not differ from the dose-response curve obtained with
native relaxin (Figure 3). Second, porcine insulin, FSH, LH and
TSH do not react in the assay system in doses up to 1 µg. Third,
when late pregnancy pig serum spiked with ^{125}I-polytyrosyl-relaxin
was filtered through a column of BioGel P-10, the immunoactive peak
coeluted with ^{125}I-polytyrosyl-relaxin, thereby indicating that
the immunoactive substance within late pregnancy pig serum and
porcine relaxin are of similar size (Sherwood et al., 1975a).

Species specificity

Presently available data indicate that the number of species
with which the homologous porcine relaxin radioimmunoassay can be
used for accurate determinations of relaxin immunoactivity levels
within the blood are limited. Employing our anti-porcine relaxin
sera, we have detected no immunoactive substance within late
pregnancy sera obtained from cows, sheep, guinea pigs, monkeys, or
human beings. Sera obtained from rats during late pregnancy contains
a substance(s) which cross reacts with several preparations of anti-
porcine relaxin sera. However, as Figure 4 shows, the rat relaxin
has a lower affinity for the anti-porcine relaxin serum than porcine
relaxin. The slopes of the regression lines obtained with highly
purified rat relaxin (Sherwood, 1979a) are approximately -0.25 and
are markedly reduced relative to the slope of porcine relaxin which
is approximately -1.00. Figure 4 also shows that relatively large
quantities of rat relaxin are required for detection in the porcine
relaxin radioimmunoassay.

Others have had more success in detecting relaxin in the blood
of species other than the pig. O'Byrne and Steinetz (1976) developed
a rabbit anti-porcine relaxin serum designated 39377 which cross

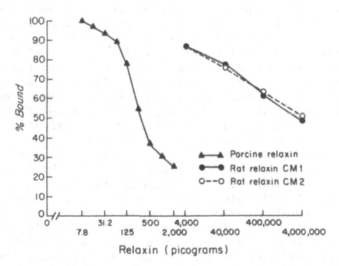

Figure 4. *Dose-response curves for porcine relaxin and rat relaxin*
preparations CM1 and CM2 in the homologous porcine relaxin
radioimmunoassay. (From Sherwood and Crnekovic, 1979).

reacts with relaxin from several species. They and their collaborators
have used that antiserum in a modified porcine relaxin radioimmunoassay to detect relaxin immunoactivity during pregnancy in the sera
of human beings, rats, mice, guinea pigs, hamsters, dogs, and baboons
(O'Byrne and Steinetz, 1976; O'Byrne et al., 1976; 1978a; Weiss et
al., 1976; 1977, 1978; Hochman et al., 1978). However, the accuracy of
quantitative estimates of relaxin immunoactivity in species other
than the pig with any porcine relaxin radioimmunoassay has not been
established since parallelism betwen the porcine relaxin standard
and multiple volumes of sera obtained from other species has not been
demonstrated.

Precision and reproducibility

The intraassay coefficient of variation ranges from approximately
8-13%. The interassay coefficient of variation of the porcine relaxin
radioimmunoassay determined by measuring the relaxin content of a
serum sample obtained from a pig during late pregnancy in nine
independent radioimmunoassays was 8.1%.

Physiological Studies with the Porcine Relaxin Radioimmunoassay

Relaxin immunoactivity in the pig

In pigs experiencing normal pregnancy and spontaneous parturition
on approximately day 114 of gestation, relaxin immunoactivity levels
(Figures 5 and 6) in peripheral plasma remain below 2 ng per ml during
the first 100 days of gestation and then rise to approximately 40 ng
per ml by 30 hours before parturition. Relaxin concentrations then
increase sharply to a mean of approximately 150 ng per ml by 14 hours
before parturition. This maximum is followed by a rapid decrease to
approximately 40 ng per ml by 2 hours preceding parturition. By one
day following parturition, relaxin levels are approximately 1 ng per
ml. Caution must be exercised in comparing relaxin levels obtained
by radioimmunoassay to relaxin levels obtained by bioassay since
the radioimmunoassay does not necessarily measure a biologically
active molecule. It seems likely, however, that the immunoactive
"substance" measured with this radioimmunoassay is, at least in part,
biologically active relaxin since the appearance of relaxin immunoactivity coincides with the high concentrations of biologically
active relaxin measured in sow ovarian vein plasma within 2 days
preceding parturition (Belt et al., 1971). The elevated levels of
relaxin observed during late pregnancy in pigs is consistent with the
long-held view that relaxin may have physiological effects associated
with parturition.

Studies employing bioassays (Belt et al., 1971), histological
techniques (Belt et al., 1971; Kendall et al., 1978), and radioimmunoassays (Sherwood et al., 1977a) indicate that it is the corpora lutea

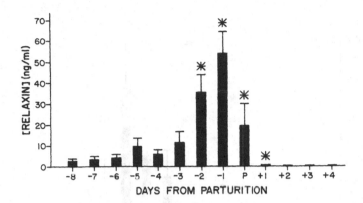

Figure 5. Relaxin concentrtations obtained daily from P-8 through P + 4. P = Day of parturition. Means of 6 animals and their standard errors (SE) are shown. Asterisks (*) denote those mean relaxin concentrations which differ significantly (P < 0.05) from those of the preceding day. (From Sherwood et al., 1975b).

of pregnancy in the pig which produce, store, and secrete relaxin. In the pig the corpora lutea are also the primary source of progesterone which is required for maintenance of pregnancy. Since the corpora lutea are undergoing functional regression, as judged by a rapid fall in progesterone levels during the two days preceding parturition (Molokwu and Wagner, 1973; Killian *et al.*, 1973), it was evident that the prepartum surge in peripheral plasma relaxin levels might be associated with the regression of the corpora lutea. In order to gain further information concerning this possibility, we utilized a series of experiments which involved surgical or pharmacological treatments which might influence luteal function during late pregnancy (Sherwood *et al.*, 1976, 1977a,b, 1978, 1979).

In one study the normal utero-ovarian relationship was altered so that there were no direct utero-ovarian connections (Figure 7). Luteolysis, parturition (Martin *et al.*, 1978), and the prepartum relaxin surge (Sherwood *et al.*, 1977b) occurred at the expected time. It, therefore, appears that the factor(s) which brings about the prepartum surge in relaxin can be carried in the systemic circulation.

The nature of the factor(s) which brings about the prepartum surge in relaxin levels is not known. However, we have evidence that prostaglandins (PG) may be involved with the relaxin surge and

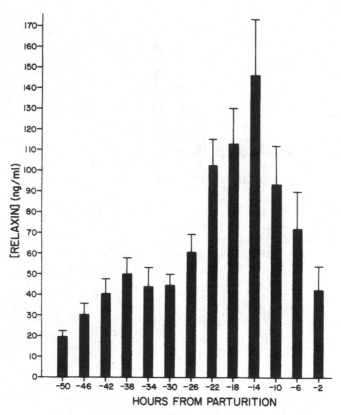

Figure 6. Relaxin concentrations obtained a 4 hr intervals immediately preceding parturition. Means + SE of 6 animals are shown. (From Sherwood et al., 1975b).

luteolysis. Figure 8 shows that the infusion of sufficient $PGF_2\alpha$ on day 110 of gestation to induce parturition on day 111 of gestation (Nara and First, 1977) brought about a surge in relaxin levels and a drop in progesterone levels in peripheral sera (Sherwood *et al.*, 1979). Additionally, injection of the prostaglandin synthesis inhibitor indomethacin from day 109 to day 116 of gestation delayed the relaxin surge (Figure 9) and parturition, which normally occurs from day 112 to day 115 of gestation until 2-4 days after the termination of indomethacin administration on day 116 of gestation. The drop in progesterone levels in indomethacin treated pigs was also delayed and occurred concurrently with the surge in relaxin levels on approximately day 119 of gestation (Figure 10B).

Peripheral blood levels of progesterone influenced parturition in the pig. Several workers (Curtis *et al.*, 1969; First and

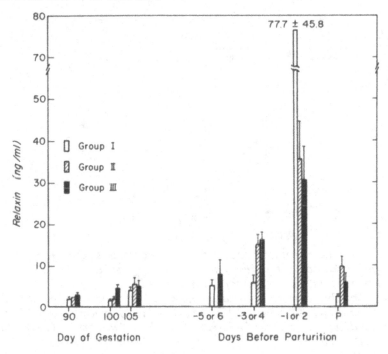

*Figure 7. Mean relaxin concentrations + SE obtained during late preg-
nancy. Group I, 7 gilts in which the ovaries were transplanted to the adjacent uterine horn. Group II, 3 gilts in
which the ovaries were transplanted to the exterior abdominal
wall. Group III, 4 gilts in which one uterine horn and its
contralateral ovary were removed. P = day of parturition.
(From Sherwood et al., 1977b).*

Staigmiller, 1973; Minar and Schilling, 1970; and Nellor *et al.*,
1975) have demonstrated that parturition can be delayed by the
administration of a progestin during late pregnancy and beyond the
expected time of parturition in pigs. In order to determine whether
the prepartum surge in relaxin is influenced by the administration
of sufficient progestin to delay parturition, an experiment was
conducted in which progesterone was administered to pregnant pigs
for six days during late gestation (Figure 11, Sherwood *et al.*,
1978). Although gestation length was prolonged in progesterone
treated animals (118.1 vs 113.8 days for controls), the time of
occurrence of the surge in relaxin levels in the peripheral sera was
not influenced (progesterone treated = 112.6 $\pm$ 0.6 SE days; controls =
113.0 $\pm$ 1.0 SE days). With this experiment there was an unusually
prolonged interval between the time of maximum relaxin concentration
and parturition. It was concluded that the surge in relaxin levels,
which occurs in pigs treated with progesterone for six days, is not
sufficient in and of itself to initiate parturition. The mechanism

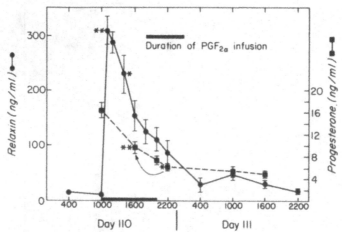

Figure 8.   *Mean relaxin and progesterone concentrations ± SE in 5 pigs infused with prostaglandin $F_{2\alpha}$ at a rate of 0.5 mg per hour over a 10 hr period on day 110 of gestation.   Asterisks denote those mean hormone concentrations which differ significantly   (*, P< 0.05; **, P <0.01) from those immediately preceding or those indicated with an arrow.   (From Sherwood et al., 1979).*

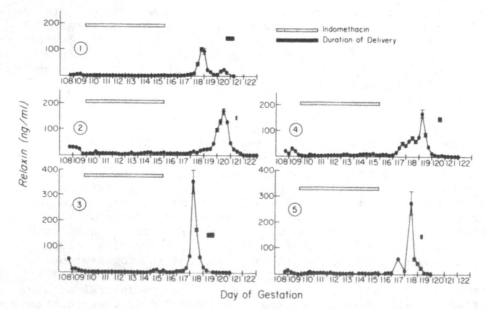

Figure 9.   *Relaxin concentrations ± SE at 6 hr intervals from 1600 hr on day 108 of gestation through 24 hr after parturition in 5 pigs injected i.m. twice each day with indomethacin at a dose of 4 mg per Kg from days 109-116 of gestation. (From Sherwood et al., 1979).*

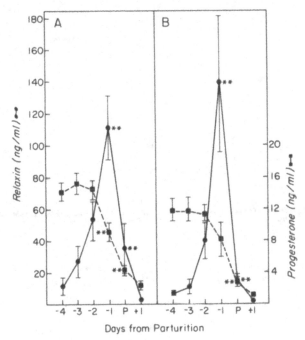

Figure 10. *Mean relaxin and progesterone concentrations ± SE in
control (A) and indomethacin treated (B) groups. The time
of the initiation of delivery for control and the indomethacin group were 114.9 ± 0.5 SE and 120.1 ± 0.4 SE days,
respectively. Asterisks denote those mean hormone concentrations which differ significantly (**, P< 0.01) from
those immediately preceding. P = Day of parturition.
(From Sherwood et al., 1979).*

whereby progesterone delays parturition in pigs is not completely
understood. Whatever the mechanism, it appears that progesterone
does not interfere with the early events which lead to the massive
release of relaxin from the corpora lutea on approximately day 113
of gestation.

Relaxin immunoactivity in species other than the pig

Relaxin immunoactivity has been detected in the blood of several
species during pregnancy with the modified porcine relaxin radioimmunoassay of O'Byrne and Steinetz (1976). Relaxin immunoactivity
has been reported to be present in the plasma of women within 14
to 21 days of conception (Quagliarello *et al.*, 1979) and to remain
elevated throughout nearly all of gestation (O'Byrne *et al.*, 1978a).
However, unlike the pig, levels do not increase during late gestation

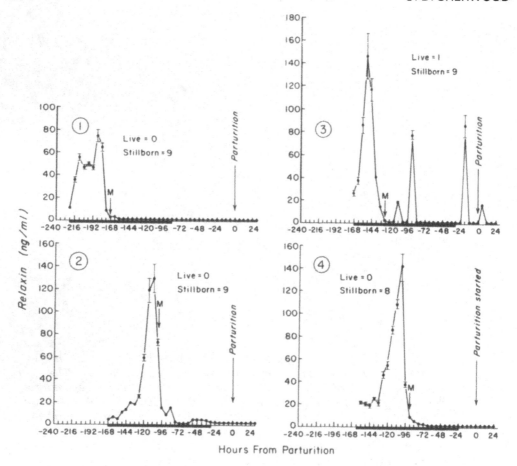

Figure 11. Mean relaxin concentrations + SE in four pigs treated with progesterone (25 mg, 4 times/day) for 6 days, from day 110 through 115 of gestation. Duration of progesterone treatment is indicated by dark bars along abscissas. (From Sherwood et al., 1978).

(Figure 12). The human corpus luteum appears to be the primary source of relaxin since relaxin biological and immunological activity are present in extracts of human corpora lutea of pregnancy (O'Byrne *et al.*, 1978b; Weiss *et al.*, 1978), and relaxin immunoactivity is higher in the ovarian vein draining the ovary containing the corpus luteum of pregnancy than in the peripheral circulation or the vein draining the contralateral ovary (see Figure 13A from Weiss *et al.*, 1976). Unlike the pig, infusion of sufficient $PGF_2\alpha$ to induce parturition during late gestation does not influence serum levels of relaxin (see Figure 13B from Hochman *et al.*, 1978).

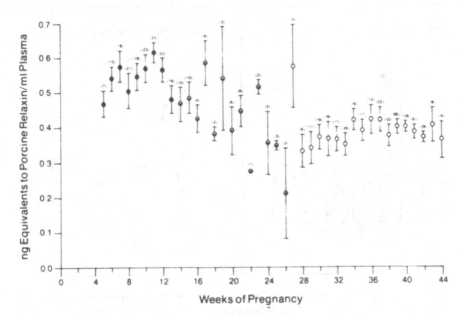

*Figure 12. Relaxin immunoactivity in plasma of women throughout ges-
tation. Numbers in parentheses indicate the numbers of
women sampled at each time interval. Vertical bars indicate (+) SE. ● first trimester; ◓ second trimester; ○ third
trimester. (From O'Byrne et al., 1978a).*

Relaxin immunoactivity has also been detected in the serum of
rats, mice, hamsters, and guinea pigs (O'Byrne and Steinetz, 1976;
O'Byrne *et al.*, 1976) during the last half of pregnancy. The increasing levels of relaxin have been shown to precede the increase
in cervical dilatability, a physiological effect which has been
attributed to relaxin, which occurs in rats (Figure 14), mice, and
hamsters during late gestation (Schwabe *et al.*, 1978).

RAT RELAXIN RADIOIMMUNOASSAY

Development of the Rat Relaxin Radioimmunoassay

As previously noted (Figure 4), the slope of the dose-response
curve obtained with rat relaxin is lower than the slope of the dose-
response curve obtained with porcine relaxin in the porcine relaxin
radioimmunoassay; and relatively large quantities of rat relaxin are
required for detection. In order to enable rigorous quantitative
determinations of rat relaxin in our physiological studies, rat
relaxin was isolated; and a homologous rat relaxin radioimmunoassay
was developed.

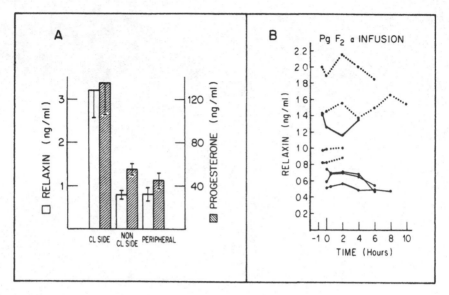

Figure 13A.   *Relaxin immunoactivity in serum from patients after*
             luteectomy at midtrimester. (From Weiss et al., 1976).

Figure 13B.   *Serum relaxin immunoactivity during labors induced by*
             infusion of PGF₂α. Broken lines represent induced labors
             that terminated in vaginal delivery and solid lines
             represent labors which failed to result in vaginal
             delivery. (From Hochman et al., 1978).

Radioiodination of rat relaxin

Equal quantities of the two highly purified forms of rat relaxin
isolated according to the procedure of Sherwood (1979a), which are
described in Chapter 3, were pooled and used for all aspects of the
development of the rat relaxin radioimmunoassay.

Rat relaxin was radioiodinated according to a modification of
the method of Bolton and Hunter (1973). With this method, rat
relaxin is radioiodinated through conjugation to a ^{125}I-labeled
3-(4-hydroxyphenyl) propionamide group. The specific radioactivity
of the ^{125}I-labeled rat relaxin obtained by this procedure ranges
from 100-130 µCi/ug. From 30-60% of the ^{125}I-labeled rat relaxin is
precipitable in excess antibody and the ^{125}I-labeled rat relaxin may
be used for at least 5 weeks without repurification.

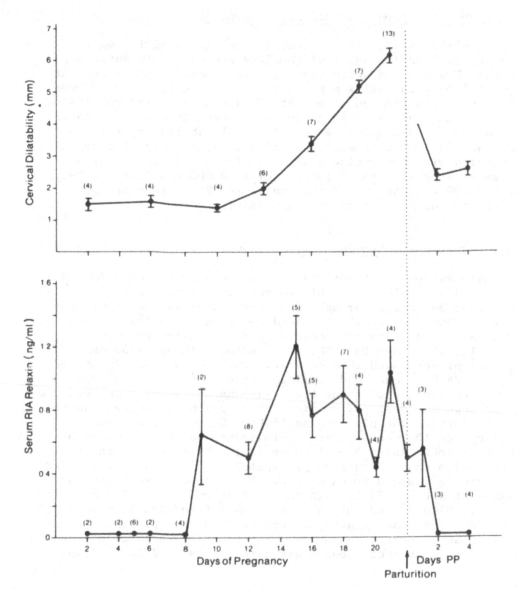

Figure 14. Relaxin immunoactivity and cervical dilatability
during pregnancy in rats. Redrawn from Steinetz et al.
(1959) and O'Byrne and Steinetz (1976). From Schwabe
et al. (1979).

Preparation of rabbit anti-rat relaxin sera

Rat relaxin antigen was prepared by emulsifying 1.0 mg rat relaxin in 1 ml of 0.9% saline and 1 ml complete Freund's adjuvant. Two adult male New Zealand white rabbits were immunized at 3-week intervals with 500 µg rat relaxin by intradermal injections into seven or eight sites in the medial aspect of each thigh. The rabbits were bled from a lateral ear vein 1 week after each immunization injection. Antisera were frozen until tested with ^{125}I-labeled rat relaxin for titer. Within four months of the initial injection of rat relaxin, both rabbits produced antisera suitable for use in the relaxin radioimmunoassay at final dilutions of 1:10,000 (antiserum 259-5) and 1:100,000 (antiserum 267-5). Antiserum 267-5 is routinely used for the rat relaxin radioimmunoassays.

Rat relaxin radioimmunoassay procedures

Double antibody rat relaxin radioimmunoassays are conducted in 12 x 75 mm disposable glass culture tubes. Quantities of rat relaxin, ranging from 8-4,000 pg or unknowns, are placed in each tube; and sufficient PBS-1% ovalbumin is added to bring the volume to 500 µl. Two hundred microliters of rabbit anti-rat relaxin serum 267-5 (Diluted 1:20,000 in 0.05 M EDTA-PBS and containing 1:300 male rabbit serum) are added to each tube. The contents are incubated at 4°C for 24 hr. One hundred microliters of ^{125}I-labeled rat relaxin (prepared by diluting the ^{125}I-labeled rat relaxin obtained from the Sephadex G-25 column with PBS-1% ovalbumin so that on the day of iodination 100 µl contains 55,000-60,000 cpm) are added to each tube, and the contents are again incubated at 4°C for 24 hr. Twenty-four hours later 200 µl sheep anti-rabbit γ-globulin, at a dilution which enables maximum precipitation of bound ^{125}I-labeled rat relaxin, are added to each tube. The contents are mixed and incubated at 4°C for 72 hr. Three milliliters of cold PBS are then added to each tube, and the tubes are centrifuged for 30 min at 1,000 x g at 4°C. The supernatants are decanted and the precipitates are counted in an automatic γ-counter. Rat relaxin standard and unknown serum or tissue extract samples are normally assayed in quadruplicate.

Characterization of the Rat Relaxin Radioimmunoassay

Sensitivity

A typical standard curve obtained with the rat relaxin radioimmunoassay is shown in Figure 15. The "least detectable dose" (Feldman and Rodbard, 1971) which is consistently measured is 32 pg. When logit and log transformations (Rodbard and Lewald, 1970) are used, a linear regression is obtained from 32 to 1,000 pg. Figure 15 also shows that volumes of 10 µl or less or 200 µl serum obtained

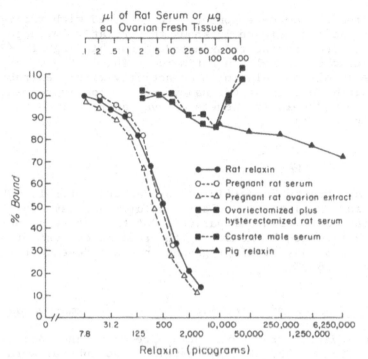

Figure 15. *Dose-response curves for rat relaxin, pregnant rat serum, pregnant rat ovarian extract, ovariectomized plus hysterectomized adult rat serum, castrate adult male rat serum, and porcine relaxin in the homologous rat relaxin radioimmunoassay. (From Sherwood and Crnekovic, 1979).*

from castrate adult males or ovariectomized plus hysterectomized adult rats did not affect the binding of ^{125}I-labeled rat relaxin to the rat relaxin antiserum. However, a slight, but reproducible inhibitory effect, was detected when volumes of rat sera ranging from 25-100 μl were used. During the last half of pregnancy, rat relaxin levels are normally determined with multiple volumes of plasma or sera ranging from 1 to 5 μl; and, therefore, this slight inhibitory effect presents no problem.

Hormone specificity

Available evidence indicates the rat relaxin radioimmunoassay is specific for relaxin. First, the slopes of the dose-response curves obtained with multiple volumes of both late pregnancy rat serum and an extract of ovaries obtained on day 16 of pregnancy did

not differ from the dose-response curve obtained with rat relaxin
(Figure 15).   Second, Figure 15 shows that relatively large quantities
of highly purified porcine relaxin reduce the binding of ^{125}I-labeled
rat relaxin to the rat relaxin antiserum.   Third, the occurrence
and relative levels of relaxin immunoactivity within extracts of ·
ovaries obtained throughout pregnancy are in close agreement with
the occurrence and relative levels of ovarian relaxin biological
activity (Figure 16A).

Precision and reproducibility

The mean intraassay coefficient of variation for 14 unknown
samples within a typical rat relaxin radioimmunoassay was 10.2%.
The interassay coefficient of variation of the rat relaxin radioimmunoassay determined by measuring the relaxin content of a serum
sample obtained on day 19 of pregnancy in six independent radioimmunoassays was 6.9%.

Physiological Studies with the Rat Relaxin Radioimmunoassay

Relaxin levels in rat sera during pregnancy and early lactation
are shown in Figure 16B.   Relaxin levels in peripheral sera obtained
from day 11 to day 18 of pregnancy from anaesthetized rats bled by
heart puncture were in good agreement with those obtained from
unanaesthetized rats bled by indwelling jugular cannula.   Clearly
detectable levels of relaxin (1 to 3 ng/ml) were not obtained until
day 10 of pregnancy.   Mean relaxin levels increased over the next
four days and generally ranged from 50 to 90 ng/ml from day 14 through
day 20 of pregnancy.   Relaxin levels then increased sharply reaching
maximal levels of 152 and 140 ng/ml on days 21 and 22 of pregnancy,
respectively.   By day 1 of lactation, relaxin levels dropped to 12 ng/
ml.   The occurrence and relative levels of relaxin activity within
the sera throughout pregnancy (Figure 16B) coincided with the
occurrence and relative levels of relaxin biological and immunological
activity within ovarian extracts (Figure 16A).

The advantage of the homologous rat relaxin radioimmunoassay
over the porcine relaxin radioimmunoassay for quantitative determination of relaxin immunoactivity is obvious.   The levels of relaxin-
immunoactivity in the sera of rats during late pregnancy obtained
with the homologous rat relaxin radioimmunoassay (Figure 16B) are
100-fold greater than the levels of relaxin reported when the
modified porcine relaxin radioimmunoassay was employed (Figure 14).

The homologous rat relaxin radioimmunoassay is sufficiently
sensitive to enable the determination of relaxin levels within small
samplings of blood obtained at frequent intervals from pregnant rats.
In order to obtain a more complete understanding of relaxin immuno-

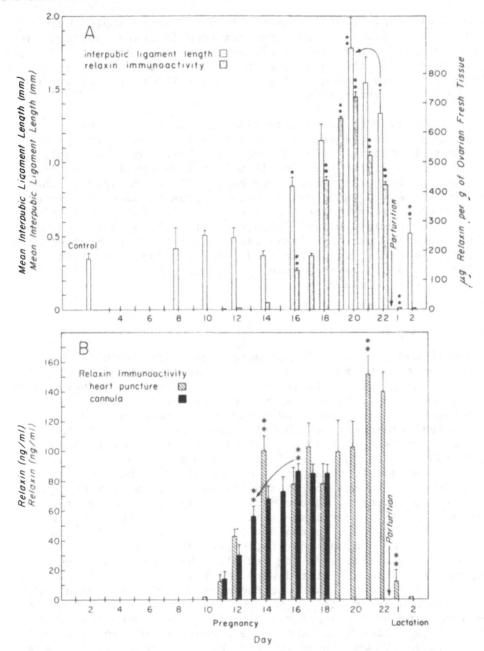

Figure 16A. Relaxin immunological and biological activity in ovarian extracts obtained from rats on each of the days shown.

Figure 16B. Relaxin levels in peripheral sera were obtained from rats via heart puncture and indwelling jugular cannula.

activity levels during late pregnancy in rats, sera samples were
obtained via indwelling jugular cannulas from 14 unanesthetized rats
at 6 hr intervals from day 19 of pregnancy until parturition. Figure
17 demonstrates that the rat, like the pig, experiences a surge in
relaxin to concentrations generally exceeding 100 ng per ml during
the day preceding parturition.

The sensitivity of the rat relaxin radioimmunoassay also enabled
the determination of the rate at which relaxin immunoactivity is
cleared from the blood. Relaxin levels were determined in small
samples of sera obtained via indwelling jugular cannulas from four
rats following bilateral ovariectomy on day 21 of gestation. The
rate of decline shown in Figure 18 demonstrates characteristics of
a multiexponential curve. The mean clearance t1/2 from 30 to 180 min
was 56 $\pm$ 7 min (standard error). Figure 18 also shows that clearance
rate obtained with porcine relaxin was similar to that obtained with
rat relaxin. When 250 µg of purified porcine relaxin was injected
intreavenously to an ovariectomized gilt, the clearance t1/2 from
60 to 180 min was 72 min.

SUMMARY

A homologous porcine relaxin radioimmunoassay which is sufficiently sensitive to measure 32 pg of relaxin has been developed.
We have used the porcine relaxin radioimmunoassay for the measurement
of relaxin immunoactivity levels in the peripheral blood of pigs
experiencing normal pregnancy and a variety of surgical and
pharmacological treatments which influence parturition. In the
pig, relaxin levels in the peripheral plasma remain low throughout
the first 100 days of the approximately 114 day gestation period
and then rise gradually to about 40 ng per ml 30 hr before parturition. A prepartum surge in relaxin levels to concentrations generally over 100 ng per ml occurs during the day which precedes
parturition. Relaxin levels are maximal approximately 14 hr before
parturition and then decline rapidly during the hours which immediately
precede parturition. By one day following parturition, relaxin
levels drop to approximately 1 ng per ml. The prepartum surge in
relaxin appears to be associated with the regression of the corpora
lutea. There is evidence that the factor(s) which bring about the
relaxin surge can be carried to the ovaries systemically and do not
require normal nerve or vascular connections. Although the nature
of the factor(s) which bring about the prepartum relaxin surge and
luteolysis is not known, there is evidence that prostaglandins may
be involved. Relaxin immunoactivity has been detected throughout
nearly the entire gestation period in the human being with the
modified porcine relaxin radioimmunoassay described by O'Bryne and
Steinetz. With that radioimmunoassay, relaxin immunoactivity has
also been detected during the last half of pregnancy in the sera of
rats, mice, guinea pigs, and hamsters.

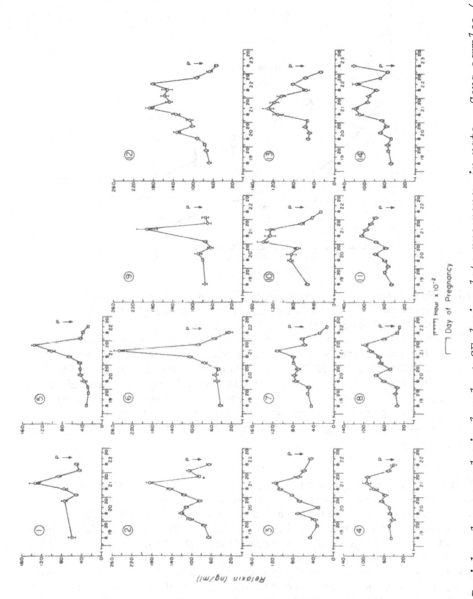

Figure 17. Peripheral sera relaxin levels + SE during late pregnancy in rats. Sera samples (≤200 μl) were obtained at 6 hr intervals from 14 unanaesthetized rats via indwelling jugular cannulus.

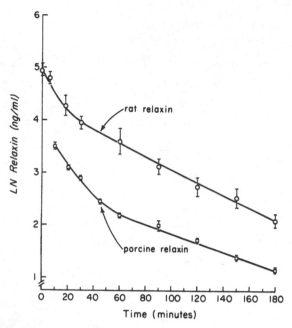

Figure 18.   *Rat relaxin immunoactivity levels in blood samples*
              obtained via indwelling jugular cannula following
              bilateral ovariectomy of four rats on day 21 of gestation.
              Rat relaxin immunoactivity levels were determined with
              the homologous rat relaxin radioimmunoassay (Sherwood
              and Crnekovic, 1979).   Porcine relaxin immunoactivity
              in blood samples obtained via indwelling jugular cannula
              following a single intravenous injection of 250 μg of
              highly purified porcine relaxin into a 250-pound
              ovariectomized gilt.   Means ± SE shown.

     A homologous radioimmunoassay for rat relaxin has also been
developed. This radioimmunoassay, which will detect 32 pg of rat
relaxin, is sufficiently sensitive to enable the determination of
relaxin levels within small samplings of blood obtained at frequent
intervals via indwelling cannulas from pregnant rats. The homologous
rat relaxin radioimmunoassay has been employed for the measurement
of peripheral sera relaxin levels in rats throughout normal pregnancy.
In the rat, relaxin is first detected on day 10 of the 22 or 23
gestation period. Relaxin levels then rise markedly to generally
range between 50 and 90 ng per ml from day 14 through day 20 of
gestation. During the day or two preceding parturition, there is a
further increase in relaxin to maximal levels which, like the pig,
are generally over 100 ng per ml. Relaxin levels decline during the
12 to 24 hr which precede parturition.

The stage of gestation in which relaxin immunoactivity in the peripheral blood is elevated varies among species. Pigs experience high levels of relaxin only during the last approximately 15 days of the 114 day gestation period. In rodents (rat, mouse, hamster, guinea pig) relaxin immunoactivity is elevated throughout the last half of the gestation period. With women relaxin immunoactivity is elevated throughout nearly all of gestation. The regulatory mechanisms responsible for the release of relaxin remain poorly understood.

REFERENCES

Becker, R. R. and Stahmann, M. A. (1953). Protein modification by reaction with N-carboxyamino acid anhydrides. J. Biol. Chem. 204:745.

Belt, W. D., Anderson, L. L., Cavazos, L. F. and Melampy, R. M. (1971). Cytoplasmic granules and relaxin levels in porcine corpora lutea. Endocrinology 89:1.

Bolton, A. E. and Hunter, W. M. (1973). The labelling of proteins to high specific radioactivities by conjugation to a ^{125}I-containing acylating agent. Application to the radioimmunoassay. Biochem. J. 133:529.

Bryant, G. D. (1972). The detection of relaxin in porcine, ovine and human plasma by radioimmunoassay. Endocrinology 91:1113.

Bryant, G. D. and Chamley, W. A. (1976a). Changes in relaxin and prolactin immunoactivities in ovine plasma following suckling. J. Reprod. Fert. 46:457.

Bryant, G. D. and Chamley, W. A. (1976b). Plasma relaxin and prolactin immunoactivities in pregnancy and at parturition in the ewe. J. Reprod. Fert. 48:201.

Bryant, G. D., Panter, M. E. A. and Stelmasiak, T. (1975). Immunoreactive relaxin in human serum during the menstrual cycle. J. Clin. Endocrinol. Metab. 41:1065.

Bryant, G. D., Sassin, J. F., Weitzman, E. D., Kapen, S., and Frantz, A. (1976). Relaxin immunoactivity in human plasma during a 24-hr period. J. Reprod. Fertil. 48:389.

Chamley, W. A., Stelmasiak, T. and Bryant, G. D. (1975). Plasma relaxin immunoactivity during the oestrus cycle in the ewe. J. Reprod. Fert. 45:455.

Curtis, S. E., Rogler, J. C. and Martin, T. G. (1969). Neonatal thermostability and body composition in piglets from experimentally prolonged gestations. J. Anim. Sci. 29:335.

Feldman, H. and Rodbard, D. (1971). Mathematical theory of radioimmunoassay. In: Principles of Competitive Protein-Binding Assays. O'Dell, W. D. and Daughaday, W. H., ed., Lippincott, Philadelphia.

First, N. L. and Staigmiller, R. B. (1973). Effects of ovariectomy, dexamethasone, and progesterone on the maintenance of pregnancy in swine. J. Anim. Sci. 37:1191.

Hochman, J., Weiss, G., Steinetz, B. G. and O'Byrne, E. M. (1978).
    Serum relaxin concentrations in prostaglandin- and oxytocin-
    induced labor in women. Am. J. Obstet. Gynecol. 130:473.
Hunter, W. M. and Greenwood, F. C. (1962). Preparation of iodine-
    131-labeled human growth hormone of high specific activity.
    Nature 194:495.
Kendall, J. Z., Plopper, C. G., Bryant-Greenwood, G. D. (1978).
    Ultrastructural immunoperoxidase demonstration of relaxin in
    corpora lutea from a pregnant sow. Biol. Reprod. 18:94.
Kwok, S. C. M., McMurtry, J. P. and Bryant, G. D. (1976). The
    relationship between relaxin and prolactin immunoactivities in
    various reproductive states: physicochemical and immunobio-
    logical studies. In: Growth Hormone and Related Peptides.
    A. Pecile and E. E. Miller, eds. Oxford. Excerpta Medica,
    Amsterdam.
Killian, D. B., Garverick, H. A. and Day, B. N. (1973). Peripheral
    plasma progesterone and corticoid levels at parturition in the
    sow. J. Anim. Sci. 37:1371.
Marchalonis, J. J. (1969). An enzymatic method for tract iodination of
    immunoglobulins and other proteins. Biochem. J. 113:299.
Martin, P. A., BeVier, G. W. and Dziuk, P. J. (1978). The effect
    of disconnecting the uterus and ovary on the length of gestation
    in the pig. Biol. Reprod. 18:428.
Minar, M. and Schilling, E. (1970). Die beeinflussing des geburt-
    stermins beim schwein durch gestagene hormone. Deutsche
    Tieraertzl. Wschr. 77:428.
Molokwu, E. C. I. and Wagner, W. C. (1973). Endocrine physiology
    of the puerperal sow. J. Anim. Sci. 36:1158.
Nara, B. S. and First, N. L. (1977). Effect of indomethacin and
    prostaglandin $F_2\alpha$ on porcine parturition. 69th Annual Meeting
    of the American Society of Animal Science, Madison, WI Abst. 477.
Nellor, J. E., Daniels, R. W., Hoefer, J. A., Wildt, D. E. and
    Dukelow, W. R. (1975). Influence of induced delayed parturition
    on fetal survival in pigs. Theriogenology 4:23.
O'Byrne, E. M. and Steinetz, B. G. (1976). Radioimmunoassay (RIA)
    of relaxin in sera of various species using an antiserum to
    porcine relaxin. Proc. Soc. Exp. Biol. Med. 152:272.
O'Byrne, E. M., Sawyer, W. K., Butler, M. C. and Steinetz, B. G.
    (1976). Serum immunoreactive relaxin and softening of the
    uterine cervix in pregnant hamsters. Endocrinology 99:1333.
O'Byrne, E. M., Carriere, B. T., Sorensen, L., Segaloff, A., Schwabe,
    C., and Steinetz, B. G. (1978a). Plasma immunoreactive relaxin
    levels in pregnant and nonpregnant women. J. Clin. Endocrinol.
    Metab. 47:1106.
O'Byrne, E. M., Flitcraft, J. F., Sawyer, W. K., Hochman, J., Weiss,
    G., and Steinetz, B. G. (1978b). Relaxin bioactivity and
    immunoactivity in human corpora lutea. Endocrinology 102:1641.
Qualiarello, J., Steinetz, B. G. and Weiss, G. (1979). Relaxin
    secretion in early pregnancy. Obstet. Gynecol. 53:62.

Rodbard, D. and Lewald, J. E. (1970). Computer analysis of radio-
    ligand assay and radioimmunoassay data. In: Second
    Karolinska Symposia on Research Methods in Reproductive
    Endocrinology. E. Diczfalusy ed., Bogtrykkeriet Forum,
    Copenhagen.
Schwabe, C., Steinetz, B., Weiss, G., Segaloff, A., McDonald, J. K.,
    O'Byrne, E., Hochman, J., Carriere, B. and Goldsmith, L.
    (1978). Relaxin.   Rec. Prog. Horm. Res. 34:123.
Sherwood, O. D. (1979a). Purification and characterization of
    rat relaxin. Endocrinology 104:886.
Sherwood, O. D. (1979b). Relaxin. In: Methods of Hormone
    Radioimmunoassay. B. M. Jaffe and H. R. Behrman, eds.,
    Academic Press. New York.
Sherwood, O. D. and O'Byrne, E. M. (1974). Purification and
    characterization of porcine relaxin. Arch. Biochem. Biophys.
    160:185.
Sherwood, O. D. and Crnekovic, V. E. (1979). Development of a
    homologous radioimmunoassay for rat relaxin. Endocrinology
    104:893.
Sherwood, O. D., Rosentreter, K. R., and Birkhimer, M. L. (1975a).
    Development of a radioimmunoassay for porcine relaxin using
    ^{125}I-labeled polytyrosyl-relaxin. Endocrinology 96:1106.
Sherwood, O. D., Chang, C. C., BeVier, A. W. and Dziuk, P. J.
    (1975b). Radioimmunoassay of plasma relaxin levels throughout
    pregnancy and at parturition in the pig. Endocrinology 97:834.
Sherwood, O. D., Chang, C. C., BeVier, G. W., Diehl, J. R. and
    Dziuk, P. J. (1976). Relaxin concentrations in pig plasma
    following the administration of prostaglandin $F_2\alpha$ during late
    pregnancy. Endocrinology 98:875.
Sherwood, O. D., Martin, P. A., Chang, C. C. and Dziuk, P. J. (1977a).
    Plasma relaxin levels in pigs with corpora lutea induced during
    late pregnancy. Biol. Reprod. 17:97.
Sherwood, O. D., Martin, P. A., Chang, C. C. and Dziuk, P. J.
    (1977b). Plasma relaxin levels during late pregnancy and at
    parturition in pigs with altered utero-ovarian connections.
    Biol. Reprod. 17:101.
Sherwood, O. D., Wilson, M. E., Edgerton, L. A. and Chang, C. C.
    (1978). Serum relaxin concentrations in pigs with parturition
    delayed by progesterone administration. Endocrinology 102:471.
Sherwood, O. D., Nara, B. S., Crnekovic, V. E. and First, N. L.
    (1979). Relaxin concentrations in pig plasma after the
    administration of indomethacin and prostaglandin $F_2\alpha$ during
    late pregnancy. Endocrinology 104:1716.
Steinetz, B. G., Beach, V. L., and Kroc, R. L. (1959). The physio-
    logy of relaxin in laboratory animals. In: Recent Progress
    in the Endocrinology of Reproduction. C. H. Lloyd, ed., Academic
    Press, New York.
Steinetz, B. G., Beach, V. L., and Kroc, R. L. (1969). Bioassay of
    relaxin. In: Methods in Hormone Research. Vol. 2A. R. I.
    Dorfman, ed. Academic Press, New York.

Weiss, G., O'Byrne, E. M., and Steinetz, B. G. (1976). Relaxin: A product of the human corpus luteum of pregnancy. Science 194:948.

Weiss, G., O'Byrne, E. M., Hochman, J. A., Goldsmith, L., Rifkin, I., and Steinetz, B. G. (1977). Secretion of progesterone and relaxin by the human corpus luteum at mid pregnancy and at term. Obstet. Gynecol. 50:679.

Weiss, G., O'Byrne, E. M., Hochman, J. A., Steinetz, B. G., Goldsmith, L. and Flitcraft, J. G. (1978). Distribution of relaxin in women during pregnancy. Obstet. Gynecol. 52:569.

DISCUSSION FOLLOWING DR. O. D. SHERWOOD'S PAPER

Dr. Greenwood
     (University of Hawaii). David, you did prostaglandins. Did you
try any of the many varieties and derivatives of prostaglandins in the
system?

Dr. Sherwood
     No. At this point, we have not.

Dr. Greenwood
     Did you try any other hormones or steroids? Was that the only
thing you looked at?

Dr. Sherwood
     In a collaborative study with Dr. Lee Edgerton and Mark Wilson
of the University of Kentucky we determined the effect of the
administration of progesterone during late pregnancy on serum relaxin
concentrations (Sherwood *et al.*, *Endocrinology* 102:471, 1978). The
progesterone caused a delay in parturition but did not influence the
relaxin immunoactivity levels.

Dr. Greenwood
     David, first of all, let me thank you very much for your carefully
chosen words. You said, quite rightly, in the Bryant assay "the
nature of the material measured is not clearly defined."

     Now, I'm going to ask you the same question: Have you defined
the plasma materials making up the inhibition curve? You made one
statement of what you might be measuring the plasma, and that is, in
part, biologically active relaxin. We are actually in agreement. You
don't know what you are measuring, nor do we, nor does anybody, not
precisely. And I would have to add that parallelism is useful data
to obtain for an assay. But it tells us nothing on specificity. The
parallel effect from plasma means that the sum of the plasma immunoactivities is parallel to the standard curve and therefore can be
expressed in terms of the standard. As you rightly point out for the
rat heterologous assay, when it is not parallel you cannot quantify
the results. We are more in agreement than not. These are general
comments on radioimmunoassay. I have one highly specific question.
In the experiments on spiking plasma with labeled relaxin and then
showing by gel filtration identity between the peaks of radioactivity
and endogenous immunoactivity it seems to me that relaxin is the first
and only hormone that everybody has ever worked on in which people,
specifically you, are claiming homogeneity of a plasma hormone. Now,
that is a precedent not set for all the other plasma hormones. When
we fractionate plasma on sephadex and monitor for endogenous relaxin
by RIA, we get the usual heterogeneity. That is with a CMa[1] antiCMa'
assay. The only difference in our approach is that we tend to increase

our sensitivity during those experiments in order to maximalize the plasma immuno-heterogeneity.

You get a single solitary peak. We don't see that and we have never seen it on any other hormone that we have measured.

Dr. Sherwood

The difference between the porcine relaxin radioimmunoassay which we have described (Sherwood *et al., Endocrinology* 96:1106, 1975) and that of Dr. Bryant (Bryant, *Endocrinology* 91:1113, 1972) is that we have employed highly purified, biologically active porcine relaxin (Sherwood and O'Byrne, *Arch, Biochem. Biophys.* 160:185, 1974) as immunogen, radioligand, and standard whereas the Bryant assay employed relatively impure porcine relaxin. We have not claimed nor implied that the immunoactivity which we detect within rat serum with the rat relaxin radioimmunoassay is confined to molecules with a molecular weight of approximately 6,000. We have not, at this point, determined the apparent size(s) of the molecules which are detected in rat serum. Therefore, I acknowledge the possibility that we may be detecting not only molecules which have a molecular weight of 6,000 but also some which are larger. We have determined the elution profile for the relaxin immunoactivity in pregnant pig serum (Sherwood, *et al., Endocrinology* 96:1106, 1975). Most of the relaxin immunoactivity coeluted with radiolabeled highly purified porcine relaxin which has a molecular weight of approximately 6,000. However, a small portion of the immunoactive material eluted from that column had an apparent molecular weight which was somewhat greater than 6,000.

Dr. Greenwood

We have data on that for porcine relaxin. Some of the high molecular weight materials that Dr. Kwok reported yesterday are quite parallel to the standard. Unless the fractions are homogenous we cannot quantitate the results.

The other comment is that the long switchoff of endogenous rat relaxin is really fascinating because that is really a very long half-life. What is that half life of the first peak?

Dr. Sherwood

The clearance of rat relaxin immunoactivity from sera is multi-exponential. We found the mean clearance t1/2 from 0 to 30 min to be 22 ± 3 min standard error of the mean and the t1/2 from 30 to 180 min to be 56 ± 7 min standard error of the mean. It was my expectation that relaxin immunoactivity levels would decline rapidly within 5 min of ovariectomy on day 21 of gestation. However, that was not the case. The mean serum relaxin immunoactivity levels in 4 rats was approximately 165 ng per ml immediately before ovariectomy and approximately 145 ng per ml 5 min following ovariectomy.

Dr. Greenwood
     Well, certainly in lactation in the pig, we're talking about a
half life of a minute, obtained with a homologous assay, so that is
another variable.

Dr. Steinetz
     I have a couple of questions regarding the interpretation of
the role of prostaglandins in the stimulation of relaxin secretion.
As Lloyd Anderson pointed out yesterday, oxytocin also seems to cause
relaxin secretion in late pregnancy in the pig. The only thing these
two substances would appear to have in common would be a stimulation
of uterine contractions.

     Is there any possible way of sorting out these effects? For
example, could one look at oxytocin in indomethacin treated pigs to
see if it indeed were releasing prostaglandins?

     Another thing, the corpus luteum can be rescued from luteolysis
by temporary progesterone treatment, at least in rodents. I wonder
if that sort of thing has been tried in the pig.

Dr. Sherwood
     Bernie, we did conduct one experiment in which we found that the
administration of progesterone to pigs during late pregnancy did not
delay luteolysis as judged by the occurrence of a normal surge in
relaxin immunoactivity levels (Sherwood *et al.*, *Endocrinology* 104:
471, 1978).

Dr. Steinetz
     Would progesterone, administered at the time you give the
PGF_2alpha, have any effect on the relaxin surge?

Dr. Soloff
     (Medical College of Ohio): It has been shown in the ewe and in
the mare that oxytocin is luteolytic and McCracken and Roberts, among
others, have shown that oxytocin causes the release of prostaglandins
from sheep endometrium during the estrous cycle. But I don't think
any studies have been done in late pregnancy.

Dr. Steinetz
     Has that been shown in the pig?

Dr. Soloff
     I don't believe so.

Dr. L. L. Anderson
     (Iowa State University) Several years ago, we gave oxytocin to
pigs during the estrous cycle and luteolysis did not result. Of
course, in the cow, you can also induce luteal regression with

oxytocin during the estrous cycle.   But the same protocol does not
fit for the pig.

Dr. Frieden
      (Kent State University): Have you looked at the possibility of
cross-reaction between any of your antisera and relaxin in the guinea
pig at various stages of gestation or following the administration of
estrogen and progesterone.

Dr. Sherwood
      We have not done an extensive study of the possible cross-reactivity
of our rabbit anti-rat relaxin sera with relaxin from species other
than the rat.

Dr. Kendall
      (University of Texas): Is this related to the cross-reactivity
data? Do you think that you are getting cross-reactivity in the rat
relaxin assay with the porcine? That curve you showed could have
been an extension of a nonspecific substance you were getting with
the rat.

Dr. Sherwood
      The nonspecific effect which was described was obtained with
selected volumes of castrate male or ovariectomized plus hysterectomized female rat sera.   The relatively shallow dose-response line
obtained with porcine relaxin in the rat relaxin radioimmunoassay was
obtained with increasing quantities of highly purified porcine relaxin.

Dr. Kendall
      There was no volume effect?

Dr. Sherwood
      No, no volume phenomenon there at all, Dr. Kendall.

Dr. Kendall
      Have you extended any of those studies in the rats to other
stages? For example, there was some talk on the non-pregnant animal.

Dr. Sherwood
      Our studies of relaxin levels in nonpregnant animals are just
beginning.

Dr. Jeffrey
      I was intrigued with the correlation between the relaxin levels
in the rat as pregnancy progressed with the progression of cervical
dilitation.   Conventional wisdom seems to say that dilation doesn't
begin quite so early. Have you done this same experiment in the pig
and is the same correlation present there, where the dilation begins
and really fundamentally follows the time courses that the cervix
in the rat does?

Dr. Sherwood
    Could I defer that question to you, Dr. Anderson? The question
that is being asked is whether there is a similar correlation in the
time of occurrence in the dilation of the cervix in the pig as Dr.
Stenietz picked up with the rat; that is to say, when does one begin
to see cervical dilation in the pig? What has been your experience
with that?

Dr. L. L. Anderson
    I have two slides I could show, if you would like to see them
in terms of regular *in situ* cervical development of the animals, and
the effects of relaxin on cervical development during late pregnancy.
In situ in the intact nontreated animal, the cervical diameter increases only the last two or three days before parturition. Before
I answer that, may I ask you this question that Dr. Kendall is
probably getting to: In the rats with deciduomata in which the life
span is approximately 22 days, what is the relaxin pattern like?

Dr. Sherwood
    These studies are just beginning and therefore I cannot be very
specific. However, we have sufficient data to be certain that relaxin
levels are higher in extracts of ovaries of pseudopregnant rats than
in cycling rats.

Dr. Jeffrey
    When does the relaxin begin to appear in the pig plasma as a
function of its gestation life?

Dr. Sherwood
    In the pig there is approximately a 114 day gestation period.
Relaxin immunoactivity levels remain low (less than 2 ng per ml)
throughout the first 100 days of gestation and then increase to
approximately 10 ng per ml on day 110 of gestation. A surge in
relaxin immunoactivity to levels generally exceeding 100 ng per ml
occurs during the day which precedes parturition. It is my view that
the relatively low levels of relaxin experienced beween days 100 to
112 of gestation may play an important role in preparing the uterus
for parturition. The relaxin surge obtained immediately before
parturition may, at least in part, reflect a mechanism which eliminates
a molecule which is no longer needed.

Dr. Kendall
    Could I ask just about a couple of experimental details about
the half life? Were the rats anesthetized when you did this or were
they taken from cannulated rats?

Dr. Sherwood
    These were cannulated animals.

Dr. Kendall
    And the pig was cannulated in the ear vein?

Dr. Sherwood
    They were both unanesthetized.

Dr. L. L. Anderson
    In a series of experiments when we gave relaxin during the last part of the pregnancy to pigs, we wanted to see the effects on the cervical diameter, on the time of parturition, and on the time required for the delivery of all the fetuses.

    The lower panel shows the profiles of cervical diameter increase during normal pregnancy in the pig with delivery indicated by the arrows. There is a gradual increase in cervical diameter that becomes marked just a few hours before delivery, and then a rapid cervical regression occurs after parturition.

    To test this experimentally, we wanted to push back the time for delivery in pigs. To accomplish that, we luteectomized animals at day 110. With the luteectomy at this time, you cause delivery, or you might define it as abortion, occuring within 36 hours.

    In saline injected-lutteectomized animals, the fetuses are delivered in 36 hours, and the cervix regresses markedly thereafter.

    Notice that the cervical diameter is very low during this prepartum phase.

    In pregnant gilts, given relaxin daily for several days before the time of luteectomy on day 110, the cervical diameter increases earlier and of course the maximal amount that dilation occurs for expulsion of the fetuses is the same in all three groups.

    These luteectomized pigs given relaxin deliver significantly earlier than those given saline, by about 26 hours versus 36 for the controls. Furthermore, the time required for the delivery process is significantly reduced in relaxin-injected gilts that were luteectomized. We are talking about a litter-bearing species that requires several hours to deliver those piglets. This is shortened significantly in relaxin treated pigs, as contrasted to those that were given saline and luteectomized at this time.

    In another series we injected relaxin into pigs not luteectomized, that were allowed to deliver at the normal time. We did not see too much of an effect on cervical increase in time for the delivery process in those animals. Only in the experimental situation where it was forced back a few days by luteectomy could we demonstrate that the cervix indeed does respond to relaxin in late pregnancy in this species.

THE EFFECTS OF RELAXIN ON CYCLIC-AMP AND

ORNITHINE DECARBOXYLASE LEVELS IN TARGET TISSUES

Sylvia A. Braddon

U.S. Department of Commerce
National Oceanic and Atmospheric Administration
National Marine Fisheries Service, SEFC
Charleston Laboratory
Charleston, S.C. 29412

INTRODUCTION

The ovarian peptide hormone relaxin causes distinct changes of the birth canal before parturition in most mammals (Hisaw, 1926; Hisaw and Zarrow, 1950). Rapid widening of the pubic symphysis and increased dilatability of the cervix are notable changes which accompany administration of relaxin to several species (Hisaw and Zarrow, 1950; Steinetz *et al.*, 1957; Kroc *et al.*, 1959; O'Byrne *et al.*, 1976). These changes are a reflection of the profound effect that relaxin has on the connective tissues of the pubic symphysis and uterus. RIA data confirm that serum levels of this hormone in the pig, mouse, rat and guinea pig increase significantly within hours of parturition and drop sharply thereafter (Sherwood *et al.*, 1975; 1975; O'Byrne and Steinetz, 1976). Recently several studies have confirmed that relaxin binds in a specific manner to its target tissues (Cheah and Sherwood, 1979; McMurtry *et al.*, 1978). In a quest to better understand the biochemical events which follow relaxin treatment and precede the known biological changes, two specific cellular responses were chosen for study: changes in cAMP concentrations and stimulation of ornithine decarboxylase activity.

To place these cellular responses in proper perspective a short review of the biochemical events in the mechanism of action of a protein hormone is necessary. Figure 1 summarizes a general scheme of the biochemical events that may occur once a specific hormone approaches its target tissue cell. Upon binding to its membrane bound receptor the hormone may elicit immediate cellular changes via the alteration of local membrane permeability. The

255

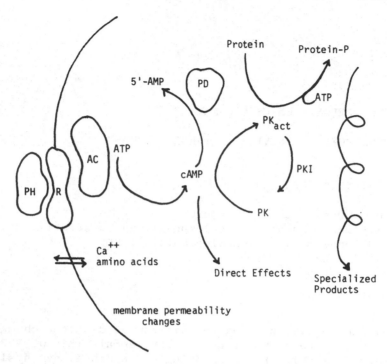

Figure 1. A general scheme for protein hormone action on a target
cell. PH, protein hormone; R, protein hormone receptor;
AC, adenylate cyclase; PK, cAMP-dependent protein kinase;
PD, phosphodiesterase; PKI, protein kinase inhibitory
protein.

concentration of specific ions or amino acids may alter significantly.
Binding of the hormone to its receptor can also lead to stimulation
of adenylate cyclase and subsequently to increased cAMP levels.
Changes in cAMP-dependent protein kinase activity is an often observed
occurrence followed by phosphorylation of a specific protein substrate
for that target tissue. cAMP may exert its effects via pathways not
requiring the action of protein kinase. In a little understood interaction there is a direct relationship between changes in intracellular
cAMP levels and the activation of ornithine decarboxylase. The sum
total of these events is expressed eventually by changes in enzyme
activities and changed levels of specific metabolic products. The
mechanism is deactivated by the action of phosphodiesterases and
protein kinase inhibitory protein.

    A quick inspection of the general scheme for protein hormone
action described above shows that the two cellular events selected

for investigation represent separate stages in the scheme. Measurement of cAMP concentration changes was chosen as a means of monitoring an early event in the mechanism of action of relaxin. Increases in relaxin-dependent cAMP levels were predicted to occur based on the knowledge that other peptide hormones (eg. LH, ACTH, TSH) (Schriber, 1974) are known to act through an elevation of cAMP levels. In addition, increases in cAMP levels indirectly infer the activation of adenylate cyclase following hormone binding.

Studies on cells in culture, and an *in vivo* study on rat liver, suggest that there is a relationship between increases in cellular cAMP levels and ornithine decarboxylase induction (Bachrach, 1975; Yamasaki and Ichihara, 1976; Oka and Perry, 1976; Byers and Russell, 1975). When cultured cells are treated with cAMP levels, an induction of ornithine decarboxylase occurs (Bachrach, 1975; Oka and Perry, 1976). Based on these studies, and the knowledge that both steroidal and protein hormones induce ornithine decarboxylase activity in their respective target tissues (Morris and Fillingame, 1974), it seemed possible that an increase in ornithine decarboxylase activity is an intermediate step in the mechanism of relaxin action. Additional support for seeking ornithine decarboxylase in relaxin target tissues arises from the knowledge that the enzyme activity is found in pelvic cartilage (from chick embryo), costal cartilage (from young rat, rabbit and human fetus) (Oka and Perry, 1976) and in cultured human and chick fibroblasts (Buehler *et al.*, 1977; Haselbacher and Humbel, 1976). The chick derived activity was tested and found to be hormone sensitive. In light of these studies measurement of ornithine decarboxylase activity in relaxin target tissues was undertaken to monitor a later biochemical event in the scheme of protein hormone action.

RESEARCH PROTOCOL

Details of the experimental regime for the results discussed herein have been previously described (Braddon, 1978a,1978b). Relaxin used was purified from a porcine ovarian acid-acetone extract (Braddon, 1978a) to a high purity (ca. 2500 U/mg). cAMP was extracted from target tissues utilizing an acid extraction followed by anion exchange chromatography as described previously (Braddon, 1978a). Assay of cAMP was conducted by a modification of the Gilman competitive protein binding method (Braddon, 1978a; Gilman, 1970). Assay of ornithine decarboxylase activity was accomplished via a modification of the method of Russell and Snyder (Braddon, 1978b; Russell and Snyder, 1968).

RELAXIN-DEPENDENT cAMP CONCENTRATION CHANGES

Biological Response

Before embarking on specific biochemical measurements with purified relaxin, it was tested in a biological assay system. The
purified relaxin preparation induced separation of the pubic bones
in two different strains of mice. The treated animals had pubic
ligaments four times longer than the control animals (Table 1).
The biological effect of relaxin was abolished by antibody preparations
against relaxin (Table 1).

Increasing responses in pubic symphysis separation were observed when increasing doses of relaxin were administered as single
injections (Table 2). The log dose-response relationship was linear.
Treatment of relaxin with dithiothreitol (DTT) was performed in
order to inactivate the hormone. Injection of 12 µg DTT-treated
relaxin did not increase the length of the interpubic ligament over
that of the control.

Effect of Relaxin on cAMP Levels in the Pubic Symphysis

Significant increases in cAMP levels were observed in mouse
pubic symphyses following the administration of relaxin (Tables 3
and 4). Initially intact mature mice were used for the experiments.
Because of a high degree of variability in the resulting cAMP deter-

Table 1.   *EFFECT OF RELAXIN ON THE LENGTH OF THE PUBIC
SYMPHYSIS LIGAMENT (18 hr POSTINJECTION).*

Treatment	n	Charles River mice; interpubic ligament length (mm $\pm$ SE)	n	Flow mice; interpubic ligament length (mm $\pm$ SE)
Control	5	0.36 $\pm$ 0.08	5	0.62 $\pm$ 0.23
BP	6	0.49 $\pm$ 0.08		*
BP + R	6	1.73 $\pm$ 0.25	5	2.56 $\pm$ 0.33
AR + BP + R	6	0.53 $\pm$ 0.08		*
AS + BP + R		*		

Each intact immature mouse was primed with 5 µg $E_2\beta$ in 0.1 ml
sesame oil, 3 days before treatment. Treatments were: BP, 0.1 ml 1%
BP (sc)/mouse; R, 1 µg relaxin; AR, 50 µg purified antibody to
relaxin in 0.2 ml phosphate buffer, pH 7.0 (ip) 30 min before relaxin
injection; and AS, antiserum, 100 µl rabbit antiserum to porcine
relaxin (ip) 30 min before relaxin injection. n, Number of mice used
to obtain the mean value (reproduced from Braddon, 1978). *Value
not determined.

Table 2. *DOSE-RESPONSE STUDY: THE EFFECTS OF VARIOUS DOSES OF RELAXIN ON THE LENGTH OF THE PUBIC SYMPHYSIS LIGAMENT*

Relaxin (µg)	n	Interpubic ligament length (mm $\pm$ SE)
0	5	0.45 $\pm$ 0.08
0.5	5	1.23 $\pm$ 0.22
1.0	5	1.39 $\pm$ 0.19
3.0	5	1.58 $\pm$ 0.22
6.0	4	1.86 $\pm$ 0.13
12.0	5	1.86 $\pm$ 0.26
12.0 $\pm$ DTT	5	0.41 $\pm$ 0.04

Each intact mature mouse was primed with 5 µg $E_2\beta$ in 0.1 ml sesame oil. The specified doses of purified relaxin were given in 0.1 ml 1% BP and the animals were killed 18 h after treatment. Relaxin that had been pretreated with excess DTT was injected at the 12 µg dose level. n, Number of mice used to obtain the mean value. (reproduced from Braddon, 1978).

Table 3. *cAMP LEVELS IN MOUSE PUBIC SYMPHYSIS*

Treatment	n	$\dfrac{\text{pmol cAMP}}{\text{mg protein}}$ $\pm$ SE
Ovariectomized mature mice		
Control	6	121 $\pm$ 9.2
BP	6	134 $\pm$ 9.6
BP + R	6	266 $\pm$ 35.1
Intact immature mice		
Control	5	167 $\pm$ 34.1
BP	5	186 $\pm$ 6.0
BP + R	5	428 $\pm$ 31.3

Each mouse was primed with 5 µg $E_2\beta$ in 0.1 ml sesame oil, 3 days before treatment. All animals were killed 30 min after treatment. Treatments were: BP, 0.1 ml 1% BP (sc)/mouse; and R, 1 µg relaxin. n, Number of mice used to obtain the mean value. (reproduced from Braddon, 1978).

Table 4. *cAMP LEVELS UNDER VARIOUS CONDITIONS*

Treatment	n	$\frac{\text{pmol cAMP}}{\text{mg protein}} \pm SE$	n	$\frac{\text{pmol cAMP}}{\text{mg protein}} \pm SE$
		Study 1		
Intact mature mice; pubic symphyses				
E_2	5	118 ± 8.0		
E_2 + BP + R	5	492 ± 51.5		
BP + R	5	286 ± 17.4		
E_2 + saline	5	140 ± 7.1		
E_2 + saline + R	5	336 ± 11.2		
E_2 + BP + insulin	5	153 ± 7.6		
		Study 2A		Study 2B
Ovariectomized mature mice; pubic symphyses				
BP		*	5	96 ± 5.3
BP + R		*	5	210 ± 11.2
E_2 + BP	5	154 ± 11.4		*
E_2 + BP + R	5	266 ± 7.1		*
E_2 + BP + insulin	5	211 ± 20.3		*
E_2 + saline + insulin	4	145 ± 19.0		*
E_2 + saline + R	4	304 ± 29.2		*
		Study 3A		Study 3B
Intact immature mice; pubic symphyses				
E_2	5	102 ± 7.9		*
E_2 + BP	5	232 ± 13.6		*
E_2 + BP + R	5	358 ± 18.9		*
BP		*	5	210 ± 8.1
BP + R	5	448 ± 37.9	5	320 ± 11.7

Table 4. Continued

Treatment	n	$\dfrac{\text{pmol cAMP}}{\text{mg protein}} \pm$ SE		
		Study 4		
Intact mature mice; liver				
$E_2\beta$ + BP	5	23.7	$\pm$	1.2
$E_2\beta$ + BP + R	5	18.1	$\pm$	1.1
$E_2\beta$ + BP + glucagon	5	65.3	$\pm$	7.3
Pubic symphyses				
$E_2\beta$ + BP	5	211	$+$	19.9
$E_2\beta$ + BP + R	5	394	$+$	28.9
$E_2\beta$ + BP + glucagon	5	213	$\pm$	15.4

All animals were killed 30 min after treatment. Treatments were $E_2\beta$ 5 µg $E_2\beta$ in 0.1 ml sesame oil/mouse, 3 days before treatment; BP, 0.1 ml 1% BP (sc)/mouse; R, 3 µg relaxin/mouse; saline, 0.1 ml 0.9% NaCl solution (sc)/mouse; insulin, 3 µg porcine insulin/mouse; and glucagon, 50µg porcine glucagon/mouse. n, Number of mice used to obtain the mean value. (reproduced from Braddon, 1978). *Value not determined.

minations, both intact immature and ovariectomized mature mice were tested. Each group of mice responded similarly to relaxin treatment; symphyseal cAMP levels were significantly increased over control values when relaxin was injected 30 min prior to measurement. Interestingly, these changes in symphyseal cAMP levels were diminished and in most cases completely abolished by prior ip injection of antibodies to relaxin (Figure 2).

As was the case in the biological response to relaxin, symphyseal cAMP levels were dependent upon the dose of relaxin (Table 5). In the studies conducted 3 µg was the lowest dose that consistently produced cAMP levels significantly greater than control values (Table 5). When DTT was used to reduce the relaxin molecule and thereby render it inactive the results were equivocal. The cAMP level was significantly lower than that produced by an equivalent amount of intact relaxin (Table 5) but was above the control levels. A possible explanation is that some of the relaxin was reoxidized before injection.

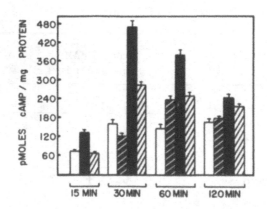

*Figure 2.   cAMP levels in pubic symphyses of ovariectomized mice as a
function of time.   Ovariectomized mice were primed with
$E_2\beta$ in sesame oil.   At the specific times after treatment,
the mice were killed and the pubic symphyses removed for
extraction and assay.   Each time represents a single study.
Each value is an expression of the mean ($\pm$ SE) of five
symphyses.   The treatments were: $E_2\beta$, 5 μg $E_2\beta$ in 0.1 ml
sesame oil (sc)/mouse; BP, 0.1 ml 1% BP (sc)/mouse; R,
3 μg relaxin; and AR, 0.1 ml (50 μg protein) antibody
to relaxin (ip) 30 min before relaxin injection. □
$E_2\beta$; ▨ , $E_2\beta$ + BP; ▓ , $E_2\beta$ + BP + R; ▨ ,
$E_2\beta$ + AR + BP + R.   (reproduced from Braddon, 1978).*

Relaxin-Stimulated cAMP Levels as a Function of Time .

Presuming that the serum level of relaxin would increase to a
maximum and then decrease following hormone injection, it was of
interest to determine the pattern of cAMP concentration changes with
time.   Utilizing ovariectomized mice, cAMP levels were measured on
symphyseal tissue at various time intervals (15, 30, 60 and 120
minutes) after relaxin injection (Figure 2).   The largest increase
in cAMP levels was observed at 30 minutes following hormone injection
(Figure 2).   While no significant difference was observed at 2 h, both
15 min and 60 min treatment groups showed significantly elevated
cAMP levels over control values.   Under like conditions intact mature mice showed a similar temporal relationship (Figure 3).

It is appropriate at this point to note that on occasion, benzo-
purpurin-treated mice had symphyseal cAMP levels different from $E_2\beta$-
treated control mice.   These differences reflect biological variability and are not statistically significant.   Though necessary for
the biological effect of relaxin, there is no apparent requirement

Table 5.   *THE EFFECTS OF VARIOUS DOSES OF RELAXIN ON cAMP LEVELS*
              IN MOUSE PUBIC SYMPHYSIS (PS).

g relaxin	n	$\frac{\text{pmol cAMP}}{\text{PS}}$ $\pm$ SE	n	$\frac{\text{pmol cAMP}}{\text{PS}}$ $\pm$ SE
		Study 1		Study 2
0	5	31.2 $\pm$ 2.0	5	43.2 $\pm$ 2.8
0.5		*	5	42.8 $\pm$ 7.8
1.0	5	37.5 $\pm$ 5.0	5	36.6 $\pm$ 1.8
3.0	5	88.8 $\pm$ 10.3	5	120 $\pm$ 3.0
6.0	5	168.4 $\pm$ 14.9	5	280 $\pm$ 26
12.0		*	5	368 $\pm$ 26
12.0 $\pm$ DTT		*	5	157 $\pm$ 12

Each mouse was primed with 5 μg $E_2\beta$ in 0.1 ml sesame oil. The specified doses of purified relaxin were given in 0.1 ml 1% BP and the animals were killed 30 min after treatment. Relaxin that had been pretreated with excess DTT was injected at the 12 μg dose level. n, Number of mice to obtain the mean value. (reproduced from Braddon, 1978). *Value not determined.

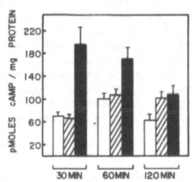

Figure 3.   *cAMP levels in pubic symphyses of intact mature mice as a*
              function of time. Intact mature mice were primed with $E_2\beta$
              in sesame oil. At the specified times after treatment,
              the mice were killed and the pubic symphyses removed for
              extraction and assay. All the intervals were studied in
              the same experiment. Each value is an expression of the
              mean ($\pm$ SE) of five symphyses. The treatments were $E_2\beta$,
              5 μg $E_2\beta$ in 0.1 ml sesame oil (sc)/mouse; BP, 0.1 ml 1%
              BP (sc/mouse); and R, 3 μg relaxin. □ , $E_2\beta$; ▨ , $E_2\beta$ +
              BP; ▮ , $E_2\beta$ + BP + R. (reproduced from Braddon, 1978).

for the respiratory agent benzopurpurin-4B in order to elicit a cAMP concentration change. Data in Table 4 (Study 1 and 2A) indicate that benzopurpurin may exert a qunatitative effect on symphyseal cAMP levels.

A Question of Estrogen

Apparently the hormonal controls in the mechanism of action of relaxin exert their influence at various stages of the response. The overall biological response requires the presence of estrogen and growth hormone. Yet the data from these studies indicate that estrogen priming of immature and ovariectomized mature mice is not necessary for a relaxin induced cAMP response. Increases in symphyseal cAMP levels over control values in unprimed relaxin-treated mice (Table 4, Studies 2B and 3B) were comparable to those observed in estrogen-primed relaxin-treated mice. It is possible that estrogen enhances the cAMP response, but it appears to be a quantitative effect since relaxin administered in the total absence of estrogen still elicited a cAMP response.

Specificity of Relaxin-Stimulated cAMP Increases

The specificity of relaxin action was determined by measuring the effect of two other protein hormones on the pubic symphysis, whereas in another study the possible stimulation by relaxin of a non-target tissue was examined. Porcine insulin, a protein similar to relaxin in molecular weight and structure (James *et al.*, 1977), did not elicit a significant increase in cAMP levels over control values in mature, intact, or ovariectomized mice [Table 4, Studies 1 and 2A ($P > 0.05$)]. Glucagon increased cAMP levels in the liver ($P = 0.05$), as expected, but did not alter symphyseal cAMP levels ($P > > 0.05$) (Table 4, Study 4). In addition, 3 μg relaxin did not increase cAMP levels in mouse liver, a non-target organ (Table 4, Study 4).

Relaxin-Related Ornithine Decarboxylase Stimulation

Relaxin stimulates ornithine decarboxylase activity in two of its target tissues, the mouse pubic symphysis and uterus (Tables 6 and 7). Stimulation was observed at both 4 and 6 hours for each of the tissues. Stimulation of ornithine decarboxylase activity in the uterus is observed as early as 2 hours following relaxin treatment and is sustained for several hours thereafter. This temporal relationship is similar to that observed in other instances of hormonal stimulation of ornithine decarboxylase activity (Morris and Fillingame, 1974). Estrogen was not required for the response

Table 6. *ORNITHINE DECARBOXYLASE ACTIVITY IN THE PUBIC SYMPHYSES OF MICE.*

Test Group		pmoles CO_2 released/h 5 pubic symphyses		
		Hours after treatment		
		2	4	6
Immature Mice:	Control	23	27	27
	Relaxin	36	47	51
Estrogen Primed	Control	14	19	--
Immature Mice:	Relaxin	18	52	--
Intact Mature	Control	--	25	--
Mice:	Relaxin	--	72	--
Estrogen Primed	Control	--	41	--
Intact Mature Mice:	Relaxin	--	86	--
Ovariectomized	Control	--	23	--
Mature Mice:	Relaxin	--	160	--

The mice were treated as described in Research Protocol. The assay for each treatment group was performed on the supernatant obtained from 5-pooled pubic symphyses and was done in triplicate. Estrogen primed mice were given 5 µg of estradiol benzoate in 0.1 ml sesame oil 3 days prior to treatment. (reproduced from Braddon, 1978). The treatments were: Control, 0.1 ml of 1% Benzopurpurin 4B; Relaxin, 3 µg of relaxin in 0.1 ml of 1% Benzopurpurin 4B.

in either tissue since non-primed ovariectomized mice showed significant increases in enzyme activity over control values.

Increases in ornithine decarboxylase activity are noted in many hormonally stimulated tissues as well as those systems which involve rapid cell proliferation. Either the enzyme itself or the polyamine products of the metabolic pathway in which it functions may be involved in the processes of DNA, RNA and protein synthesis, and it therefore may act as an intermediary in eliciting a biological response to hormones in target tissues.

Table 7.   ORNITHINE DECARBOXYLASE ACTIVITY IN THE UTERI OF MICE

		pmole CO released/h uterus		
Test Group		Hours after treatment		
Estrogen Primed Immature Mice:	Control	76 + 7	52 + 3	46 + 5
	Relaxin	119 + 17	166 + 15	90 + 12
Ovariectomized Mature Mice:	Control	----	27 + 3	27 + 4
	Relaxin	----	110 + 19	247 + 44

The mice were treated as described in Research Protocol. The assay was performed in duplicate on individual whole uteri and the value given represents the mean of 4 mice + the standard error of the mean. Estrogen primed mice were given 5 µg of estradiol benzoate in 0.1 ml sesame oil 3 days prior to treatment. (reproduced from Braddon, 1978). The treatments were: Control, 0.1 ml of 1% Benzo-purpurin 4B; Relaxin, 3 µg of relaxin in 0.1 ml of 1% Benzopurpurin 4B.

SUMMARY

Relaxin, a protein hormone of pregnancy, acts on its target tissues to elicit responses which are similar to those brought about by other protein and peptide hormones in their target tissues. Both increases in cAMP target tissue concentration and stimulation of ornithine decarboxylase activity in extracts of target tissues have been observed for several protein hormones, including relaxin. These observations provide evidence about the sequence of biochemical events that follow relaxin treatment. Specific binding of relaxin to its target tissues (Cheah and Sherwood, 1979; McMurtry *et al.*, 1978) is closely followed by an observed tissue increase in cAMP concentration (Cheah and Sherwood, 1979; Braddon, 1978a). These early events are followed after a lage period of 2-4 h by the elevation of ornithine decarboxylase (Braddon, 1978b). This enzyme activity remains elevated for several hours. The temporal pattern in ornithine decarboxylase activity is similar to that observed in the response of other target tissues to their hormone.

Apparently none of the early events in the biochemical mechanism of action for relaxin have an absolute requirement for estrogen. The level of each of the responses may be enhanced by the presence of estrogen, although there is no conclusive evidence to support this idea. Because estrogen is an absolute requirement for the remodeling of the interpubic ligament by relaxin, it appears that estrogen is necessary in a later phase of the overall process.

REFERENCES

Bachrach, U. (1975). cAMP-mediated induction of ornithine decarboxylase of glioma and neuroblastoma cells. Proc. Natl. Acad. Sci. USA 72:3087.

Braddon, S. A. (1978a). Relaxin-dependent adenosine 3':5'-monophosphase concentration changes in the mouse pubic symphysis. Endocrinolgoy 102:1292.

Braddon, S. A. (1978b). Stimulation of ornithine decarboxylase by relaxin. Biochem. Biophys. Res. Commun. 80:75.

Buehler, B., Wright, R., Schott, S., Darby, B. and Rennert, O. M. (1977). Ornithine decarboxylase and S-adenosyl methionine decarboxylase in skin fibroblasts of normal and cystic fibrosis patients. Pediat Res. 11:186.

Byus, C. V. and Russell, D. H. (1975). Ornithine decarboxylase activity: control by cyclic nucleotides. Sciences 187:650.

Cheah, S. H. and Sherwood, O. D. (1979). Target tissues for relaxin in the rat: Tissue distribution of injected ^{125}I-labeled relaxin and tissue changes in cyclic AMP levels after *in vitro* relaxin incubation. 61st Annual Meeting of the Endocrine Society, Annaheim, CA, 217.

Conroy, P. D., Simms, D. M. and Pointon, J. J. (1977). Occurrence of ornithine decarboxylase and polyamines in cartilage. Biochem. J. 162:347.

Gilman, A. G. (1970). A protein binding assay for adenosine 3':5'-cyclic monophosphate. Proc. Natl. Acad. Sci. USA. 67:305.

Haselbacher, G. K. and Humbel, R. E. (1976). Stimulation of ornithine decarboxylase activity in chick fibroblasts by non-suppressible insulin-like activity (NSILA), insulin and serum. J. Cell Physiol. 88:239.

Hisaw, F. L. (1926). Experimental relaxation of the pubic ligament of the guinea pig. Proc. Soc. Exp. Biol. Med. 23:661.

Hisaw, F. L. and Zarrow, M. X. (1950). The physiology of relaxin, Vitam. Horm. 8:151.

James, R., Niall, H., Kwok, S. and Bryant-Greenwood, G. (1977). Primary structure of porcine relaxin: homology with insulin and related growth factors. Nature 267:544.

Kroc, R. L., Steinetz, B. G., and Beach, V. L. (1959). The effects of estrogens, progestagens, and relaxin in pregnant and non-pregnant laboratory rodents. Ann. NY Acad. Sci. 75:942.

McMurtry, J. P., Kwok, S. C. M. and Bryant-Greenwood, G. D. (1978). Target tissues for relaxin identified *in vitro* with I-labelled porcine relaxin. J. Reprod. Fert. 53:209.

Morris, D. R. and Fillingame, R. H. (1974). Regulation of amino acid decarboxylation. Ann. Rev. Biochem. 43:303.

O'Byrne, E. M. and Steinetz, B. G. (1976). Radioimmunoassay (RIA) of relaxin in sera of various species using antiserum to porcine relaxin. Proc. Soc. Exp. Biol. Med. 152:272.

O'Byrne, E. M., Sawyer, W. K., Butler, M. C. and Steinetz, B. G. (1976). Serum immunoreactive relaxin and softening of the uterine cervix in pregnant hamsters. Endocrinology 99:1333.

Oka, T. and Perry, J. W. (1976). Studies on regulatory factors of ornithine decarboxylase activity during development of mouse mammary epithelium *in vitro*. J. Biol. Chem. 251:1738.

Russell, D. and Snyder, S. H. (1968). Amine synthesis in rapidly growing tissues: ornithine decarboxylase activity in regenerating rat liver, chick embryo, and various tumors. Proc. Natl. Acad. Sci. USA 60:1420.

Schreiber, V. (1974). Adenohypophysial hormones: regulation of their secretion and mechanisms of their action. In: MTP International Review of Science, Biochemistry of Hormones, H. V. Rickenberg (ed.) Vol. 8, University Park Press, Baltimore, MD. p. 61.

Sherwood, O. D., Rosentreter, K. R. and Birkhimer, M. L. (1975). Development of a radioimmunoassay for porcine relaxin using ^{125}I-labeled polytyrosyl-relaxin. Endocrinology 96:1106.

Sherwood, O. D., Chang, C. C., BeVier, G. W., Diehl, J. R. and Dziuk, P. J. (1976). Relaxin concentrations in pig plasma following the administration of prostaglandin $F_2\alpha$ during late pregnancy. Endocrinology 98:875.

Steinetz, B. G., Beach, V. L. and Kroc, R. L. (1957). The influence of progesterone, relaxin and estrogen on some structural and functional changes in the preparturient mouse. Endocrinology 61:271.

Yamasaki, Y. and Ichihara, A. (1976). Induction of ornithine decarboxylase in cultured mouse L cells I. Effects of cellular growth, hormones, and actinomycin D. J. Biochem. 80:557.

DISCUSSION FOLLOWING DR. S. A. BRADDON'S PAPER

Dr. Frieden
   (Kent State University): How long after ovariectomies were your experiments done with ovariectomized animals?

Dr. Braddon
   We rested the animals for a week before we either estrogen primed them or started them on the sequence. So hopefully, they were depleted.

Dr. Bradshaw
   (Washington University): I would like to make a couple of comments on this paper. In your summary of the mechanism of action of hormones, I think it is only fair to point out that that is really not a complete picture because certainly not all hormones act through adenyl cyclase, as your slide might have implied. In fact, there are really two classes of hormones in a very general subdivision: Those which apparently do directly interact with adenyl cyclase with a receptor and those which don't. And insulin, which is, as we heard yesterday, closely related to relaxin, is clearly in that second category. That makes your results even more interesting.

   One statement you made which I have to take issue with, when you said in 120 minutes you felt your receptors were saturated and that is why there was no further production, that is in complete contrast to the way adenyl cyclase hormones work. As long as they are sitting on the receptor, they stimulate the cyclase and only when you take the hormone off the receptor do they stop producing it. So that interpretation of the result, if it is working directly through cyclase, can't possibly be right.

   Now, more to the point, Sutherland, who is clearly the father of this field, set up four very clear criteria for defining hormones that work through adenyl cyclase. Your data only meet one of those criteria, namely the apparent intercellular production of cyclic AMP. The other three criteria, the stimulation of adenyl cyclase, the mimicing of the activity in question by cyclic AMP, and the artificial raising of intercellular cyclic levels by phosphodiesterase inhibitors, you didn't discuss.

   Do you have anything that would add to that?

Dr. Braddon
   I agree entirely that the general mechanism I showed did not include the internalization mechanism. I was in error not to point that out.

I think that to study the other phases demonstrating that
the hormone works through adenyl cyclase, one needs to get into a
cell system, either actual cell culture or explant. I don't believe
that working in the animal the way I was, that you would be very
successful. And I think the mouse pubic symphysis was probably not
the best model to work with. It is too small. It's limiting.
I think that possibly the guinea pig may be better; it has much
more tissue. I think it would be good if we could get into a cell
system, either tissue culture or explants. I have measured after-
the-fact cyclic AMP increases just in a Krebs-Ringer buffer, with this
emphasis, and I got much more repeatable results, which was good.
I was misled in the beginning when we were doing the work because
we had so much trouble with the mice and with the cyclic AMP assay.
I thought it was due to the fact that the tissue would not respond
in vitro, and instead it was due to the actual assay system. I
never returned to the *in vitro* system. But one gets definite and
very good responses *in vitro*. That would be a much better place
to work.

Dr. Bradshaw
Yes. I think it is probably worth noting that in these two
classes of hormones, those which clearly work include cyclic AMP,
or at least as far as we appreciate them, such as glucagons, which
you were using as a nice control, and those which apparently don't
work directly. Even in those cases, though, there are observed
transient increases oftentimes in cyclic AMP. But they are clearly
distinguishable intelluctually, because they are not proportional
to the hormone receptor complex being formed. Since they do generate
a lot of metabolic stimulation, they are basically anabolic stimulators
or are atypic activators, to use the late Norman Thompson's nomenclature. They do affect cyclic AMP levels, but it is a transient
level, obviously acting through some secondary stimulation of cyclases
present in the cell.

I guess my principal question that I was driving at with the
Sutherland criteria is: Do you have any evidence at all that cyclic
AMP, or one of its derivatives, can cause or mimic any known action
of relaxin?

Dr. Braddon
I didn't have a system I could test that on.

Dr. Bradshaw
Cyclic AMP will mimic the action of relaxin in the uterine
preparation. Does anybody know if it will do anything with the
symphysis?

Dr. Braddon
I think that if I were to go back and put the symphysis in
Krebs-Ringer buffer and treat it with cyclic AMP, probably there I

couldn't do it. You just can't do that on the symphysis.

Dr. Bradshaw
   It is difficult, certainly.

Dr. Braddon
   I really need to go to the actual measurements of the adenylic
cyclase and to look for protein kinase. That brings up the question:
What would be the substrate for the protein kinase? If we had a
clear idea of the molecular process in the target tissues, it would
help us to seek the actual mechanism better.

Dr. Jeffrey
   I think it is very clear that it is almost impossible to satisfy
the Sutherland conclusions in the *in vitro* system, and the point
really is that this at least affords you the sort of permissive
indication that there may well be an involvement of the hormone in
cyclic AMP production, and as Barbara points out, the next step
is clearly to get to a better system. One could treat an animal with
dibutyl cyclic AMP.

Dr. Bradshaw
   I agree with what you are saying, John, but it's a classic tenet
of endocrinology that you must link the effect that you are measuring
with the effect of the hormone, and all we have here are data that
say if you inject relaxin into the properly prepared animal model
in a punitive target tissue, you see a rise in cyclic AMP. You
cannot connect the two.

Dr. Braddon
   I think you're making a mandate for more research and I think
that's good.

Dr. Sanborn
   How long does it take you to kill the animal and take out the
pubic symphysis?

Dr. Braddon
   Under 30 seconds.

Dr. Sanborn
   I wondered if you had ever tried to anesthetize the animal and
run the whole **experiment** under anesthesia?

Dr. Braddon
   No, I did not.

Dr. Greenwood
   The second tenet in endocrinology is what is the target tissue.
Do you know the target tissue or the target cell you are working on?

Dr. Braddon

No, I do not.

Dr. Greenwood

These are short-term *in vivo* experiments; cyclic AMP in the pubic symphysis at 30 minutes, I understand, and in the uterus, two to four hours. Do you see any changes in protein in the two-to-four-hour experiment? Obviously, you couldn't expect one in 30 minutes, but you know there could be some effects on protein.

Dr. Braddon

No. In fact, there were no obvious changes in the tissue visually or histologically at 15 and 30 minutes.

One of the questions I was asked when I was writing the paper was how would I know exactly where to cut and what tissue I was after. So I tried to maximize the size of the piece of tissue I took. I took about a 10 millimeter section, which included the pubic caps and the ligament. There was a lot of inert tissue involved in the incubation.

Dr. Greenwood

So the milligrams of total protein contain inert protein. I was wondering whether it might be advisable to express it in terms of picomoles per cyclic AMP per unit of DNA, to get an index of the cellularity. Certainly one sees a change in cellularity after estrogen treatment in the pubic symphysis.

Dr. Braddon

I think that would be a good way to express it, or at least it would give us an additional piece of information.

Dr. Rosalia Mercado-Simmen

(University of Hawaii): You mentioned working on ovariectomized and immature mice. I was just wondering how you could explain why you need estrogen binding for biological response and you don't need any for cyclic AMP?

Dr. Braddon

I wish I could answer that question. I cannot explain it. We thought long and hard about it. I was hoping that estrogen might be required for receptor production, but I don't believe that is true because eventually the receptors would disappear if you held your ovariectomized animals long enough. We still had good responses, so I don't believe it was that. I think that question is entirely up in the air. It is just an observation that it was not required. It is a very interesting one. I did later treat animals with progesterone and could prevent the increase in cyclic AMP levels from control.

EFFECT OF PORCINE RELAXIN ON CYCLIC NUCLEOTIDE LEVELS AND SPONTANEOUS CONTRACTIONS OF THE RAT UTERUS*

B. M. Sanborn[+], H. S. Kuo[+], N. W. Weisbrodt[++], and O. D. Sherwood[#]

Departments of Reproductive Medicine and Biology[+] and Physiology[++], The University of Texas Medical School at Houston, Houston, TX 77025 and Department of Physiology and Biophysics[#], School of Basic Medical Sciences, University of Illinois, Urbana Illinois 71801

INTRODUCTION

Relaxin has been known for some time to inhibit spontaneous uterine contractions in a number of species (Schwabe et al., 1978). Furthermore a number of studies have indicated that circulating factors in addition to steroid hormones regulate uterine contractility and responsiveness during pregnancy (Porter, 1972; Korenman et al., 1974; Porter and Downing, 1978). In the human, serum relaxin levels are elevated early in pregnancy, suggesting that this hormone may play a role in maintaining uterine quiescence during that period (Quagliarello et al., 1979).

One mechanism by which various agents effect uterine relaxation has been postulated to involve changes in tissue cyclic AMP (cAMP), but this does not appear to be the case in all instances (Harbon et al., 1978; Diamond, 1977; Andersson and Nilsson, 1977; Korenman and Krall, 1977; Sanborn et al., 1980). Nonetheless, cyclic AMP and its analogs as well as phosphodiesterase inhibitors relax uterine strips. Furthermore, the majority of the evidence points to an involvement of cAMP in at least one component of the mechanism by which β-adrenergic agents relax the uterus. Release of epinephrine has been suggested as the mechanism by which relaxin exerts its effect

*This work was supported in part by NIH Grants HD09618(BMS) and HD08799(ODS). Research Career Development Awards 5-K04-H000126(BMS), 1-K04-HD000019(ODS) and DA-00022(NWW) are acknowledged.

on the uterus (Rudzik and Miller, 1962a,b). It is therefore of
interest to consider whether relaxin elevates uterine cAMP and
whether catecholamines are mediators in this process.

MATERIALS AND METHODS

Uteri were removed from 150–200 g Long Evans female rats
which had been primed with estradiol benzoate (50 µg/day in sesame
oil, sc). Uteri were slit, scraped to remove endometrium, cut into
$\sim$ 100 mg strips, and suspended isometrically at $\sim$ 1 g tension in the
buffer of Diamond and Hartle (1976) as described in detail
elsewhere (Sanborn et al., 1980). After treatment, the strips
were frozen with chilled tongs, stored in liquid N_2, and assayed
for cAMP and cGMP by radioimmunoassay (Sanborn et al., 1980; Heindel
et al., 1978). Protein was determined by the method of Lowry
(Layne, 1957).   All data are reported as the mean $\pm$ SE of 4
determinations unless otherwise indicated. Data were analyzed by one
way analysis of variance and Duncan's multiple range test. Relaxin
preparations employed were NIH-R-P1(442 GPU(Guinea pig units/mg),
ODS-R-15(2500-3,000 GPU/mg), and NIH-RXN-P1(3,000 GPU/mg). Unless
otherwise indicated, ODS-R-15 was used.

RESULTS AND DISCUSSION

Effect of Relaxin on Spontaneous Activity

Relaxin preparations NIH-R-P1 and ODS-R-15 suppressed
spontaneous contractile activity in the absence of phosphodiesterase
inhibitors. As illustrated in Figure 1, purified relaxin markedly
decreased the maximal force generated, the frequency of the contractions, and the area parameter which is a reflection of energy
expended (Korenman et al., 1974; Sanborn et al., 1980) at concentrations below 0.4 µg/ml. Under these conditions, there was no
observable change in cAMP or cGMP levels, measured 20 minutes after
exposure of uterine strips to relaxin.

Effect of Relaxin on Uterine Cyclic Nucleotide Levels

Relaxin preparations NIH-R-P1, ODS-R-15 and NIH-RXN-P1 all
elevated uterine cAMP levels when phosphodiesterase inhibitors were
present in the medium (Sanborn et al., 1980). The effect was
maximal by 20 minutes (Figure 2) and was dose-related, with a
maximum at approximately 1 µg/ml (Figure 3). No changes in
cGMP levels were observed under these conditions.

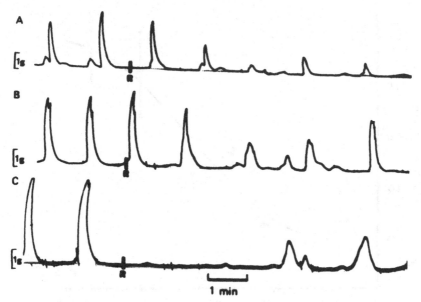

Figure 1. Representative tracings of spontaneous contractions and
response of uterine strips to treatment with relaxin.
A, 0.064 µg/ml; B, 0.3 µg/ml; C, 0.96 µg/ml

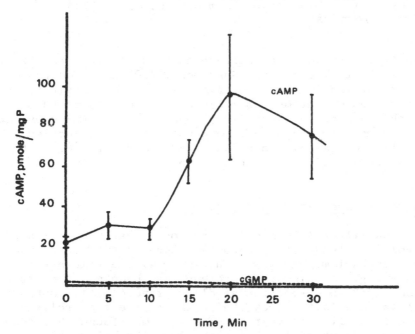

Figure 2. Cyclic nucleotide levels in isometrically suspended uterine
strips measured as a function of time after exposure to
0.4 µg/ml relaxin. From Sanborn et al.(1980) with
permission.

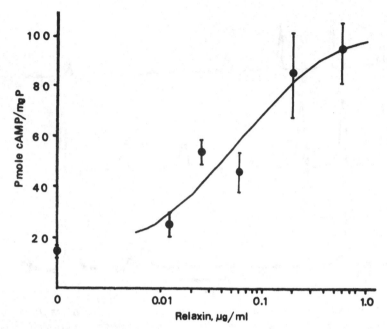

*Figure 3.   Dose-related elevation of uterine cAMP levels in
response to relaxin.   From Sanborn et al. (1980)
with permission.*

    The ability of relaxin to elevate cAMP was limited to the uterus
and cervix (Table 1).   Cheah and Sherwood (1980) have independently
reached a similar conclusion.   Together these data constitute the
first *in vitro* demonstrations of a biochemical effect of this
hormone on the uterus.   Braddon (1978) has reported cAMP elevation
in the pubic symphysis region of the mouse.   This evidence suggests
that the ability of relaxin to elevate cAMP is restricted to those
tissues known to be affected by the hormone.

Role of Catecholamines in Relaxin Action

    Rudzik and Miller (1962a,b) had proposed that the action of
relaxin involved release of epinephrine which in turn acted via a
β-adrenergic mechanism.   As shown in Figure 4, the relaxant action
of the β-adrenergic agonist isoproterenol was blocked by pretreatment
of the tissue with the β-antagonist dl-propranolol.   In contrast,
propranolol was unable to block the relaxant effect of relaxin.
This finding is similar to that of Paterson, who found that pro-
nethalol, also a β-antagonist, did not block the relaxant effect of
relaxin on the uterus (Paterson, 1965).   The data suggest that
catecholamines do not serve as obligatory intermediates in this
action of relaxin.

Table 1. *TISSUE SPECIFICITY OF THE RESPONSE TO RELAXIN*

Tissue	cAMP/ pmoles/mg P	
	Control	Relaxin
Uterus[a]	22 ± 7	$73 \pm 6**$
Cervix[b]	38 ± 2	$164 \pm 50**$
Ileum[a]	7 ± 1	9 ± 1
Vas deferens[a]	33 ± 9	52 ± 5
Testicular capsules[b]	44 ± 9	42 ± 5
Epididymis[b]	5 ± 1	6 ± 2

The first three tissues were obtained from female rats and the rest from adult male rats. [a]*Isometrically suspended,* [b]*unrestrained. Different from control at $P < 0.01$, **, $P < 0.05$, *.*

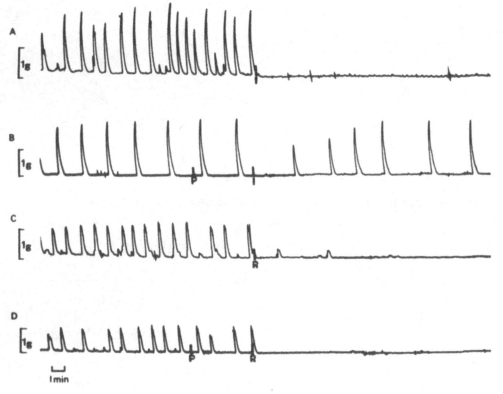

Figure 4.   The effect of 5 μM propranolol on uterine relaxation
produced in response to 0.36 μg/ml relaxin or 60 μM isoproterenol.   A: Effect of isoproterenol (I) on spontaneous
activity.   B: Effect of addition of propranolol (P) and isoproterenol (I) in succession on spontaneous activity.   C:
Effect of relaxin (R) on spontaneous activity.   D: Effect
of addition of propranolol (P) and relaxin (R) in succession
on spontaneous activity.   From Sanborn et al. (1980) with
permission.

   In the presence of phosphodiesterase inhibitors, propranolol was
able to suppress the ability of isoproterenol to elevate urine cAMP
(Table 2).   However, propranolol did not block the elevation of cAMP
in response to relaxin indicating that this action was also not
mediated by catecholamines.

Effect of Relaxin on Adenylate Cyclase Activity

   In order to determine whether relaxin elevated cAMP by direct
means, the effect of the hormone on myometrial membrane adenylate
cyclase was studied.   Preliminary experiments indicate that relaxin
can indeed increase adenylate cyclase activity in the presence of

Table 2. THE EFFECT OF PROPRANOLOL ON THE ABILITY OF ISOPROTERENOL
AND RELAXIN TO ELEVATE UTERINE CYCLIC NUCLEOTIDE LEVELS

Treatment Sequence	cAMP pmoles/mg P	cGMP pmoles/mg P
Control	21 ± 6	2.0 ± 0.3
Propranolol (5 µM)	21 ± 3	2.0 ± 0.4
Isoproterenol (10 µM)	724 ± 1[a,b,c]	2.6 ± 0.3
Propranolol + Isoproterenol	40 ± 4[c]	2.4 ± 0.2
Relaxin (0.36 µg/ml)	100 ± 17[a,b]	2.1 ± 0.1
Propranolol + Relaxin	107 ± 8[a,b]	2.3 ± 0.5

Propranolol was added 5 minutes before addition of isoproterenol or
relaxin and tissues were frozen 20 minutes after introduction of these
agents. Different at P < 0.01 from: a, control or propranolol; b,
propranolol + isoproterenol; c, propranolol + relaxin. From Sanborn
et al. (1980) with permission.

the nonhydrolyzable GTP analog Gpp(NH)p. The magnitude of the effect
is significant but relatively small in an assay under linear conditions
(Figure 5). However, the stimulation is of the same order of mangitude
as exhibited by isoproterenol. These data, coupled with reports of
specific binding to uterine tissue (Cheah and Sherwood, 1980; McMurtry
et al., 1978; Bryant-Greenwood *et al.*, 1981) suggest that relaxin
exerts its effects on the uterus by direct interaction. One result of
this interaction appears to be to increase adenylate cyclase activity.

CONCLUSIONS

The ability of purified relaxin preparations to relaxin rat
uterine strips has been confirmed and the ability of these preparations to elevate uterine cAMP has been established. It appears that
neither of these actions requires obligatory β-adrenergic intermediates, since propranolol was unable to block them while inhibiting
the effect of isoproterenol. The target organ specificity of the cAMP
response correlates well with other reports of direct binding (Cheah and
Sherwood, 1980; McMurtry *et al.*, 1978; Bryant-Greenwood *et al.*, 1981)
and correlates well with earlier reports of observable relaxin effects.

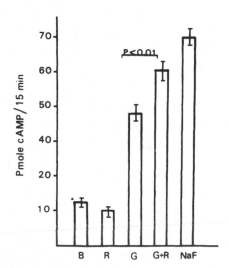

*Figure 5.   Effect of relaxin (r, 50 µg/ml) on adenylate cyclase
              activity in the absence and presence of Gpp(NH)p(G, 40 µM)
              in 2,000 x g uterine membranes assayed in the system of
              Thompson et al. (1973) at 30° in the presence of 0.2 mg/
              ml myokinase. Nucleotides were separated by Dowex and
              alumina chromatography (Salomon et al., 1974). B, basal
              activity, NaF, activity in the presence of 10 mM NaF.*

Since cAMP increases could only be observed in the presence of phosphodiesterase inhibitors and relaxin-mediated relaxation occurred in the absence of any apparent change in tissue cAMP, it is not possible at the present time to implicate cAMP in the mechanism by which relaxin causes uterine relaxation. If these two parameters are casually related, it may be that rapid, compartmentalized changes in cAMP which would not have been detected by the methods employed are involved. On the other hand, the elevation of cAMP may be unrelated to the relaxant effect, but nonetheless part of the total sequence of events whereby relaxin influences the uterus. Since relaxin may play some part in regulating uterine contractility during pregnancy, it is of critical importance to understand the mechanisms by which this hormone influences the uterus.

ACKNOWLEDGEMENTS

The authors wish to thank Mr. S. H. Cheah for fruitful discussions during the latter part of this work and the National Pituitary Agency for providing NIH-R-P1 and NIH-RXN-P1 relaxin.

REFERENCES

Andersson, R. G. G. and Nilsson, K. B. (1977). Role of cyclic nucleotides: Metabolism and mechanical activity in smooth muscle. In: The Biochemistry of Smooth Muscle", N. L. Stephans, ed., University Park Press, Baltimore, MD. p. 263.

Braddon, S. A. (1978). Relaxin-dependent adenosine 3',5'-monophosphate concentration changes in the mouse pubic symphysis, Endocrinology 102:1292.

Bryant-Greenwood, G, Mercado-Simmen, Rosalia, Yamamoto, Sandra Y., Arakaki, R. F., Uchima, F. D. A. and Greenwood, F. C. (1981). Relaxin receptors and a study of the physiological roles of relaxin. 15th Midwest Conference on Endocrin. and Metab.

Cheah, S. H. and Sherwood, O. D. (1980). Target tissues for relaxin in the rat: Tissue distribution of injected ^{125}I-labeled relaxin and tissue changes in cyclic AMP levels after in vitro relaxin incubation. Endocrinology 106:1203

Diamond, J. (1977). Evidence for dissociation between cyclic nucleotide levels and tension in smooth muscle. In: "The Biochemistry of Smooth Muscle". H. L. Stephans, ed., University Park Press, Baltimore, MD. p. 343.

Diamond, J. and Hartle, K. D. (1976). Cyclic nucleotide levels during carbachol-induced smooth muscle contractions. J. Cycl. Nucleotide Res. 2:179.

Harbon, S., Vesin, M. F. , Khac, L. D. and Leiber, D. (1978). Cyclic nucleotides in the regulation of rat uterus contractility. In: Molecular Biology and Pharmacology of Cyclic Nucleotides, G. Folco and R. Paolette, eds., Elsevier, Holland. p. 279.

Heindel, J. J., Hintz, M. I., Steinberger, E. and Strada, S. J.
(1978). The effect of FSH on cyclic nucleotide levels in
testicular tissue from rats of various ages: Non correlation
with cyclic nucleotide phosphodiesterase activity. Endocrine
Res. Commun. 4:6.

Korenman, S. G., Bhalla, R. C., Wortsman, J., Stevens, R., Wells,
L. and Carpenter, L. (1974). Hormonal regulation of uterine
contractility: The role of the adenylate cyclase system. J.
Steroid Biochem. 5:905.

Korenman, S. G. and Krall, J. F. (1977). The role of cyclic AMP
in the regulation of smooth muscle cell contraction in the
uterus. Biol. Reprod. 16:1.

Layne, E. (1957). Protein estimation with the Folin-Ciocalteu
method, In: Methods in Enzymology. S. P. Colowick and N.
O. Kaplan, ed. Vol. III, Academic Press, NY p. 448.

McMurtry, J. P., Kwok, S. C. M. and Bryant-Greenwood, G. D. (1978).
Target tissues for relaxin identified *in vitro* with ^{125}I-
labelled porcine relaxin. J. Reprod. Fert. 52:209.

Paterson, G. (1965). The nature of the inhibition of the rat uterus
by relaxin. J. Pharm. Pharmacol. 17:262.

Porter, D. G. (1972). Myometrium of the pregnant guinea pig:
The probable importance of relaxin. Biol. Reprod. 7:458.

Porter, D. G. and Downing, S. J. (1978). Evidence that a humoral
factor possessing relaxin like activity is responsible for
uterine quiescence in the late pregnant rat. J. Reprod.
Fert. 52:95.

Quagliarello, J., Steinetz, F. G. and Weiss, G. (1979). Relaxin
secretion in early pregnancy. Obstet. Gyn. 53:62.

Rudzik, A. D and Miller, J. W. (1962a). The mechanism of uterine
inhibitory action of relaxin-containing ovarian extracts.
J. Pharmacol. Exp. Ther. 138:82.

Rudzik, A. D. and Miller, J. W. (1962b). The effect of altering
the catecholamine content of the uterus on the rate of contractions and the sensitivity of the myometrium to relaxin.
J. Pharmacol. Exp. Ther. 138:88.

Salomon, Y., Londos, C. and Rodbell, M. (1974). A highly
sensitive adenylate cyclase assay. Analyt. Biochem. 58:541.

Sanborn, B. M., Heindel, J. H. and Robison, G. A. (1980). The
role of cyclic nucleotides in reproductive processes. Ann.
Rev. Physiol. 42 (in press).

Sanborn, B. M., Kuo, H. S., Weisbrodt, N. W. and Sherwood, O. D.
(1980). The interaction of relaxin with the rat uterus.
I: Effect on cyclic nucleotide levels and spontaneous contractile activity. Endocrinology 106:1210.

Schwabe, C., Steinetz, B., Weiss, G., Segaloff, A., McDonald, J. K.,
O'Bryne, E., Hochman, J., Carriere, J. and Goldsmith, L. (1978).
Relaxin. Recent Prog. Horm. Res. 34:123.

Thompson, W. J., Williams, R. H. and Little, S. A. (1973). Studies
on the assay and activities of guanyl and adenyl cyclase of
rat liver. Arch. Biochem. Biophys. 159:206.

DISCUSSION FOLLOIWNG DR. B. M. SANBORN'S PAPER

Dr. Ralph Bradshaw
  (Washington University): I was particularly interested in one slide, which showed the time course of cyclic AMP production. There was about a 20 minute lag followed by the rise, and then it started to decay. However, the data didn't extend beyond 30 minutes.

Dr. Sanborn
  Yes.

Dr. Bradshaw
  My first question is: Why the lag? Adenyl cyclase-dependent systems classically do not show a lag. Rather there is usually an instantaneous response when the hormone binds to the receptor.

  Secondly, if you extend the experiment another 30 minutes, does the concentration of cAMP return to the base line value?

Dr. Sanborn
  O.K. May I have that slide back. Cyclic AMP levels are maximal by 20 minutes. You can detect it at 15. You can detect by 10 minutes, but there seems to be a lag between zero and 10 minutes. I'm not absolutely sure where the lower limit is, because we haven't gone back to define that in great detail. I'm not sure at the moment what that indicates. Since we know that there are effects of guanyl nucleotides on the cyclase, it may be that we don't have the proper constitutents in the buffer, to see what would happen in a physiological state. I don't know. You are right that we really should see an effect by five minutes.

Dr. Bradshaw
  You should see it faster than five minutes.

Dr. Sanborn
  We see an effect of relaxin on adenylyl cyclase in less than five minutes. When we're talking about total tissue cyclic AMP, that is a combination of a number of things. We have not gone back systematically to explore that.

Dr. Bradshaw
  The magnitude of the response and the fact that it goes up and comes right back down again are consistent with the class of hormones that don't act by directly stimulating adenyl cyclase, but rather stimulate other aspects of the metabolism in the cell. Although one of the things you see in these systems is some activation of the cyclase, the profile you get with hormones such as glucagon that act through cyclase is not very different. The magnitude of the stimulation is much greater in these cases than what you are seeing.

Dr. Sanborn

Well, if you notice the isoproterenol stimulation was greater than that of relaxin.

Dr. Bradshaw

Quite a bit greater.

Dr. Sanborn

We are in the process of looking at the interaction between those two agents with respect to whether they are interacting with the same cyclase. It is still possible that relaxin is releasing local catecholamines that aren't blocked by the beta-adrenergic agents. We have some experiments in progress which involve depleting the local concentrations of adrenergic agents to rule out this possibility.

Dr. Bradshaw

But I thought your results were very convincing.

Dr. Sanborn

With respect to the time course of the reaction, I think I differ a little with you on the interpretation (Author's insert: Bhalla, Korenman and I noted some time ago (*Endocrinology* 92:429, 1973) that in a similar uterine strip assay, isoproterenol elevated tissue cAMP with a time course in general terms similar to the one I showed for relaxin, i.e., a rise to a plateau and then a decline. The only difference was that the rise was more rapid (within 2 minutes) and the decline occurred by 20 minutes. Several workers have shown that isoproterenol acts directly by stimulating adenylyl cyclase in this system). If you look in an isolated cell system you do see a rapid increase and then a decrease with time (for example, T. Haga *et al.*, *Proc. Natl. Acad. Sci. USA* 74:2016, 1977). Dr. G. A.Robison in the Department of Pharmacology, UTMSH, has been doing some computer modeling based on the regulation of cAMP levels by hormonal stimulation of adenylyl cyclase (*Fed. Proc.* 38:532, 1979).

Dr. Bradshaw

With which hormone?

Dr. Sanborn

I believe it is glucagon (Author's note: BHK cells and epinephrine were used to obtain data for the modeling).

Dr. Bradshaw

Yes, but glucagon is destroyed by enzymes in the membrane very quickly which is the main reason why it tails off. The half life of glucagon on the surface of the hepatocyte is something like 10 minutes.

Dr. Sanborn

Well, there are other instances.

Dr. Bradshaw

   If you keep adding glucagon, the levels of cAMP do not decay,
they stay up. As long as you have glucagon receptors occupied, the
adenyl cyclase stimulation remains. However, if you put in only a
single bolus of glucagon, it will go up and then come back down.

Dr. Sanborn

   Well, under certain conditions, he can restimulate. Beyond
a certain point, you do get a desensitization reaction which can
occur even while you are looking at the cyclic AMP under the same
time course (R. Barber *et al., Adv. Cyc. Nucl. Res.* 9:507, 1978).

Dr. Niall

   (University of Melbourne): I just wanted to comment that Dr.
Bruce Kemp, in our lab, has done some studies recently on the effects
of relaxin on cyclic AMP dependent protein kinase in the uterus.
So far, he has not been able to see any immediate effect of relaxin
on the cyclic AMP dependent kinase.

Dr. Sanborn

   On total activation of soluble kinase?

Dr. Niall

   Yes. This is total activation; however, these are preliminary
results and a lot more sorting out needs to be done.

Dr. Roberts

   (University of Kansas): The effects that both of these papers
have described are interesting. I think they show a trend. But one
of the things that disturbs me is the magnitude of the increase in
enzyme levels, that is, the cyclic AMP level increase, since if, in
fact, it's mechanism of action is to bind to other proteins or
enzymes, such as kinase. In the case of a number of other hormones
that work by cyclase, the effects are much larger in magnitude. Their
order of magnitude is larger, because it is the sort of thing you
would expect to see if you were going to significantly affect the
state of occupancy of a binding site on a protein that is going to
be affected. So I am disturbed by the order of the total cyclic AMP
that you are accumulating in the cell. I wonder if you would comment
on that.

Dr. Sanborn

   Well, as Drs. Beavo, Bechtel and Krebs noted a number of years
ago (*Proc. Natl. Acad. Sci. USA* 71:3580, 1974) one would predict
on the basis of the basal levels of cyclic AMP and the activation
constant for cAMP-dependent protein kinases that essentially all the
enzyme would be activated with basal cAMP levels. This prediction
doesn't hold true, probably because the actual cellular concentrations
of protein kinase are relatively high, which shifts the apparent

activation constant. (Author's insert: Nonetheless, using calculations similar to those of Beavo *et al*., a tissue level of 200 pmoles
cAMP/mg protein, which can be reached with relaxin and easily
exceeded with isoproterenol, would be enough to significantly activate
the kinases). Furthermore, there is evidence from a number of systems
that the cyclic AMP is sequestered and may have a very local action.
I don't think we can rule out cAMP as a second messenger for relaxin
at the present time on the basis of the order of magnitude of the
cyclic AMP elevation. In fact, in the Leydig cell system, the levels
of cyclic AMP go up markedly in response to HCG, but it only takes
a very small, almost nondetectable increase to cause major changes in
testosterone secretion.

Dr. Jeffrey
      I might make a point too, with respect to this. One thing
that you note, is you need a diesterase inhibitor to show net cyclic
AMP changes at all in the uterus. Even isoproterenol will increase
cyclic AMP when incubated with some uterine preparations. At any
rate, I don't know how ours compare, but it is very difficult to
see a net cyclic AMP increase with maximum concentrations of isoproterenol, until quite often you have plenty of diesterase inhibitor
such as MIX. Aside from the fact this is a brand new tissue and a
brand new hormone, whether or not it acts by way of the classical
pathway, is that the tissue is very different. It appears to have a
very active diesterase endogenously. The net increase is a balance
between the amount of diesterase remaining, even in the presence of
all of the MIX you can get in solution, and the total synthetic rate,
just as in any other system. Furthermore, who knows what population
of cells might be involved with relaxin? Should it be a small
fraction of the total then the order of magnitude of the response
would not be the same as what one is accustomed to seeing. I mention
these things in symphathy with someone who is subjected to these
kinds of questions, since it is really difficult to show an increase
at all. I don't think she would make any case for the final absolute
level of cyclic AMP that could be attained if all the diesterases
were considered. I also want to point out that if there is a specific
way to handle a pool of cyclic AMP produced at the behest of the
hormone, assuming that it is, then you may not see an increase at
all, but it would still be a cyclase stimulator.

      So I think it is a very difficult problem. I think it's suf-
ficient for today to have seen the kind of indications that there
are and certainly the data reported today can be looked at in much
greater length and will stimulate much more research work, which is
clearly what is needed.

Dr. Steinetz
      We really have no idea of the rate of penetration of the 6,000
molecular weight polypeptide into the tissue *in vitro*. If we had

such a measurement which would be possible with radiolabeled relaxin it might tend to resolve some of these conflicting opinions.

Dr. Francis-Dean Uchima

(University of Hawaii): I was looking at another point of view. Do you know what happens to cyclic AMP if you don't use phospho-diesterase inhibitors when you stimulate?

Dr. Sanborn

Ten or twenty minutes after exposure to relaxin, cyclic AMP levels have not changed. We haven't looked in more detail at the time course in the absence of phosphodiesterase inhibitors.

Dr. Uchima

What about isoproterenol?

Dr. Sanborn

We do get a small rise with very high concentrations of iso-proterenol in the absence of MIX, but as you noticed, isoproterenol elevated cAMP levels to a greater degree than relaxin in the presence of MIX.

Dr. Jeffrey

That is exactly my experience.

RELAXIN RECEPTORS AND A STUDY OF THE

PHYSIOLOGICAL ROLES OF RELAXIN

Gillian D. Bryant-Greenwood, Rosalia Mercado-Simmen,
Sandra Y. Yamamoto, R. F. Arakaki, F. D. A. Uchima, and
F. C. Greenwood

Departments of Anatomy & Reproductive Biology and
Biochemistry & Biophysics
University of Hawaii
Honolulu, Hawaii 96822

This paper will be divided into two sections, the first
dealing with our work on relaxin receptors and the second with the
current evidence for relaxin being a physiologically important
hormone in the non-pregnant animal.

1. *RELAXIN RECEPTORS*

a. *Pubic symphysis*

In our initial studies, we looked for evidence for the binding
of ^{125}I-labelled relaxin to target tissues in species known to be
sensitive to relaxin by their use in biological assay systems
(McMurtry *et al.*, 1978). For our first studies, Dr. McMurtry in our
laboratory used the immature female mouse weighing between 18-20 grams
treated 7 days previously with 5 μg estradiol, exactly as for the
mouse interpubic ligament bioassays (Steinetz *et al.*, 1960). Simple
homogenates of pooled mouse interpubic ligaments were incubated
with ^{125}I-labelled relaxin and the binding exhibited was time,
temperature and pH dependent as well as being specifically inhibited
by unlabelled relaxin in the ng/ml range, whereas porcine insulin,
glucagon, human FSH or epidermal growth factor had no effect on the
binding at all concentrations tested (McMurtry *et al.*, 1978). Similar
results were obtained when homogenates of pubic symphyses from
normal virgin guinea pigs were incubated with ^{125}I-labelled relaxin.
The pubic symphysis system was further studied in order to try to
define more clearly the level at which relaxin was exerting its
biological action.

b. *Fibroblasts*

Fibroblasts from pubic symphysis explants obtained from estrogen primed mice were cultured (McMurtry *et al.*, 1980). When sufficient fibroblasts were available for binding studies, they were harvested and incubated with labelled relaxin with appropriate controls. The binding of labelled hormone to these intact cells was also found to be time, temperature and pH dependent. In competition experiments, relaxin alone inhibited the binding in the ng/ml range and only porcine proinsulin showed any degree of competitive inhibition, suggesting *inter alia* some structural homologies between relaxin and proinsulin (McMurtry *et al.*, 1980). Essentially similar results were obtained when we used fibroblasts cultured from human skin biopsies (McMurtry *et al.*, 1980). This was an interesting observation since it suggests that fibroblasts may be ubiquitous in their ability to specifically bind relaxin, or that the skin, a target tissue for estrogen, might also be a relaxin target tissue. In the same study, we showed the ability of relaxin to stimulate the growth of fibro-blasts *in vitro*, differences in response were noted depending upon the site from which the cells originated. The cells from the forearm and upperarm were more sensitive to relaxin as a mitogenic agent than the cells from the nose and scalp (McMurtry *et al.*, 1980). This was the first demonstration that relaxin may have receptor activity in tissues other than the reproductive tract, and therefore may have a more general role in collagen metabolism. It also indicates that relaxin is a growth factor from its biological action as well as its structural similarity with the nerve growth factor family of peptides (Niall *et al.*, 1978).

We have extended this work on the fibroblast receptor by using it as a model system to link relaxin and its interaction with the receptor through to a biological end point--*de novo* collagen biosynthesis as judged by hydroxyproline incorporation into collagen. Using fibroblasts cultured from guinea pig cervix, preliminary work has shown that cells incubated with 100 ng/ml relaxin for 3 hours show a significant increase in total protein synthesis as well as hydroxyproline incorporation into collagen. Fibroblasts from other sites, dose dependency and the effect of longer incubation need further study.

c. *Uterus and Cervix*

Initial studies using uterine segments from estrogen primed virgin mice or mature rats, demonstrated that binding of ^{125}I-labelled relaxin was time and temperature dependent (McMurtry *et al.*, 1978). We were unable to show specific binding to rat uterine homogenates, probably due to the severity of the homogenization procedure as then used. On the other hand, homogenates of guinea pig cervix did demonstrate binding which was time dependent at $22^{\circ}C$ (McMurtry *et al.*, 1978).

Rat Uterus. The binding of ^{125}I-labelled relaxin to the rat
uterus has been further explored in depth and may be summarized as
follows. The binding activity has been localized in the membrane-
enriched particulate fraction of rat myometrium and binding has
been shown to be time and temperature dependent, reversible, of
high affinity (Ka 10^9–10^{10}/m) with a limited steady state over a
60 minutes time course (Mercado-Simmen *et al.*, 1980). Work on the
characterization of this binding has now reached a point where we
feel we can use the term "receptor" with confidence rather than
"binding protein."

The binding to the membrane-enriched particulate fraction of
rat myometrium is both tissue and ligand specific. Plasma membrane-
enriched particulate fractions from rat leg muscles, assumed not
to be a relaxin target tissue, did not exhibit any specific binding.
The degree of ligand specificity has been studied by the inhibiting
effects on the binding of labelled relaxin by a number of structurally
related peptide hormones. Proinsulin > IGF > insulin inhibited over
a concentration range 100–1000 times greater than native relaxin.
Hence the uterine receptor clearly distinguishes between relaxin and
other hormones structurally related to it. We had previously shown
that proinsulin showed the greatest inhibiting activity both in a
radioreceptor system (McMurtry *et al.*, 1980) and interestingly in
radioimmunoassays for relaxin (Bryant-Greenwood and Greenwood, 1979)
It would appear that this is more than chance and suggests greater
structural homology between proinsulin and relaxin than the other
hormones tested. The C-peptide of proinsulin had no effect in
either the radioreceptor assay (Mercado-Simmen *et al.*, 1980) or the
radioimmunoassays (Bryant-Greenwood and Greenwood, 1979).

Maximum binding of ^{125}I-relaxin to its uterine receptor occurred
at 5 minutes incubation at 27°C. The rapidiity of this binding is of
interest physiologically since the action of relaxin on the isolated
estrogen primed rat uterus is very rapid (Wiquist and Paul, 1958).
In addition, it was found that the divalent cations Mn^{2+}, Mg^{2+} and
Ca^{2+} enhanced the specific binding of the labelled hormone relative
to that observed in buffer alone or in buffer with EDTA. Binding
was facilitated to the greatest extent by Mn^{2+} at all concentrations
tested (0.52–5.20 nM) and this facilitation was concentration
dependent at early incubation times.

When ^{125}I-labelled relaxin is incubated with the membrane-
enriched particulate fraction from rat myometrium, the steady state
of the reaction is limited and is a consequence of three processes
elucidated in a number of experiments:

1) Proteolysis of the labelled relaxin occurs.

2) Some solubilization of the binding component into the medium occurs.

3) Inactivation of the labelled and unlabelled relaxin is induced by the presence of Mn^{2+}.

The solubilization of the receptor, indicates that the receptor preparation is not homogenous and that some may be only loosely attached to the plasma membranes and not embedded in the lipoprotein bi-layer. Manganese ions also cause a direct loss of immunoactivity of both labelled and unlabelled relaxin in aqueous solution independent of the presence of the membranes. This is possibly due to aggregation of relaxin by complex formation since a number of polypeptide hormones have been reported to be susceptible to ion-induced aggregation (Wahlborg and Frieden, 1965).

A critical assumption made throughout these studies is that the properties described for the interactions between labelled relaxin and its receptor are the same as for unlabelled or native relaxin and its receptor. This has been demonstrated by showing the same number of high affinity binding sites and the same association constant Ka of the particulate fractions for native, unlabelled relaxin as for the iodinated hormone. This was carried out by using the same concentration range of relaxin $10^{-12}-10^{-9}M$ and a fixed concentration of ^{125}I-relaxin for Scatchard analyses. Dissociation studies and Scatchard analyses both indicate that there are 2 types of binding sites in the pregnant and the estrogen primed animal. In the cyclic rat, only low levels of relaxin receptors occur and a straight line Scatchard plot was therefore obtained.

The characterization of the receptor has allowed more precise study of the changes in the receptor as a function of physiological state.

Table 1 shows the effect of estrogen priming, ovariectomy and ovariectomy with estrogen priming on the numer of high affinity binding sites. The results suggest that estrogen priming "sensitizes" an animal to the subsequent effects of relaxin in a bioassay by inducing relaxin receptors in particular target tissues. The absence of receptors without priming by exogenous estrogen is technical not physiological, since when a more detailed study in the cyclic animal was carried out, receptor activity was found at proestrus and estrus (Table 2), indicating, therefore, a role for relaxin in the cyclic animal. The effect of priming with exogenous estrogen, although reproducible in both the cyclic and ovariectomized animal, may be physiological or pharmacological. It is not known yet whether there is a dose dependent effect of estrogen on the relaxin receptor.

Table 2 also shows a peak of relaxin receptors on day 17 of pregnancy, thereafter declining to the time of parturition. Receptor activity in early pregnancy and just prior to parturition is still

Table 1. *BINDING AFFINITY AND NUMBER OF HIGH AFFINITY BINDING
SITES IN THE UTERINE PLASMA MEMBERANE-ENRICHED FRACTION
IN THE RAT.*

Experimental State	High Affinity Binding Sites (pmoles/mg protein)	$(Ka) \times 10^{-10}$ (m^{-1})
Cyclic	None Observable	
Cyclic + Estrogen	194 $\pm$ 29	3.9
Ovariectomized	None Observable	
Ovariectomized + Estrogen	115 $\pm$ 48	7.7

equivalent to that found in the cyclic animal. The cycle and
pregnancy are estrogen dominated events and we have attempted to
correlate the small amount of available data in Table 2. Here the
number of relaxin binding sites are recorded together with published
endogenous estrogen level in the respective physiological states
(Shaikh, 1971). It can be seen that there is no direct relationship
between endogenous estrogen level and the number of relaxin
myometrial binding sites and it would appear that factors other
than estrogen may modulate the relaxin receptor. Hence estrogen
alone and directly may not be responsible for controlling the
relaxin receptor. Estrogen and its effect on prostaglandin,
prostaglandin and its effect on relaxin may be just one possibility.
It would be surprisingly simplistic to expect that only estrogen
is responsible for the orchestration of the relaxin receptor.

Concomitant endogenous relaxin levels in the rat have yet to
be studied, however, Sherwood and Crnekovic have reported levels
at days 10, 21 and 22 during pregnancy as well as day 1 postpartum (Sherwood and Crnekovic, 1979). When these together with
relaxin receptor data and endogenous estrogen levels in serum are
examined simultaneoulsy (Table 2), it can be seen that relaxin
receptors in the myometrium bear little relationship to relaxin
levels in serum. The "surge" of relaxin in plasma as seen in
late pregnancy could be the direct cause of the actual reduction in
number of relaxin receptors or a reduction caused by an increase in
receptor occupancy by endogenous relaxin. We have not as yet been
able to distinguish between these two possibilities.

The relaxin receptors found in the membrane-enriched particulate
fraction of the rat uterus may be related to the inhibition of the

Table 2. *RELAXIN RECEPTORS, ENDOGENOUS ESTROGEN AND RELAXIN IN THE RAT.*

	Binding Sites pmoles/mg protein	Estrogen* (E_2) (pg/ml)	Relaxin** (ng/ml)
I. Cyclic			
Diestrus	None Observable	499 + 112	
Proestrus	5.3	2178 + 563	
Estrus	3.2	161 + 28	
Metestrus	None Observable	401 + 252	
II. Pregnancy			
Day 5	7	129 + 36	
Day 9		153 + 22	
Day 10	12 + 5		3
Day 17	151 + 16	179 + 27	
Day 19	31 + 10	249 + 28	
Day 20	16		
Day 21		445 + 115	160
Parturition	4	628 + 210	150

*Shaikh, 1971

**Sherwood and Crnekovic, 1979

uterine contractile response to relaxin observed both *in vivo* and *in vitro*. We have not as yet related the specific binding to this biological response but the indirect evidence adduced to date would encourage us to do this as a next step in our investigations.

d. *Mammary Gland*

Relaxin levels in blood have been shown to increase acutely on suckling in the sheep, (Bryant and Chamley, 1976), human (Bryant, 1973), and sow (Afele *et al.*, 1979) surprisingly in view of the classical role of relaxin as a pregnancy hormone. Ascribing a role or roles for the relaxin released, indeed ascribing the source itself is difficult but some light has been shed by a limited study of receptors. We have not yet studied the uterine receptor for relaxin during lactation in the rat and certainly no work has been carried out on these in the sheep, human or sow. A direct physiological effect of the released relaxin on the mammary gland is suggested by preliminary results obtained showing mammary gland binding sites were indeed present in pregnancy in the rat and on days 5 and 10 of lactation (McMurtry *et al.*, 1978). Interestingly, greatest binding activity was found from late pregnant rats (day 20) when endogenous relaxin levels are high; this in itself indicates the possibility that the decline in myometrial receptors prior to parturition is not due to receptor occupancy by endogenous hormone. Full characterization of the mammary gland receptor certainly needs to be carried out and the biological response of relaxin on the mammary gland sought. It is interesting that this demonstration makes relaxin the third ovarian hormone with mammary gland receptors, however, its role in mammary physiology, during pregnancy and lactation, clearly needs to be defined.

2. *RELAXIN: A HORMONE OF THE NON-PREGNANT ANIMAL*

Relaxin is considered to be a hormone of importance only in the pregnant animal and produced by the corpus luteum. The previous section has shown that relaxin receptors are present in the myometrium of the cyclic rat at proestrous and estrus; this strongly suggests a role for relaxin in the non-pregnant cyclic rat.

Additional evidence will show that relaxin is not merely a hormone of transitory importance in the life cycle. Like estrogen, high levels are found in blood during pregnancy in contrast with only very much lower levels during the cycle; nobody would refute the importance of estrogen in the latter situation. The term non-pregnant is also used to include the lactating post-parturient female as well as the male.

a. *Isolation of Relaxin From the Non-Pregnant Animal*

Ovaries from sows which had never cycled; i.e., prepubertal, and therefore had no corpora lutea, were extracted for relaxin by the method of Sherwood and O'Byrne (1974). The profile of the Sephadex G-50 column was scanned for absorbance at 280 nm and immunoactivity in the porcine relaxin radioimmunoassay (Afele *et al.*, 1979) the results are shown in Figure 1. There was no peak detected by absorbance over the F.2 region where relaxin from the pregnant sow ovary is eluted. However, the radioimmunoassay data shows immunoactivity detectable in a distinct peak at the elution volume of 6,300 dalton relaxin. The total yield of this peak was 4.05 mg of CM-a' immunoactivity as compared to a yield of 223 mg from the same net weight (1 Kg) of pregnant sow ovaries. However, this showed that relaxin is undoubtedly present in low amounts in sow ovaries which contain only follicles. No attempt at further isolations and purifications were made but there is no reason to believe that structurally the relaxin would be any different from that isolated from the ovaries of pregnant sows.

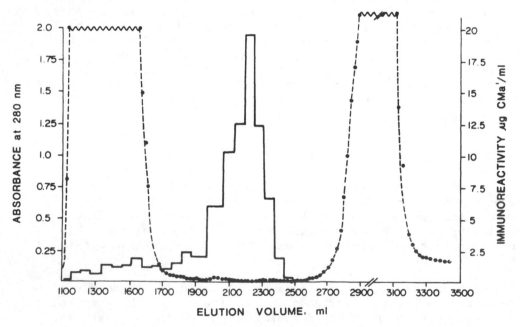

Figure 1.   *Gel filtration of an extract of prepubertal sow ovaries on Sephadex G-50 (fine). Absorbance at 280 nm and immunoactivity of eluates (histogram).*

We have carried out similar isolation studies using the boars'
testes. For this extraction we have used our modification of the
Sherwood and O'Bryne procedure (Kwok and Niall, 1980). This
entails the addition of proteinase inhibitors PMSF and sodium azide
throughout extraction in order to protect the small quantities of
relaxin present from proteolysis. In addition, a second Sephadex
G-50 (superfine) column was used for the G.2 peak prior to its
chromatography on CM cellulose. The results of radioimmunoassay
on these columns is similar to that shown in Figure 1; full details
of recoveries are to be published (Yamamoto and Bryant-Greenwood,
to be published). It is interesting to note that the yield of
relaxin from the boars' testes varies with the age of the animal,
the young animals having less relaxin. This may be an indication
of its reproductive function in the male. The final relaxin obtained
was biologically active when assayed in our rat myometrial receptor
assay (Mercado-Simmen et al., 1980) with 2.57 ng CM-a' equivalent
to each μg boars' testes relaxin (Yamamoto and Bryant-Greenwood,
to be published).

b. *Localization by Fluorescent Antibody in the Male*

The isolation studies using the boars' testes gave no indication
of tissue localization, only the presence of relaxin. Accordingly,
we have attempted to confirm the localization of relaxin shown by
Dubois and Dacheux (1978) by the fluorescent antibody technique.
Using a similar antiserum to NIH-R-P1 we obtained results identical
to those reported (Dubois and Dacheux, 1978); fluorescence was found
in the connective tissue and cells of the interstitium as well as
the Sertoli cells of the seminiferous tubules. However, the
availability of homogenous relaxin (CM-a') and an antiserum raised
to CM-a' allowed us to localize relaxin in the pregnant sow corpus
luteum where fluorescence was observed only in the cytoplasm of the
luteal cells. Adult boars' testes were then examined but this
tissue was completely devoid of fluorescence. The conclusion is
that low levels in the testis were below the sensitivity of the
fluorescent antibody method, compounded by the fact that relaxin
in the testis may not be stored in discrete granules as found in
the corpus luteum (Arakaki et al., to be published). The
fluorescence noted by Dubois and Dacheux and ourselves with
antiserum to crude relaxin is specific to the antibody directed to
a range of porcine peptides in the crude preparation and not to the
small amount of relaxin present.

c. *Radioimmunoassay Data--Relaxin in the Cycle*

Radioimmunoassays for relaxin have set points of sensitivity
adequate for measuring levels in plasma during pregnancy.

Sensitivities have not been optimized for the measurement of the lower levels of the non-pregnant animal. In a study with Dr. H. Brinkley, University of Maryland, we have found that relaxin is detectable in 20% (> 50 pg/ml) of plasma samples from 4 cyclic sows bled every 6 hours throughout the estrous cycle; with increased sensitivity, the rate of detection could be higher. The mean level detected was 570 pg/ml. This study used a porcine relaxin radio-immunoassay in the sow. When this assay is applied to human plasma samples, relaxin is undetectable. However, using our initial radioimmunoassay system based on NIH-R-P1, we were able to detect relaxin related immunoactivity in the menstrual cycle (Bryant et al., 1975). O'Byrne and Steinetz have used an assay based on a mixture of relaxin pooled from CM-cellulose purification (CM-B + CM-a + CM-a') with an antiserum raised to the crude G.2 fraction from Sephadex G-50. This assay shows an interesting wide species specificity but a low sensitivity in plasma. Hence relaxin was only rarely detectable in plasma obtained from non-pregnant women bled at weekly intervals (O'Byrne et al., 1978).

The radioimmunoassay based on CM-a' relaxin has been optimized for use in a study of relaxin during the guinea pig estrous cycle (Boyd et al., to be published). From the inhibition curves obtained, guinea pig relaxin appears to resemble porcine relaxin more closely than does human relaxin. We have used indwelling catheters in 12 animals for the collection of daily blood samples and shown that 2 small peaks of activity in blood were detectable during the follicular phase and two very much greater peaks occur in the late luteal phase (Boyd et al., to be published). Table 3 shows a summary of the radioimmunoassay data obtained on the non-pregnant cyclic animal and the assay systems which have been used. All three assay systems used for these studies are porcine relaxin and only differ in the purity of the antigen used for both label and anti-serum production. The high apparent levels of relaxin reported in plasma with our assay using NIH-R-P1 are due to the results being calculated in terms of an impure standard (NIH-R-P1). We have published the specificity of the radioimmuoassay using NIH-R-P1 in some detail in terms of the radioimmunoassay developed from highly purified relaxin. The somewhat surprising conclusion that both assays measure overlapping and unknown spectra of relaxin-related immunoactivities, including relaxin, possibly prorelaxin, big relaxin and fragments from these (Bryant-Greenwood and Greenwood, 1979).

d. Radioimmunoassay Data--Relaxin in Lactation

We have reported the suckling-induced rise of relaxin found in plasma in a number of species by radioimmunoassay. Table 4 summarizes the data and the assay systems used. Acute rises within

Table 3. RADIOIMMUNOASSAY OF RELAXIN IN THE CYCLIC ANIMAL.

SPECIES	ASSAY	SENSITIVITY	AUTHORS
GUINEA PIG	CM-a' anti CM-a'	> 50 pg/ml	Boyd, Mento, Kendall & Bryant-Greenwood. To Be Published
SHEEP	NIH-R-P1 anti NIH-R-P1	> 6.3 ng/ml*	Chamley, Stelmasiak & Bryant-Greenwood JRF 45:455 (1975).
PIG	CM-a' anti CM-a'	> 50 pg/ml	Brinkley & Bryant-Greenwood To be published.
HUMAN	NIH-R-P1 anti NIH-R-P1	> 6.3 ng/ml*	Bryant, Panter & Stelmasiak. JCEM 41:1065 (1975)
HUMAN	CM-B + CM-A anticrude relaxin	25-50 pg equivalents porcine relaxin	O'Byrne, Carrier, Sorenson, Segaloff, Schwabe & Steinetz JCEM 47:1106 (1978)

*Footnote: Results expressed in terms of the crude standard (NIH-R-P1).

Table 4. *RADIOIMMUNOASSAY OF RELAXIN IN LACTATION*

SPECIES	ASSAY	SENSITIVITY	SUCKLING EFFECT	AUTHORS
GUINEA PIG	CM-a' anti CM-a'	> 50 pg/ml	negative	Boyd, Kendall, Mento & Bryant-Greenwood. To be published.
SHEEP	NIH-R-Pl anti NIH-R-Pl	> 6.3 ng/ml*	positive acute	Bryant & Chamley. JRF 46:457 (1976).
PIG	CM-a' anti CM-a'	> 50 pg/ml	positive acute	Afele, Chamley, Dax & Bryant-Greenwood. JRF 56:451 (1979)
HUMAN	NIH-R-Pl anti NIH-R-Pl	> 6.3 ng/ml*	positive acute	Bryant. "Human Prolactin" p. 92 Excerpta Media (1973).

*Footnote: Results expressed in terms of the crude standard (NIH-R-Pl).

1-2 minutes have been measured in plasma in the sheep (Bryan and
Chamley, 1976), human (Bryant, 1973) and pig (Afele et al., 1979)
no such rise was seen in the guinea pig at either 2, 8 and 14 days
post-partum (Boyd et al., to be published).

The development of an homologous rat radioimmunoassay
(Sherwood and Crnekovic, 1979) would now permit studies on the
physiology of relaxin in the non-pregnant state. However, the
physiology of relaxin has not reached the stage (unlike FSH or LH)
where physiology can be used as a prop to the specificity of
heterologous assays. There is an obvious need for a fully homologous
and sensitive radioimmunoassay for human relaxin; the results
obtained with heterologous systems need verification with an
homologous radioimmunoassay since it is already clear that relaxin
physiology is not freely transferable from one species to another.

e. Perfusion In Vitro of the Non-Pregnant Sow Ovary

With the assistance of Dr. L. Warnes, Mr. F. Amato and Mrs.
M. M. Ralph in the laboratory of Dr. R. F. Seamark, University of
Adelaide, South Australia, we have studied the relaxin output
from the non-pregnant sow ovary perfused in vitro. A summary of
this data is shown in Table 5. Ovaries were classified according
to stage of the cycle from the appearance of the ovary. The ovary
was brought from a local slaughter house and was pre-perfused for
a period of 1 hour with recycling medium. This was then discarded
and fresh medium was used in open circulation. Venous samples were
collected at 1 minute intervals and analyzed for relaxin and steroid
hormones. At the termination of the experiment, the weights of the
stroma plus follicles and of the corpora lutea were recorded
(Warnes et al., to be published).

The role of the perfusion flow rate was examined in a late
luteal ovary (PO15) and an early luteal ovary (PO10) by varying the
flow rate imposed from 2.0-5.5 ml/min. The early luteal ovary
showed no detectable relaxin production (Table 5) whereas the late
luteal ovary showed that a production of both relaxin and progesterone which was directly related to the flow rate imposed. From
Table 5 it can be seen that the detection or not of relaxin in the
perfusate appears to be related to the mass of corpora luteal tissue
present in the perfused ovary. Hence the relaxin detected was of
corpora luteal origin, follicular relaxin either being too low to
detect or not escaping into the perfusion medium; e.g., when only
corpora albicans were present (PO12), Table 5 relaxin levels were
below the sensitivity of the radioimmunoassay (> 50 pg/ml). Not
surprisingly studies carried out on pregnant sow ovaried perfused
in vitro showed that the production rate of relaxin was several
orders of magnitude greater, as shown for plasma relaxin levels in
the sow, discussed in sections 2.c. and 2.d.

Table 5.   RELAXIN PRODUCTION FROM NON PREGNANT SOW OVARIES ISOLATED
AND PERFUSED IN VITRO

NO.	C.L. WEIGHT mg*	STROMA + FOLLICLE WEIGHT	CYCLE STAGE	FLOW RATE + ml/min	RELAXIN[†] ng/min
PO 7	3.7 (11)	2.48	LATE LUTEAL	3.1	2.55
PO 9	2.8 (6)	3.2	MID LUTEAL	?	NOT DETECTABLE
PO10	...	---	EARLY LUTEAL	3.6	NOT DETECTABLE
PO11	5.93 (10)	3.63	LATE LUTEAL	4.4	13.6
PO12	...	---	LATE FOLLICULAR	?	NOT DETECTABLE
PO14	1.48 (6)	2.76	MID LUTEAL	?	NOT DETECTABLE
PO15	8.44 (13)		LATE LUTEAL	4.5	2.6

*Number in parenthesis.

[†]Mean values in the period following the intial 1 hr pre-perfusion.

However, the production rates in perfusion suggest that relaxin production from certain ovaries is below the sensitivity of our radioimmunoassay or that relaxin is not released continuously from the non-pregnant cyclic ovary and may be present only in greatest amounts when the corpora lutea are present. The data show unequivocable evidence for the production of relaxin by the non-pregnant sow ovary.

f. Relaxin Production by the Non-Pregnant Sow Follicle In Vitro

With Dr. R. F. Seamard, University of Adelaide, we have carried out a study on the production of relaxin by the non-pregnant sow follicle isolated *in vitro* for up to 6 days.

We have shown that relaxin levels are high in follicular fluid collected from pregnant sow ovaries and cystic sow follicles (Bryant-Greenwood *et al.,* to be published). Levels are an order of magnitude lower in follicular fluid from cyclic sows but do show considerable fluctuations with the time of the cycle. Highest levels were found in the late luteal phase (6.8 ng/ml mean of 5 fluid pools from 5 different animals), still high in the preovulatory period (1.6 ng/ml mean of 3 animals), and low in the early luteal and late follicular phases.

Whole porcine follicles were cultured from a single luteal phase ovary (N = 7) for 6 days, the medium changed daily and relaxin, progesterone, estradiol and androstenedione measured. The results are shown in Figure 2. Relaxin levels rose after 48 hours of culture and were sustained over the following 24 hours, thereafter falling to the same as the initial 24 hour culture period. The steroid output is very similar to the profiles obtained with ovine Graafian follicles in culture (Moor, 1977).

Similar cultures have been carried out using follicle wall segments; relaxin production was 50 times greater and progesterone production 10 times greater than from whole follicles cultured *in vitro*. It has been shown that little luteinization occurs in whole follicles in culture whereas it occurs readily after approximately 48 hours *in vitro* in follicle wall explants. It is possible that relaxin production is much higher from whole follicles than is actually measured in the medium since it may only escape from the follicular fluid by diffusion. *In vivo* it appears that the high levels of relaxin in follicular fluid represent production by the granulosa cells and storage within the follicle. The physiological role for this relaxin is not known.

It may be noted that levels are highest in follicular fluid in the presence of a corpus luteum (Kerin *et al.,* 1978). Therefore, the signal for relaxin biosynthesis to occur in the corpus lutuem may

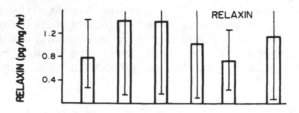

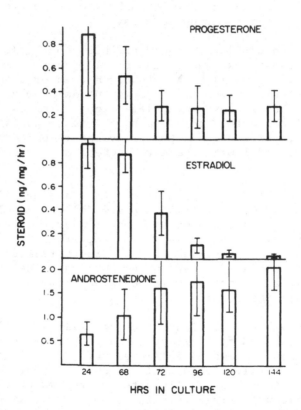

Figure 2. *Relaxin and steroid hormone production by whole Graafian follicles from a single luteal phase sow ovary (N = 7). Cultured in vitro for 6 days. Histograms represent mean ± SD.*

also affect the production of relaxin by the Graafian follicle. Nevertheless this work points to the non-pregnant follicles ability to synthesize relaxin and supports data from the isolation and perfusion studies.

COMMENT

Evidence from our laboratory has shown that relaxin is a product of the non-pregnant corpus luteum and Graafian follicle, suggestive of a physiological role for this hormone in the non-pregnant state. The data from our radioreceptor studies has shown that relaxin receptors are present in the non-pregnant animal and suggests that circulating relaxin has a physiological role. The role or roles may be different from the role of relaxin seen as a "surge" in plasma in late pregnancy in a number of species. The amounts of relaxin produced are much smaller in the cyclic female and it may represent a "local" hormone hence bypassing the need for storage in granules and large amounts circulating peripherally.

The situation in lactation may again be different; levels in plasma are elevated acutely on suckling in a number of species. The corpus luteum at this stage can be discounted as a source of relaxin, hence follicular tissue and/or the uterus may be the sources. It has been shown that exogenous oxytocin causes increased ovarian vein levels of relaxin in late pregnancy whereas relaxin in the corpora lutea remain unchanged. This data suggests also an extra corpora lutea source of the hormone.

It appears that the radioreceptor techniques for showing the presence of specific relaxin receptors in non-pregnancy are a more sensitive index for physiological roles of relaxin than the current sensitivities of radioimmunoassays. It seems important that levels are reported as below the sensitivity of those assays rather than relaxin is absent in a particular physiological state.

The evidence presented allows us to conclude that relaxin is a hormone of the non-pregnant animal. Future investigations will focus on the elucidation of the physiological roles that relaxin has in the non-pregnant female and the male.

ACKNOWLEDGEMENTS

This work was financially supported by grant HDO6633 and the Pacific Biomedical Research Center, University of Hawaii.

REFERENCES

Afele, S., Bryant-Greenwood, G. D., Chamley, W. A. and Dax, E. M. (1979). Plasma relaxin immunoactivity in the pig at parturition and during nuzzling and suckling. J. Reprod. Fert. 56:451.

Arakaki, R., Kleinfeld, R. and Bryant-Greenwood, G. G. To be published. Immunofluorescence studies using antisera to purified porcine relaxin.

Boyd, S., Mento, N., Kendall, J. and Bryant-Greenwood, G. D. To be published. Relaxin immunoactivity in the guinea pig estrous cycle, pregnancy and lactation.

Bryant, G. D. (1973). Comment and discussion, In: "Human Prolactin" J. L. Pasteels and C. Robyn, ed. Excerpta Medica Amsterdam

Bryant, G. D. and Chamley, W. A. (1976). Changes in relaxin and prolactin immunoactivities in ovine plasma following suckling. J. Reprod. Fert. 46:457.

Bryant, G. B., Panter, M. E. A. and Stelmasiak, T. (1975). Immunoreactive relaxin in human serum during the menstrual cycle. J. Clin. Endo. Metab. 41:1065.

Bryant-Greenwood, G. D. and Greenwood, F. C. (1979). Specificity of radioimmunoassay for relaxin. J. Endocr. 31:239.

Bryant-Greenwood, G. D. and Greenwood, F. C. (1979). Specificity of radioimmunoassays for relaxin. J. Endocr. 81:239.

Bryant-Greenwood, G. D., Jeffries, R., Ralph M. M. and Seamark, R. F. To be published. Relaxin production by the porcine Graafian follicle in vitro.

Dubois, M. P. and Dacheux, J. L. (1978). Relaxin, a male hormone? Cell. Tiss. Res. 187:201.

Kerin, J., Seamark, R. F. and Bryant, G. (1978). Relaxin: a product of the human Graafian follicle? In: "Functional Morphology of the Ovary". Univ. of Glasgow Abst. 22.

Kwok, S. C. M. and Niall, H. D. (1980). Evidence for proteolysis during purification of relaxin from pregnant sow ovaries. Endo. Res. Comm. In press.

McMurtry, J. P., Kwok, S. C. M. and Bryant-Greenwood, G. D. (1978). Target tissues for relaxin identified in vitro with ^{125}I-labelled porcine relaxin. J. Reprod. Fert. 52:209.

McMurtry, J. P., Floersheim, G. L. and Bryant-Greenwood, G. D. (1980). Characterization of the binding of ^{125}I-labelled succinylated porcine relaxin to human and mouse fibroblasts. J. Reprod. Fert. In press.

Mercado-Simmen, R. C., Bryant-Greenwood, G. D. and Greenwood, F. C. (1980). Characterization of the binding of ^{125}I-relaxin to rat uterus. J. B. C. In press.

Moor, R. G. (1977). Sites of steroid production in ovine Graafian follicles in culture. J. Endocr. 73:143.

Niall, H. D., Bradshaw, R. A. and Bryant-Greenwood, G. D.   (1978).
    Relaxin: An insulin-related growth factor, Proceedings of the
    ICN-UCLA Symposium on Transmembrane Signally, Keystone, Colorado.
O'Byrne, E. M., Carrier, B. T., Sorensen, L., Segaloff, A., Schwabe,
    C. and Steinetz, B. G.   (1978). Plasma immunoreactive relaxin
    levels in pregnant and non-pregnant women. J. Clin. Endo.
    Metab. 47:1106.
Shaihk, A. A. (1971). Estrone and estradiol levels in ovarian venous
    blood from rats during the estrous cycle and pregnancy. Biol.
    Reprod. 5:297.
Sherwood, O. D. and Crnekovic, V. E.   (1979). Development of a
    homologous radioimmunoassay for rat relaxin. Endocrinol.
    104:893.
Sherwood, O. D. and O'Byrne, E. M.   (1974). Purification and
    characterization of porcine relaxin. Arch. Biochem. Biophys.
    160:185.
Steinetz, B. G., Beach, V. L., Kroc, R. L., Stasilli, N. R., Nussbaum,
    R. E., Nemith, R. J. and Dun, R. K. (1960). Bioassay of
    relaxin using a reference standard. A simple and reliable method
    utilizing direct measurement of interpubic ligament formation
    in mice. Endocrinol. 67:102.
Wahlborg, A. and Frieden, E. (1965). Comparative interaction of
    thyroxine and analogues with Cu (11). Arch. Biochem. Biophys.
    111:702.
Warnes, L., Amato, F., Ralph, M. M., Bryant-Greenwood, G. D.,
    Greenwood, F. C. and Seamark, R. F. To be published. The
    production of relaxin and steroid hormones by the isolated
    porcine ovary perfused in vitro.
Wiquist, N. and Paul, K. G. (1958). Inhibition of the spontaneous
    uterine motility in vitro as a bioassay for relaxin. Acta
    Endocr. Copenh. 29:135.
Yamamoto, S. and Bryant-Greenwood, G. D. To be published. Isolation
    of relaxin from the boars' testes.

DISCUSSION FOLLOWING DR. G. D. BRYANT-GREENWOOD'S PAPER

Dr. Sherwood

(University of Illinois): Several years ago, we measured the
levels of relaxin immunoactivity within the blood of 6 cycling pigs.
We detected relaxin immunoactivity levels consistent with those you're
suggesting i.e. less than one nanogram per milliliter. In all
cases, the levels were highest during the luteal phase.

Have you looked at the biological activity of the material
that you're getting following gel filtration and ion exchange
chromatography from the testes?

Dr. Bryant-Greenwood

No, we haven't. We are currently using the radioimmunoassay
with the radio-receptor assay system as an indication of biological
activity. But certainly before publication, we'll have a look at
that. But I expect from our present data that it will be of low
biological activity, which may be of some physiological significance
to the male.

Dr. Sherwood

But you're getting yields sufficient to explore that question?

Dr. Bryant-Greenwood   .

Yes. We don't want to use it for anything else. I don't think
there is much point in looking at the amino-acid sequence of
testicular relaxin. I don't see why it would be any different from
the female corpus luteum hormones.

Dr. Frieden

(Kent State University): You're quite right. The boar relaxin,
quote, may very well be very similar to that of the sow. But many
years ago Herman Cohen found biologically detectable quantities of
relaxin, as I remember, in rooster testes. And it would be
extremely interesting, both chemically and biologically, to find out
if an avian relaxin shares any of the similarities that we've been
finding in rat, for example, and sow relaxins.

You haven't looked, I suppose, at these?

Dr. Bryant-Greenwood

No, we haven't.

Dr. Bradshaw

(Washington University): I was fascinated with the experiment
that showed the loss of receptors with increased concentration of
relaxin. I would certainly like to believe that that is a classic
case of receptor down-regulation, that is, as you expose the tissue

to increasing amounts of hormones it takes more and more receptors inside, presumably by endocytosis. This has been shown with many other systems. However, I guess it is premature to conclude that for sure.

Dr. Bryant Greenwood
    That would be nice.

Dr. Bradshaw
    I want to ask you two questions about your receptor binding data. What was your nonspecific binding? I presume that it was substracted from the data before you showed it.

Dr. Bryant-Greenwood
    Yes, it was all subtracted.

Dr. Bradshaw
    What kind of levels were you getting?

Dr. Bryant-Greenwood
    Can I call on Rosalia? She's the one that actually carried out the experiments. I think she can handle the nitty-gritty details.

Dr. Mercado-Simmen
    (University of Hawaii): At first, when I started with my project, I usually got a very high nonspecific binding. Now I'm getting about one to two percent of the total binding.

Dr. Bradshaw
    Your nonspecific binding is now one to two percent of the total binding. You can't argue with that.

    Can I ask you another question, Gil? Your Scatchard analysis was faintly reminiscent of a few I have seen before such as insulin and nerve growth factor. However, you didn't say anything about the possiblility of ligand-induced negative cooperativity, which has been postulated on both insulin and NGF. The usual test for this is the De Meyts kinetic test. Have you done such an experiment?

Dr. Mercado-Simmen
    I carried out the concentration dependence studies of the binding of labeled relaxin to uterine fractions and got non-linear Scatchard plot. The curvilinear Scathcard plot indicated two classes of binding sites or negative cooperactivity among relaxin sites. I then carried out dissociation studies where I did dissociation of relaxin binding in the presence or absence of CMa[1]. I found that the dissociation profiles of labeled relaxin were the same under both conditions; the half-time dissociations were the same. So I figured the non-linear Scatchard plot was due to two classes of

binding sites. Moreover, we did the dissociation studies and then looked at the integrity of the dissociated product by immunoprecipitation. We found that the product which was released from its binding to uterine fractions in the earlier times of the dissociation was less intact than the product at the later stages of the dissociation. So I think that could explain two different classes of binding sites.

Dr. Bradshaw

If I understood you correctly, you said that in the association-dissociation experiment, you observed proteolysis of the dissociated product?

Dr. Mercado-Simmen

Yes, the immunoprecipitability of the dissociated product at the earlier stages of the dissociation is less than that at the longer dissociation times.

Dr. Bradshaw

So there is some destruction of the relaxin tracer when it is occupying the receptor?

Dr. Greenwood

(University of Hawaii): That is one interpretation. The other interpretation is that the radioreceptor, like an antibody, will bind "damaged" hormone.

Dr. Bradshaw

You said that the damaged hormone came off faster, which is consistent with what is seen in other systems.

Dr. Bylander

(Kent State University): I notice that in your analysis using estrogen priming, you looked only at the high affinity binding sites. Did you look at the low affinity binding sites after estrogen priming?

Dr. Mercado-Simmen

Actually, yes. After estrogen priming, I found two classes of sites, the high affinity and the low affinity binding sites. I calculated that the high affinity binding sites are about 125 picomoles per milligram protein.

I also calculated the low affinity binding sites, from estrogen-primed rats which is about 300 picomoles/mg protein. But when I did the different stages of pregnancy, I didn't calculate the number of low affinity binding sites.

Dr. Bylander
      The reason I mention this is because of data which showed
that whereas estrogen is synergistic with relaxin in building up
the glycogen content, it doesn't increase the threshold.

Dr. Mercado-Simmen
      I was just thinking, too, that probably the two classes of
binding sites are involved in different functions and that the
increase in uterine glycogen that you showed earlier could be with
a second class of binding sites and that the high affinity binding
sites could be involved in the relaxation of uterine contractions.

Dr. Soloff
      (Medical College of Ohio): I couldn't help notice a striking
similarity between some aspects of the relaxin receptor and the
oxytocin receptor. First of all, there is a manganese requirement
for the oxytocin receptor. Parenthetically, you might try cobalt,
because at least with oxytocin, that is equally as effective as
manganese. There are no enzymes that I know of that demonstrate
this metal ion specificity.

      The second thing, of course, is that the receptor is in the
myometrium and is estrogen responsive. Estrogen stimulates the
appearance of oxytocin receptors and they are maximal during proestrus and estrus.

      I was also struck by the similarity in the structure of oxytocin
with its six-membered ring and the intrachain disulfide bridge of
relaxin.

Dr. Bryant-Greenwood
      Are you suggesting that perhaps we're looking at the binding
of relaxin on an oxytocin receptor or vice versa?

Dr. Soloff
      Another thing you saw was that you found an increase in
plasma relaxin in the blood after suckling. Was the relaxin measured
by the radioreceptor assay?

Dr. Bryant-Greenwood
      No, that was by radioimmunoassay. They have two distinct
actions on the uterus: oxytocin contracting the uterus and relaxin
causing relaxation and abolishing the contractions.

Dr. Soloff
      You can also look at it from the point of view that relaxin
relaxes the uterus, but if you have oxytocin, it overrides the
relaxin effect. You might wonder, if that is due to a displacement
of relaxin from the oxytocin receptor site.

So what I would ask: Have you looked at the ability of oxytocin to
compete with relaxin for the relaxin receptors?

Dr. Bryant-Greenwood
    No, we haven't looked at that.

    Fred, do you want to comment?

Dr. Greenwood
    I was thinking of oxytocin. Dr. Chamley established that there
were separate receptors and that oxytocin could override the action
of relaxin. When we gave relaxin intravaginally at the end of
pregnancy, we suddenly had cold feet. The uterus would no longer
respond to oxytocin. Then we remembered the data on the isolated
rat uterus that had been done in our lab; oxytocin would override
or would be independent of any relaxin receptor. However, we have
certainly never looked at whether oxytocin would compete *in vitro*
with relaxin for the relaxin receptor.

Dr. Hugh Niall
    (University of Melbourne): On the possibility mentioned by
the last speaker of a role of the cystine bridge in binding to
receptors, I think that probably is a little farfetched, in that it
is very likely, from the structure of insulin and also the structure
of relaxin, that the intrachain bridge is buried.

    I just wanted to mention a very interesting observation on the
possible role of manganese in binding. Neil Isaacs and Guy Dodson
have been trying hard to crystallize relaxin. In the course of these
experiments, they have looked at the interaction of a whole range
of divalent cations with relaxin and have found that all are capable
of aggregating and precipitating it in a presumably rather nonspecific
way. The models show that there are a number of glutamic acid residues
scattered over the surface, which are probably associated with
neighboring positive charges from adjacent basic residues; and I
imagine that the divalent cations are interacting with these acidic
groups.

    I wonder whether you found, in fact, what order of difference
there was between manganese and other divalent cations?

Dr. Bryant-Greenwood
    I think we have only looked at calcium and magnesium, as you
saw on the slide, they did have some effect, but not nearly the
effect of manganese.

Dr. Michael Gast
    (Washington University): Gillian, I wonder, did you look at
relaxin levels in control tissues in the pigs that you had in the

early follicular stages; in other words, your immature, noncycling
pigs? I wonder if, as a negative control, you looked at uterus, liver,
whatever you could grab as the pig went down the line--to compare
levels in those tissues and to see if perhaps you weren't measuring
some sort of base line contaminant cross reacting with your antiserum. The work was very pretty, but I think that is the one thing
that I had a question about, based on my own experience with identical
early follicular preparations.

Dr. Bryant-Greenwood
     We have only looked at plasma levels in prepubertal pigs and
they are all extremely low. So it is unlikely that the level of
relaxin in the prepubertal ovaries is from the blood content. We
haven't actually worked on batches of liver or anything else. By
simple calculation, we know that it is not blood relaxin.

     Now, I suppose we should go back and do what you suggest, but
it is a very time-consuming thing, but, as you say, a rather
important negative type of experiment to do.

Dr. Gast
     The question I suppose we are addressing is: What is the
stimulus for relaxin production? Is it there all the time or is
luteinization in some form the stimulus? Your work can answer that,
I think, with the addition of that type of control.

Dr. Bryant-Greenwood
     Well, I believe that relaxin is coming from the follicles in
the prepubertal ovaries. As I showed, it is present in follicular
fluid and probably the granulosa cells in the follicle are capable
of its production. So my guess is that it is follicular in origin.

Dr. Gast
     Along that same line, have you looked at histological prepar-
ations of the ovaries that you used and examined them for the
presence of luteinization in some of the larger follicles? With human
ovaries, as you increase follicular size toward the preovulatory
period, where in your work with the sow we first see significant
rises in relaxin levels, you begin to see luteinizing of the theca
and granulosa cell layers in those ovaries. I wonder if that may
be the time we're beginning to see the rises in RIA data.

Dr. Bryant-Greenwood
     No. We haven't looked at them histologically, but w did some
work sometime back with Drs. Kerin and Seamark in the hum r
culturing follicles from both ovaries. We found significantly higher
amounts of relaxin production from the follicles of the ovary which
contained the corpus luteum than from the other ovary. It appears
that the stimulus, whatever it is, to the corpus luteum to produce

relaxin also affects the follicles on that particular side, which is
an interesting observation.

Dr. Sanborn

(Texas Medical School): I was very interested in your receptor
data. I wonder what the pattern looks like during pregnancy, if you
express it per uterus or per DNA as well as per milligram of protein.
Is it a similar pattern?

Dr. Bryant-Greenwood

Yes. I think it would be similar. We have not actually plotted
it like that.

Dr. Greenwood

Hugh, a comment on that manganese effect. When I was in Adelaide
I phoned Neil Isaacs, and I said "Neil, I've got a paper from Rosie
on manganese. What could manganese have to do with relaxin in pure
solution?"

He said, "Of course, you should know that," and it was he who
postulated, which I passed on to Rosie, that the manganese was
forming the complex between relaxin and the receptor, and therefore,
enhancing binding. Also, that you would get a relaxin:manganese
aggregate, which would then, as Rosie was able to show, cause a loss
of immunoactivity. This is a loss in pure solution, as Gill mentioned.

EFFECT OF A PURIFIED PORCINE RELAXIN UPON GLYCOGEN AND PROTEIN IN THE RAT UTERUS

Edward H. Frieden, Peter Vasilenko, III and Walter C. Adams

Departments of Chemistry and Biological Sciences
Kent State University, Kent, OH 44242

The recent isolation (Sherwood and O'Byrne, 1974; Frieden *et al.*, 1980) and characterization of porcine relaxin as a two-chain polypeptide bearing a distinct structural similarity to insulin (Schwabe and McDonald, 1977; James *et al.*, 1977) has revived interest in an earlier report (Steinetz *et al.*, 1950) that relaxin can exert glycogenic and protein anabolic effects in ovariectomized, estrogen-treated rats. Since the relaxins used in these early experiments were of relatively low specific activity (10-150 GPU/mg), we have examined the metabolic effects of purified, electrophoretically homogenous porcine relaxin as well as NIH-relaxin.

MATERIALS AND METHODS

Relaxin used in these experiments was isolated from a porcine relaxin concentrate (R-P-1, 440 GPU/mg) obtained from the National Institutes of Health. The purification procedure consisted of gel filtration on Bio-Gel P-10 at pH 5.0 followed by electrophoresis at pH 9.0 on a column of Sephadex G-25 (Frieden *et al.*, 1980). This process results in the separation of three electrophoretically distinct fractions with relaxin activity (Figure 1). The fraction used in our experiments is identified as relaxin B; its specific activity, determined by guinea pig symphyseal relaxation assay (Frieden and Hisaw, 1950) was 1750 GPU/mg and its electrophoretic behavior and amino acid composition closely resembled that of the fraction CM-B of Sherwood and O'Byrne (1974).

Thirty-day-old Sprague-Dawley rats were ovariectomized and divided into two groups. One week after ovariectomy, the animals in one group were given an intramuscular injection of 5 µg estradiol benzoate in sesame oil; the others were given sesame oil

315

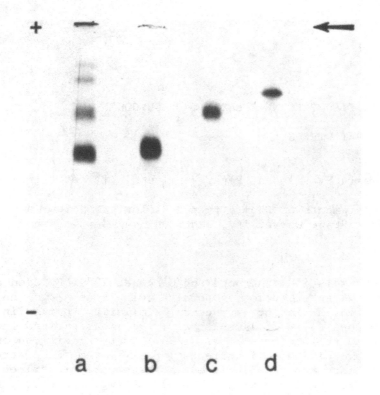

Figure 1.   *Polyacrylamide gel electrophoresis of purified relaxins in*
            NH$_4$OAc buffer, pH 5.0. The arrow indicates the point of
            application of the same. a) Gel-filtered NIH relaxin;
            b) Relaxin A; c) Relaxin B; d) Relaxin C. (Reproduced,
            by permission from Frieden et al., 1980).

alone.   After an additional week, both groups were given either two
injections of relaxin in 0.2 ml of 1% benzopurpurine 4B, or vehicle
alone, twelve hours apart.   Food was withdrawn after the second
relaxin injection.   Twelve hours later the animals were sacrificed,
and uterine wet and dry weights, glycogen (Walaas, 1952; Seifter *et
al.*, 1950) and total nitrogen were determined.   In some experiments
blood glucose and diaphragm glycogen were also determined.

For incorporation experiments, uterine segments from control of
NIH-relaxin-treated (NIH-R-P-1, 0.1 mg) rats were removed 3 or 12
hours after injection, suspended in 2 ml Krebs-Ringer phosphate buffer
containing glucose-U-^{14}C (5.5 mM; 1 µCi/ml) and incubated at 36.5°
for 1 hour.   Diaphragms were obtained from animals at 12 hours and
similarly treated.   The tissues were then rinsed and digested in
30% KOH at 100° for 30 minutes.   Ten mg carrier glycogen were added
to the digest, and the glycogen repeatedly precipitated with ethanol

until the filtrate was free of radioactivity. The glycogen was then dissolved in water and its concentration determined by the anthrone method (Walaas, 1952). Aliquots of the glycogen solution were dissolved in Bray's counting solution (Bray, 1960) and counted in a scintillation counter.

RESULTS

One-tenth mg (175 GPU) of Relaxin B increased mean uterine weight and glycogen concentration of estrogen-primed rats by 40% and 42%, respectively (Table 1). Unexpectedly, significant increases in both parameters (40% and 19%) were also observed in unprimed, ovariectomized rats. As shown in Table 1, the increase in uterine weight reflected true uterine hypertrophy, since increases in uterine nitrogen paralleled increases in uterine weight in both groups of relaxin-treated animals, whereas uterine water content was unchanged. In consequence of increases in both uterine mass and glycogen concentration there occurred a marked increase in total uterine glycogen.

In order to establish threshold and dose-response relationships of relaxin, 1 to 30 μg of relaxin B was administered, also in divided doses, to both unprimed and estrogen-primed, ovariectomized rats. In unprimed animals as little as 3 μg (5 GPU) of the relaxin elicited a significant response in both the glycogenic and uterotrophic effects (Figure 2), but neither response was enhanced beyond that achieved with the 10 μg dose. In estrogen-primed animals both responses were linear with the logarithm of the dose from 3 to 30 μg, and the slope was greater than in the relaxin-treated, unprimed animals.

In contrast to its effect on glycogen and protein accumulation in the uterus, 0.1 μg of relaxin B had no effect upon diaphragm glycogen or blood glucose in fasted rats (Table 1). Moreover, the rates of incorporation of labeled glucose into glycogen of rat uterine segments or diaphragm muscle 3 or 12 hours after exposure to NIH relaxin were not significantly different from those of control (estrogen-primed) uteri or diaphragms (Table 2).

DISCUSSION

Our data indicate that in addition to its ability to induce symphyseal relaxation in guinea pigs and mice, relaxin possesses intrinsic capabilities to influence glycogen and protein metabolism, which are, however, confined to the reproductive tract. Furthermore, in contrast to some of its other actions, the uterotrophic responses to relaxin can occur in the absence of prior exposure to estrogen, although the steroid clearly plays a synergistic role in these phenomena. The observation that estrogen pretreatment enhances the higher doses of relaxin to a greater extent than the threshold doses

TABLE 1.   INFLUENCE OF PORCINE RELAXIN (FRACTION B) ON UTERINE WEIGHT AND
            COMPOSITION IN COMPARISON TO DIAPHRAGM GLYCOGEN AND BLOOD
            GLUCOSE.   FIGURES REPRESENT MEANS ± SEM

	Unprimed		Estrogen Primed[a]	
	Vehicle	Relaxin[b]	Vehicle	Relaxin[b]
Number of Rats				
Uterus				
Wet Weight--mg	47.5 ± 2.5	66.4 ± 3.2	88.9 ± 6.1	123.8 ± 10.9
Dry Weight--mg	7.3 ± 0.4	11.8 ± 0.9	14.6 ± 1.1	21.4 ± 1.8
Glycogen Conc.-- µg/g	960 ± 59	1134 ± 81	839 ± 59	1192 ± 100
Total--µg	44.5 ± 2.6	74.5 ± 5.8	73.9 ± 6.8	143.3 ± 13.4
Water--%	84.5 ± 0.7	82.0 ± 1.3	83.6 ± 0.5	82.7 ± 0.6
Nitrogen Total--mg	1.05 ± .04	1.38 ± .10	2.20 ± .13	3123 ± .38
Diaphragm				
Glycogen Conc--µg/g	1052 ± 133	1029 ± 69	824 ± 86	1004 ± 103
Blood				
Glucose Conc--mg/dl	75.5 ± 9.9	64.8 ± 6.8	82.9 ± 3.0	80.7 ± 5.4

[a]Estradiol benzoate administered 5 µg in 0.2 ml sesame oil 7 days after
ovariectomy and 7 days prior to sacrifice.

[b]Total dose of relaxin B administered as 0.05 mg 24 hours and 0.05 mg 12
hours prior to sacrifice; 0.2 ml of 1% benzopurpurine 4B as vehicle.

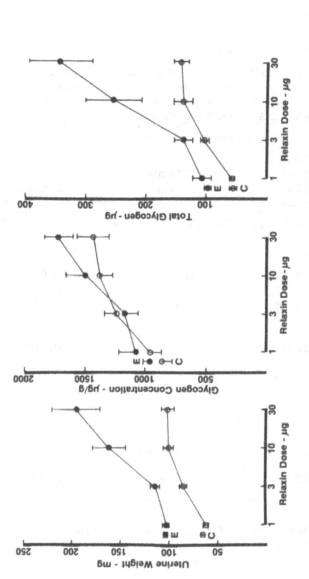

Figure 2.   Dose-response effect of relaxin B on uterine weight and glycogen content in estrogen-primed (closed circled) and unprimed (open circles) ovariectomized rats. Vertical lines represent S.E.M.   See text for experimental details. (Reproduced by permission from Vasilenko et al., 1980).

Table 2.   IN VITRO INCORPORATION OF GLUCOSE-U-^{14}C INTO GLYCOGEN
OF UTERI AND DIAPHRAGMS FROM ESTROGEN-PRIMED,
OVARIECTOMIZED RATS TREATED WITH NIH-RELAXIN (0.1 mg)[a].
FIGURES REPRESENT MEANS ± SEM.

	Time Following Relaxin Injection	Tissue Weight mg	Glucose-U-^{14}C Incorporation uMoles/g/hr
Uterus			
Control	3 hr	122 ± 15	0.077 ± .006
Relaxin	3 hr	124 ± 10	0.071 ± .009
Control	12 hr	115 ± 9	0.103 ± .008
Relaxin	12 hr	150 ± 21	0.125 ± .018
Diaphragm			
Control	12 hr	220 ± 26	0.536 ± .077
Relaxin	12 hr	224 ± 25	0.456 ± .068

[a]NIH-R-P-1, 0.1 mg administered as single dose s.c. in 0.2 ml benzopurpurine 4B. Controls received 0.2 ml vehicle.

suggests that estrogen may regulate the concentration of relaxin receptors in the uterus, and although relaxin binding to reproductive tissues does not require the presence of estrogen nevertheless binding is enhanced by priming (McMurtry *et al.*, 1978).

If the apparent inability of relaxin to affect the rate of formation of glycogen *in vitro* reflects a similar situation in the intact animal, the relaxin-induced increase in glycogen content of the uterus must then be due to a glycogen-sparing action of the hormone. Although the glycogen content of the rat uterus has been reported to decline during early pregnancy (Demers *et al.*, 1972), its concentration rises again from day 16 to parturition (Sherwood and Crnekovic, 1979). Coincidentally, significant concentrations of relaxin are detectable in rat ovaries during this period. Thus, the available evidence suggests a direct role for relaxin in uterine growth during the final stages of gestation involving carbohydrate and protein storage similar in some respects to that induced systemically by insulin (Vasilenko *et al.*, 1980).

This research was supported in part by Biomedical Research Support Grant SO7 RR-07182 awarded by the Division of Research Resources, National Institutes of Health.

REFERENCES

Bray, G. A. (1960). A simple efficient liquid scintillator for counting aqueous solutions in a liquid scintillation counter. Anal. Biochem. 1:279.

Demers, L. M., Yoshinaga and Greep, R. O. (1972). Uterine glycogen metabolism of the rat in early pregnancy. Biol. Reprod. 7:297.

Frieden, E. H. and Hisaw, F. L. (1950). The purification of relaxin. Arch. Biochem. 29:166.

Frieden, E. H., Rawitch, A. B., Wu, L. C. C. and Chen, S. W. C. (1980). The isolation of two proline-containing relaxin species from a porcine relaxin concentrate. Proc. Soc. Exp. Biol. Med. 163:521.

James, R., Niall, H., Kwok, S. and Bryant-Greenwood, G. D. (1977). Primary structure of porcine relaxin: homology with insulin and related growth factors. Nature 267:544.

McMurtry, J., Kwok, S. and Bryant-Greenwood, G. D. (1978). Target tissues for relaxin identified *in vitro* with ^{125}I-labelled porcine relaxin. J. Reprod. Fertil. 53:209.

Schwabe, C. and McDonald, J. K. (1977). Relaxin, a disulfide homolog of insulin. Science 197:914.

Seifter, S., Dayton, S., Novie, B. and Muntwyler, E. (1950).
    Estimation of glycogen with the anthrone reagent. Arch.
    Biochem. 25:191.

Sherwood, O. D., and O'Byrne, E. M. (1974). Purification and
    characterization of porcine relaxin. Arch. Biochem. Biophys.
    160:185.

Sherwood, O. D., and Crnekovic, V. E. (1979). Development of a
    homologous radioimmunoassay for rat relaxin. Proc. Soc.
    Exp. Biol. Med. 104:893.

Steinetz, B. G., Beach, V. L., Blye, R. P. and Kroc, R. L. (1950).
    Changes in the composition of the rat uterus following a
    single injection of relaxin. Endocrinology 61:166.

Vasilenko, P., III, Frieden, E. H. and Adams, W. C. (1980). Effect
    of purified relaxin on uterine glycogen and protein in the
    rat. Proc. Soc. Exp. Biol. Med. 163:245.

Walaas, O. (1952). Effect of estrogen on the glycogen content of
    the rat uterus. Acta Endocrinol. (Copenhagen). 10:175.

DISCUSSION FOLLOWING DR. E. H. FRIEDEN'S PAPER

Dr. L. L. Anderson
    (Iowa State University): Have you looked at uterine growth
in response to estrogen and relaxin in terms of the RNA or DNA?

Dr. Frieden
    No, we don't have any data on either DNA or RNA content.

Dr. Gast
    (Washington University): Along those same lines, have you taken
a look at the histology of the myometrium and the endometrium in
these animals? Do you see increases in the cellularity? Do you
see simply increases in the size of the existing cells? Does this
differ from simple estrogen treatment? Secondly, in endometrium,
do you notice changes in the glands, which are important glycogen-
producing organs, and do you see any differences in the vascularity
of the uterine bed?

Dr. Frieden
    I would like to refer that question, if I may, to Professor
Adams.

Dr. Adams
    (Kent State University): No, we have not pursued any of the
histology, although the question is certainly a very valid one. We
need to know the balance in the growth of the two parts of the organ
as well. In our future experiments, we are going to be separating
the myometrium and the endometrium in terms of both the growth
effects and the effects on glycogen storage. Right now, we don't
really know the answers to the questions as to the histological
changes.

Dr. Kendall
    (University of Texas): Could you tell us what the changes in
glycogen content are in the uterus during pregnancy?

Dr. Frieden
    I'm not familiar with them. Perhaps Dr. Steinetz recalls?

Dr. Kendall
    I was trying to fit this into the physiology of pregnancy.
Could someone tell me what the changes in uterine glycogen content
are during pregnancy in the rat?

Dr. Steinetz
    (CIBA-GEIGY, Corporation): You're taxing my memory to about
20 years ago. There are definitely changes in both the myometrium

and the endometrium. There is an increase in total glycogen toward
the end of pregnancy in the rat. The measurements have all been done
on total uterine glycogen, but histochemically, you can definitely
see big increases in endometrial glands during pregnancy. I have
a comment regarding the possible mechanism here. As I recall, again
from 20 years ago, Janet Schmidt, who was with Sam Leonard at
Cornell, reported a paper in *Endocrinology* where they found a
definite increase in phosphorylase A in rats treated with relaxin.
They thought this might account for the increase in glycogen.

Dr. Frieden
If I could comment on that point, Schmidt and Leonard did
show increases in total phosphorylase. Later on, this problem was
studied further by Teynard, who, I think, was also a student of
Leonard's, and who came to the conclusion that the apparent
increase was, in fact, due to diminished destruction or diminished
rates of inactivation of phosphorylase A. This is a little hard to
fit into the data that we have, as, in fact, are the effects on
cyclic AMP, which one would expect if phosphorylase in the uterus,
as it does in the liver, has a glycogenolytic action rather than
an glycogenic action, as the equilibrium constant ought to indicate.
It's a little hard to understand why the glycogen increased.

This is one of the reasons, of course, why we were so much
interested in repeating these data.

Dr. Sanborn
(Texas Medical School): I would like to respond to your comment
concerning cAMP. You are looking, I recall, after 24 hours. That
situation may not relate to acute effects of cyclic AMP elevation.
You might see a rapid transient effect of relaxin relating to changes
in cAMP and then a secondary effect, which may be a consequence of
other actions of relaxin.

Dr. Frieden
That is one reason why we did some of our incorporation experi-
ments at different time intervals. But the shortest time interval,
I think, was three hours. That, in fact, may be too late.

Dr. Sanborn
There may also be changes in calcium levels, which may, in
themselves, affect the glycogenolysis pathway. It would be difficult
to sort that out.

Dr. Jeffrey
I have a question. I notice a substantial increase in protein
in the uterus at the behest of relaxin as well. I wonder if you
might examine the relaxin-treated uterus with respect to any
specific proteins that might have accumulated. One just happens
to have crossed my mind, collagen, for example.

Dr. Frieden

No, we haven't done that, although I understand that there are a lot of other people interested in the changes in collagen content of the uterus.

A long time ago I did look at changes in the collagen content of the guinea pig symphysis in response to an estrogen-relaxin combination. Since there were tremendous increases in water content and a few other things, we expressed the total collagen in porportion to total proteins. There were significant increases but so far, we have done nothing specific as far as the uterus is concerned.

TARGET TISSUES FOR RELAXIN

S. H. Cheah and O. D. Sherwood

Department of Physiology and Biophysics
University of Illinois
Urbana, IL   61801   USA

INTRODUCTION

Two series of experiments have been conducted to identify possible target tissues for relaxin in the rat (Cheah and Sherwood, 1980). This paper will briefly describe the results of these experiments in which we: (a) examined the distribution of radioactivity in various tissues following the injection of ^{125}I-labeled relaxin (^{125}I-relaxin) *in vivo* and (b) measured the cAMP levels in tissues following incubation with relaxin *in vitro*.

It is believed that the initial step in the mechanism of action for many polypeptide hormones involves the binding of the hormone to specific, high affinity membrane-bound binding sites or "receptors" which are found in limited quantities within the target tissue (Sands and Rickenberg, 1978). The binding of the hormone stimulates the activity of adenylate cyclase which triggers an increase in intracellular cAMP levels. The cAMP serves as an intracellular second messenger which mediates the biological response of the hormone.

The purpose of the *in vivo* studies was to identify those tissues which appear to have specific binding sites for relaxin. The approach with these studies was to inject ^{125}I-relaxin and then to identify those tissues (a) in which the concentration of radioactivity increased above blood levels and (b) in which this concentration could be inhibited with excess unlabeled relaxin. These two characteristics would indicate that these tissues may contain high affinity binding sites which are specific for relaxin and present in limited quantities. The *in vitro* experiments were done to identify those tissues, if any, which show increases in cAMP levels

327

after stimulation with relaxin. A tissue which shows characteristics
of having specific binding sites for relaxin and also demonstrates
increases in cAMP levels following incubation with relaxin would
very likely be a target for the hormone.

MATERIALS AND METHODS

Experiments were conducted with ovariectomized adult Sprague-
Dawley rats (Holtzman Co., Madison, Wisconsin). One week before use
the rats were injected subcutaneously with 10 μg 17β-estradiol
cyclopentylpropionate. Highly purified porcine relaxin (Sherwood
and O'Bryne, 1974) was used for all experiments described.

^{125}I-relaxin was prepared using ^{125}I-labeled Bolton-Hunter
reagent (Bolton and Hunter, 1973). For binding studies to be
meaningful, it is important that the labeled hormone contains biological activity. Therefore, in initial experiments the biological
property of relaxin following modification with the uniodinated
Bolton-Hunter reagent N-succinimidyl 3-(4-hydroxyphenyl) propionate
(SHPP) was tested. Modified relaxin (MR) was prepared by stirring
5 mg of relaxin dissolved in 5 ml of 0.1 M sodium borate buffer,
pH 8.5, with 1.25 mg of SHPP for 24 hr at 0-4°C. The small hydrolyzed
molecules were removed by extensive dialysis against a solution
consisting of 0.001 M $Na_2HPO_4 \cdot 7H_2O$, 0.01 M NaCl and adjusted to
pH 11 with 1 M NaOH (EB). The biological activity of the MR
preparation was determined by the mouse pubic symphysis assay
(Steinetz et al., 1969). The extent of contamination of the MR
preparation with unmodified relaxin was determined by disc gel
electrophoresis at pH 4.3 (Reisfeld et al., 1962).

The hormone iodination procedure used was a modification of
that described by Bolton and Hunter (1973). Five μg of relaxin
dissolved in 5 μl of 0.1 M sodium borate buffer, pH 8.5, were
reacted for 30 min at 0°C with 4 mCi of ^{125}I-labeled Bolton-
Hunter reagent. The reaction was stopped by the addition of 0.5 ml
of 0.2 M glycine dissolved in 0.1 M sodium borate buffer, pH 8.5.
The mixture was stirred a further 5 min. The ^{125}I-relaxin was
separated from ^{125}I-labeled 3-(4-hydroxyphenyl) propionic acid and
^{125}I-labeled glycine using a 1.4 x 25 cm Sephadex G-25 column and
EB as the eluting buffer.

In the in vivo studies, 5 μCi of ^{125}I-relaxin alone or in combination with 15 μg of unlabeled relaxin in 0.5 ml of physiological
saline were injected into the tail vein of each rat. Animals were
sacrificed by cervical dislocation at various times following injection. A blood sample was obtained from the heart; and tissues were
collected, weighed, and the level of radioactivity determined. The
"relative concentration of radioactivity" (cpm per 100 mg of tissue/
cpm per 100 μl of blood) was determined. If the result is greater

than 1, it indicates that the concentration of radioactivity in
the tissue is higher than that of blood.

In the *in vivo* studies, tissues were incubated in Krebs-Ringer
bicarbonate buffer, pH 7.4, containing 5.5 mM glucose (KRBG).   Incubations were done using 40 ml beakers in a shaking water bath at a
temperature of $37^{\circ}C$ and in an atmosphere of 95% O_2-5% CO_2.   Tissues
were first preincubated for 30 min in 23 ml of KRBG.   Theophylline,
contained in 2 ml KRBG, was then added so that the final concentration was 5 mM.   After another 5 min of incubation, relaxin dissolved in 100 µl of KRBG was administered (final concentration 4 µg/
ml.   Controls received no relaxin.   Following another 15 min of incubation, the tissues were frozen in liquid nitrogen and stored in a
$-100^{\circ}C$ freezer.   Tissues were processed for measurement of cAMP
levels by radioimmunoassay as described by Steiner (1974) with the
addition of the acetylation step described by Harper and Brooker
(Harper and Brooker, 1975).   The protein content in the trichloroacetic acid (TCA) precipitate obtained during the processing of
the tissue was determined by the Lowry protein assay (Lowry *et al.*,
1951) and the cAMP levels were expressed as pmoles/mg TCA
precipitated protein.

RESULTS

The results of the biological studies with MR show that MR contained substantial biological activity, although the slope of the
dose response curve was slightly less than that of native relaxin's
(Figure 1).

Analysis of the MR preparation by polyacrylamide disc gel
electrophoresis showed two bands of protein (Figure 2; gel 2) which
migrated toward the cathode more slowly than native relaxin (Figure 2;
gel 1).   The pattern of the bands was different than that of gel 3
(Figure 2) which was run with MR to which native relaxin was added.
Thus, the MR preparation contained little or no unmodified relaxin,
and the biological activity observed was due to MR alone.   It was
concluded that relaxin iodinated with ^{125}I-labeled Bolton-Hunter
reagent had a good chance of retaining its biological activity, and,
therefore, would be suitable for use in binding studies.

The specific radioiactivity of relaxin radiolabeled with the
[125]I-labeled Bolton-Hunter reagent ranged from 0.14 to 0.32 mCi/µg.
Of the tissues examined during the first four hours following the
injection of ^{125}I-relaxin, thyroid, kidney, liver, lung, spleen,
and uterus (horns and cervix) had relative concentrations of radioactivity greater than 1 (Figure 3).   The adrenal gland and diaphragm,
as well as skeletal muscle, intestine and pubic symphysis, failed
to concentrate radioactivity above blood levels.   The simultaneous
administration of excess native relaxin and ^{125}I-relaxin prevented

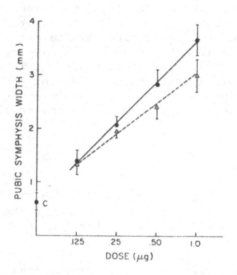

Figure 1.   Biological activities of relaxin (——————) and MR
(-----) as measured by the mouse pubic symphysis
assay (Sherwood and O'Byrne, 1974).   Each point
represents the mean ± SE from 20 mice.   C = saline
controls.

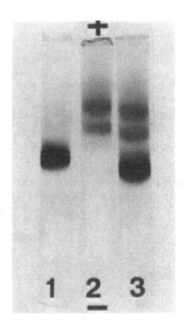

Figure 2.   Disc gel electrophoresis of MR and relaxin at pH 4.3
            using 7½% polyacrylamide (Steinetz et al., 1969).   Gel 1
            was run with relaxin, gel 2 with MR, and gel 3 with a
            mixture of MR and relaxin.   Electrophoresis was done at
            6 mA per gel for 45 min.   The protein bands were stained
            with 1% Amido-Schwarz dissolved in 7% acetic acid.

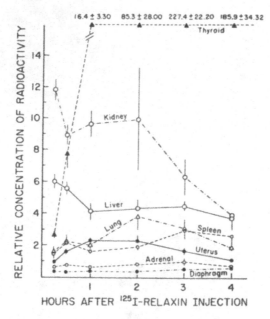

Figure 3.   Relative concentrations of radioactivity in tissues from
             rats collected at various times following intravenous
             injection of 5 µCi of ^{125}I-relaxin.   Each point is the
             mean ± SE from four rats.

the uterus from concentrating radioactivity above blood levels at
1, 2 and 3 hr after injection (Figure 4).   No inhibition of uptake
of radioactivity by excess unlabeled relaxin was observed in the
thyroid, kidney, liver, lung and spleen.   The uterus failed to concentrate radioactivity above blood levels following the injection
of ^{125}I-labeled 3-(4-hydroxyphenyl) propionic acid, ^{125}I-labeled
glycine or ^{125}I-labeled bovine serum albumin.

    Of the tissues examined in the in vitro studies, only the uterine
horns and cervix showed increases in cAMP levels following incubation
with relaxin (Figure 5).

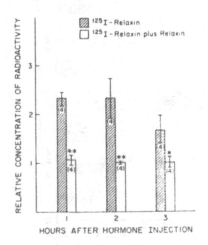

Figure 4.   Relative concentrations of radioactivity in rat   uterus
at 1, 2, and 3 hr following intravenous injection of
5 µCi of ^{125}I-relaxin, or ^{125}I-relaxin plus 15 µg of
unlabeled relaxin.   Each bar represents the mean ± SE
from four rats.   *P< 0.05; **P< 0.01.

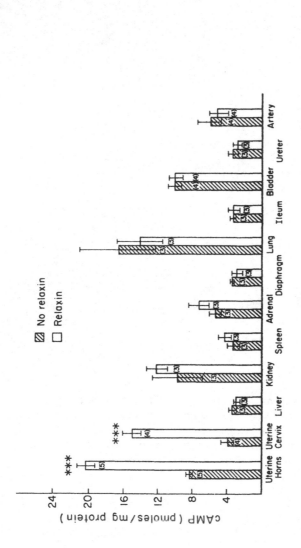

Figure 5. *Levels of cAMP in rat tissues following 15 min incubation with or without 4 µg relaxin/ml. Numbers in parentheses indicate the number of repetitions. Tissues were incubated as described in Materials and Methods. Each bar is the mean + SE. ***P< 0.001.*

DISCUSSION

The *in vivo* data suggest that the uterus may contain a finite quantity of specific high affinity binding sites for relaxin which allow the tissue to concentrate and retain the injected ^{125}I-relaxin above blood levels. That this binding is of limited quantity and specific for relaxin is suggested by the finding that excess cold hormone inhibited the concentration of radioactivity. Further evidence for the specific nature of this uptake of ^{125}I-relaxin by the uterus is the finding that the tissue failed to accumulate radioactivity above blood levels following the injection of other ^{125}I-labeled materials. The *in vitro* characterization of these apparent binding sites for relaxin has still to be accomplished.

The *in vitro* data show that relaxin may exert a biological effect on the uterine horns and cervix, and that like many poly-peptide hormones relaxin may act, at least in part, through cAMP.

The results of these experiments suggest that uterine horns and cervix are target tissues for relaxin.

(Supported by NIH Grant USPH HDO8700 and by Ford Foundation grant 7000333B).

REFERENCES

Bolton, A. E. and Hunter, W. M. (1973). The labeling of proteins to high specific activities by conjugation to a ^{125}I-containing actylating agent. Biochem. J. 133:529.

Cheah, S. H. and Sherwood, O. D. (1980). Target tissues for relxin in the rat: tissue distribution of injected ^{125}I-labeled relaxin and tissue changes in adenosine 3',5'-mono-phosphate levels after *in vitro* relaxin incubation. Endocrinology 106:1203.

Harper, J. F. and Brooker, G. (1975). Femtomole sensitive radio-immunoassay for cyclic AMP and cyclic GMP after 2'0 acetylation by acetic anhydride in aqueous solution. J. Cyclic Nuc. Res. 1:207.

Lowry, O. H., Rosebrough, N. J., Farr, A. L. and Randall, R. J. (1951). Protein measurement with the folin phenol reagent. J. Biol. Chem. 193:265.

Reisfeld, R. A., Lewis, U. J. and Williams, D. E. (1962). Disk electrophoresis of basic proteins on polyacrylamide gels. Nature 195:281

Sands, H. and Rickenberg, H. V. (1978). Assessment of the role of cyclic nucleotides as hormonal mediators. Int. Rev. Biochem. 20:45.

Sherwood, O. D. and O'Byrne, E. M. (1974). Purification and characterization of porcine relaxin. Arch. Biochem. Biophys. 160:185.

Steiner, A. L.   (1974).   Assay of cyclic nucleotides by radioimmuno-
    assay methods.   Methods Enzymol.   38:96.
Steinetz, B. G., Beach, V. L. and Kroc, R. L.   (1969).   Bioassay
    of relaxin.   In: Methods in Hormone Research.   Vol. 2A, R. I.
    Dorfman, ed., Academic Press, New York.

DISCUSSION FOLLOWING MR. S. H. CHEAH'S PAPER

Dr. Frieden
    (Kent State University): I don't think that last slide showed
the period of time that you incubated with relaxin.

Dr. Cheah
    It was 15 minutes.

Dr. Gast
    (Washington University): I was very interested to see your
data on kidney and liver, particularly in the time course of appearance
in the kidney where you had a lot of radioactivity and then very
rapidly lost that radioactivity. I would consider doing a couple
of other things, that is, looking in urine for the appearance of
radioactivity and verifying that the radioactivity is relaxin
containing radioactivity as opposed to free I-125. The second thing
is looking at the gall bladder to see if you have gotten liver
metabolism of the hormone.

Dr. Cheah
    I haven't looked at the urine. It is very likely that the kidney
is involved in the metabolism and/or excretion of the hormone.

Dr. Gast
    Did you collect any hormone?

Dr. Cheah
    No, I didn't look at the gall bladder.

Dr. Bryant-Greenwood
    (University of Hawaii): I would just like to comment that in your
in vivo situation, the first point you look at is at one hour,
whereas we have shown that within 60 minutes the dissociation of
binding has already occurred.

    I would suggest that you start looking at a shorter time scale.

Dr. Cheah
    The concentrations of radioactivity were at a maximum 60 minutes
after injection of ^{125}I-relaxin in the *in vivo* system. In a slide
presented earlier (Figure 3), the results at 15 minutes and 30
minutes postinjection were also shown. Also since we were working
with an *in vivo* system, the time course of uptake of radioactive
hormone may be different from that of an *in vitro* system.

Dr. Bradshaw
    (Washington University): Did you look at mammary glands?

Dr. Cheah
   Yes, we looked at the mammary glands in a limited number of
rats.   There was no increase in radioactivity.

Dr. Bradshaw
   No increase at all?

Dr. Cheah
   No.

Dr. Bradshaw
   What percent of the total label that you injected did you find
in the uterus?

Dr. Cheah
   I cannot recall the exact figures.

Dr. Bradshaw
   Was it one percent? A half percent? It looked like you had a
large amount in the thyroid and the kidney. Furthermore, even though
the uterus was the only tissue that showed apparent specific binding
by the displacement by unlabelled hormone experiment, it didn't look
to me like it was a very big percentage of what you injected.

Dr. Cheah
   The percentage was certainly very small, but the concentration
of radioactivity in the uterus was consistently above blood levels in
three different experiments. Also these higher levels of radioactivity
could by consistently displaced with excessive cold relaxin.

Dr. Greenwood
   (University of Hawaii): Dr. Cheah, you obviously know the
limitation of this technique. Did you try blocking the uptake
of I^{125} to any tissue by including potassium iodide? It struck me
that in your experiment of adding relaxin, you got a 50 percent
reduction in a small amount of uptake by a lot of cold relaxin. This
infers that 50 percent of that label is I^{125}. I was wondering whether
you used iodide to confirm that?

   The other thing that intrigues me about the cold experiment is
that when you inject hormone probably very little hormone ever gets
onto its target tissue. Most of it gets degraded, and the degradation
pathways of hormones really are black boxed.

Dr. Cheah
   With the cold experiments, the thyroid contained as much radioactivity as the animals given hot relaxin alone. So I think that
there was no difference in metabolism. I haven't used cold iodide in
any experiments. The levels of radioactivity left in the uterus after
displacement with cold relaxin were probably due to passive distribu-

tion of radioactive material. It is very likely therefore that any
radioactivity above these levels was due to active uptake of radioactive material, in this case, ^{125}I-relaxin by high affinity
receptors for the hormone.

Dr. Sherwood
        I think that question relative to the kidney was a very good one.
Some time ago we were interested in isolating human relaxin. (Obviously the availability of the source of the hormone is a real
problem. So we wondered if we could collect urine from pregnant women
and begin to isolate relaxin from that source. We conducted a
preliminary experiment in order to determine whether biologically
active relaxin is excreted in the urine. We used pigs for this
experiment. I think, Cheah, you will remember this experiment. On
several mornings we had a bucket brigade that went down to the pig
farms. We collected several liters of urine which we concentrated
in hopes of finding relaxin biological activity. We did not.
Our interpretation was that the molecule was not being excreted
into the urine in intact form.

EFFECT OF RELAXIN ON MAMMARY GROWTH IN THE HYPOPHYSECTOMIZED RAT[1]

Lila C. Wright and Ralph R. Anderson

Department of Dairy Science and Animal Science
Research Center
University of Missouri-Columbia
Columbia, MO 65211

INTRODUCTION

The ovarian peptide, relaxin, has long been known to modify the structures in the area of the birth canal of the pregnant animal in preparation for parturition (Hall, 1960; Hisaw, 1926; Hisaw *et al.*, 1944; Steinetz *et al.*, 1960). Since relaxin is found in abundance in the blood serum of many pregnant mammals, it seems plausible that the development of the mammary gland during gestation might be regulated in part at least by the presence of the hormone. Much work in delineating qualitative hormone requirements for mammary growth in hypophysectomized rats has been accomplished through the technique of whole mount observations (Cowie and Folley, 1947; Hamolsky and Sparrow, 1945; Kahn, Baker and Zannotti, 1965; Mixner, Lewis and Turner, 1940). In the past this technique was adapted to semiquantification by at best using some arbitrary numerical scale to assign each gland a grade for the extent of development (Kahn, Baker and Zanotti, 1965; Meites, 1965; Wrenn *et al.*, 1966). Chemical DNA determination is an acceptable method for quantification in spite of the minor complication in measuring stromal as well as parenchymal tissue, and a qualitative picture of growth is not obtained. Therefore, it was concluded that the best approach to investigating the effect of relaxin on growth and differentiation of the mammary gland was to combine previously determined DNA measurements with whole mount observations, and to develop a better method of quantification for a more valid statistical analysis.

---

[1] Contribution from the Missouri Agricultural Experiment Station, Journal Series No. 8493. Approved by the Director.

MATERIALS AND METHODS

Thirty-three hypophysectomized female albino rats weighing 76-100 g (age = 30 days) were purchased from Charles River Breeding Laboratories, Inc., Wilmington, Massachusetts. They were maintained on wire drawer cages, three per cage, Purina Lab Chow, and water *ad libitum,* at a constant room temperature of $25.5 \pm 1^{\circ}C$ with daily exposure to 14 hours of light and 10 hours of dark. The rats were weighed daily for one week to determine whether or not growth had been retarded. Those which gained over 10 g in the adjustment period were discarded from the experiment. The rats which failed to grow were randomized into 11 groups of three rats for hormone treatments. The remaining rats continued to be weighed daily until termination of the experiment. Doses of thyrotropin, relaxin, prolactin, and somatotropin were dissolved in saline and daily injected locally into the mammary gland pad. One side (3 injection sites/side) served as the treatment side while the other served as the control. Estrogen and progesterone were dissolved in oil and injected systemically to prevent accumulation of the oil in the mammary gland and subsequent interference with the whole mount procedure. All hormones were injected for 10 days. On the 11th day, the rats were sacrificed by ether asphyxiation and the abdominal inguinal mammary glands excised. Tissues were immediately prepared as whole mounts in accordance with the procedure presented by Freeman and Topper (1978) except for the slight modification of preserving the tissues in Flo-Texx (Lerner Laboratories, Stamford, CT) instead of Permount. The skull was dissected and the sella turcica examined to verify completeness of hypophysectomy.

Eleven groups of rats, three rats per group, received the following treatment combinations in a .2 ml vehicle for 10 days:

a.   Thyrotropin (bovine TSH, .3 IU).

b.   TSH + estradiol benzoate (EB, .1 µg)

c.   TSH + relaxin (porcine R, 100 GPU or 40 µg)

d.   Prolactin (bovine PRL, 1 mg NIH-P-B-2, 20 IU)

e.   TSH + R + EB

f.   EB + progesterone (P, .2 mg)

g.   TSH + R + EB + P

h.   PRL + EB

i.   TSH + PRL + EB + P

j.   TSH + PRL + R + EB + P

k.   TSH + PRL + R + EB + P + somatotropin (ovine GH, 1 mg NIH-GH-s-6, 1.6 IU).

The wholemounts were photographed and the image projected onto
a grid. Variables subjected to statistical treatment included changes
in numbers of ducts, numbers of end-buds, length of ducts, width of
ducts, and lobule-alveolar differentiation. These were statistically
analyzed by analysis of variance and Fisher's Least Significant
Difference Multiple Range Test (Snedecor and Cochran, 1976).

RESULTS

Evidence presented in Figure 1, Table 3 concludes that relaxin
significantly increases the lengthening of ducts. In Figure 1 it
is important to note the long, narrow extending ducts with few end
buds and little branching in the mammary gland under the influence
of relaxin. Relaxin also synergizes with other mammogenic hormones
to promote growth and branching of ducts into end-buds (Figure 2).
As compared to Figure 1, this picture of estrogen and progesterone
with relaxin shows more branching and an increase in end buds, which
is statistically supported by Table 1. The ducts, however, have
maintained length due to the presence of relaxin as compared to the
actions of estrogen alone (Figure 3) where ducts are shorter with
more branching into end-buds. Therefore, it may also be said that
estrogen, and estrogen with progesterone, in absence of the primary
mammogens significantly increase the number of ducts (Table 1) and
end-buds (Table 2) which can be attributed to the branching actions
of these hormones.

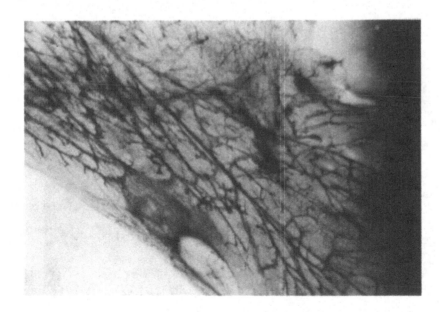

Figure 1.   TSH + Relaxin

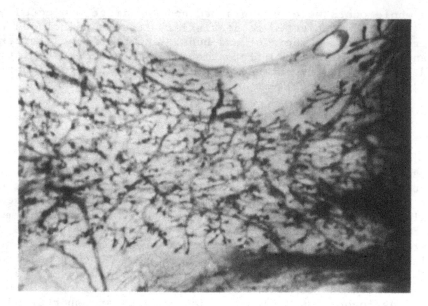

Figure 2.   TSH + Relaxin + Estrogen + Progesterone

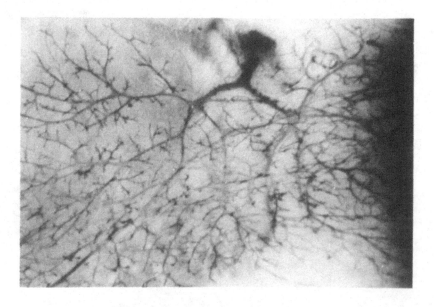

Figure 3.   TSH + Estrogen

Table 1. EFFECT OF RELAXIN AND OTHER HORMONES IN IMMATURE HYPOPHYSECTOMIZED FEMALE RATS ON NUMBERS OF MAMMARY GLAND DUCTS.

Group	Combined Mean ± SEM[a]	Group	Control Mean ± SEM	Group	Injected Mean ± SEM
9	57.0 ± 8.1a*	3	57.0 ± 8.9a	4	41.0 ± 5.6a
3	59.0 ± 5.7a	9	61.7 ± 13.0ab	9	52.3 ± 14.7a
10	61.2 ± 10.4a	10	66.3 ± 19.3ab	10	56.0 ± 16.5a
11	65.7 ± 5.3a	11	66.7 ± 9.0ab	7	57.0 ± 17.2a
4	65.7 ± 13.3a	7	88.0 ± 17.9ab	3	60.0 ± 11.2a
7	72.5 ± 12.5a	8	90.0 ± 22.5ab	11	64.7 ± 9.8a
8	78.0 ± 11.7ab	4	90.3 ± 13.2abc	8	66.0 ± 11.7a
2	110.5 ± 21.6bc	5	125.3 ± 25.3abc	2	67.3 ± 4.7a
5	112.7 ± 15.8c	6	150.3 ± 44.0bc	5	100.0 ± 26.4a
6	132.0 ± 23.46c	2	153.7 ± 9.9bc	1	101.0 ± 18.1a
1	135.3 ± 38.4c	1	169.7 ± 84.9c	6	113.7 ± 32.2a
LSD[b]	34.7		78.2		80.7

[a]SEM = Standard error of the mean
[b]LSD = Least significant difference
*Column values with different subscripts are significantly different (α = .05).
1 = TSH
2 = TSH + EB
3 = TSH + R
4 = PRL
5 = TSH + R + EB
6 = EB + P
7 = TSH + R + EB + P
8 = PRL + EB
9 = TSH + PRL + EB + P
10 = TSH + PRL + R + EB + P
11 = TSH + PRL + R + STH + EB + P

Table 2.   *EFFECT OF RELAXIN AND OTHER HORMONES IN IMMATURE*
HYPOPHYSECTOMIZED FEMALE RATS ON NUMBERS OF MAMMARY GLAND
END BUDS.

Group	Combined Mean ± SEMa	Group	Control Mean ± SEM	Group	Injected Mean ± SEM
11	130.0 ± 67.7a*	10	117.0 ± 23.3a	11	10.0 ± 25.1a
3	150.0 ± 32.0ab	3	157.0 ± 33.3a	3	142.0 ± 72.7ab
10	175.0 ± 33.4ac	7	180.0 ± 26.8ab	9	200.0 ± 43.7abc
9	195.0 ± 20.6ac	9	191.0 ± 27.3ab	1	228.0 ± 86.3bc
7	249.0 ± 77.5acd	6	234.0 ± 40.0ab	10	233.0 ± 38.0bc
5	260.0 ± 69.4acd	5	242.0 ±119.0ab	5	278.0 ± 36.6bc
6	263.0 ± 36.6acd	11	250.0 ± 84.4ab	6	293.0 ± 74.4bc
1	285.0 ± 54.4bcd	8	253.0 ± 92.8ab	2	301.0 ± 94.9bc
8	309.0 ± 47.6cd	4	297.0 ± 49.8abc	7	317.0 ± 173.0bc
4	312.0 ± 31.5cd	1	342.0 ± 79.6bc	4	327.0 ± 58.7bc
2	383.0 ± 79.1d	2	464.0 ±143.1c	8	365.0 ± 30.8c
LSDb	139.3		181.9		201.3

[a]SEM = Standard error of the mean
[b]LSD = Least significant difference
*Column values with different subscripts are significantly different
  (α = .05).
1 = TSH
2 = TSH + EB
3 = TSH + R
4 = PRL
5 = TSH + R + EB
6 = EB + P
7 = TSH + R + EB + P
8 = PRL + EB
9 = TSH + PRL + EB + P
10 = TSH + PRL + R + EB + P
11 = TSH + PRL + R + STH + EB + P

Table 3. *EFFECT OF RELAXIN AND OTHER HORMONES IN IMMATURE HYPOPHYSECTOMIZED FEMALE RATS ON LENGTH (cm) OF MAMMARY GLAND DUCTS.*

Group	Combined Mean + SEMa	Group	Control Mean + SEM	Group	Injected Mean + SEM
11	10.0 + .5a*	6	11.0 + .9a	11	8.7 + .5a
6	13.2 + .6a	11	11.2 + .8a	5	11.0 + .8ab
7	13.2 + .7a	7	12.5 + .9ab	10	13.5 + 1.1bc
5	14.2 + .8ab	9	13.9 + 1.0abc	7	14.0 + 1.2bc
10	14.6 + .7ab	8	14.0 + .9abc	6	15.3 + .9bcd
8	15.2 + .8ab	10	15.6 + .9bc	9	17.7 + 1.4cde
9	15.8 + .9b	4	16.2 + 1.1bc	8	17.7 + 1.7cde
4	18.1 + .9c	5	17.4 + 1.3cd	2	18.6 + 1.3de
2	19.4 + 1.0c	3	17.6 + 1.3cd	4	20.0 + 1.4c
1	22.3 + 1.8d	2	20.2 + 1.4de	1	21.1 + 1.5e
3	24.6 + 1.9e	1	22.6 + 3.3e	3	31.5 + 3.3f
LSD[b]	2.1		3.9		4.4

[a]SEM = Standard error of the mean

[b]LSD = Least significant difference

*Column values with different subscripts are significantly different (α = .05).

1 = TSH
2 = TSH + EB
3 = TSH + R
4 = PRL
5 = TSH + R + EB
6 = EB + P
7 = TSH + R + EB + P
8 = PRL + EB
9 = TSH + PRL + EB + P
10 = TSH + PRL + R + EB + P
11 = TSH + PRL + R + STH + EB + P

Aside from actions attributable to relaxin, it was observed
how prolactin enhanced widening of ducts (Table 4) and development
of end buds (Table 2, Figure 4). The ducts appear thicker and heavier
with less development of branching. When estrogen is added to
prolactin, however, the endbuds are nearly as numerous (Table 2).
There is a higher degree of branching (Table 1) and yet the ducts
have maintained their width as seen in Figure 5, Table 4. Finally,
growth hormone in synergism with thyrotropin, prolactin, relaxin,
estradiol, and progesterone greatly accelerates development of
lobule-alveolar structures as seen in Figure 6. No other group
responded with lobule-alveolar differentiation.

From the tables and figures five basic conclusions have been
established:

1. Estradiol with progesterone and estradiol in absence of
the primary mammogens prolactin and growth hormone greatly increase
numbers of ducts.

2. Numbers of end-buds are promoted by estradiol, prolactin
and estradiol in synergism with prolactin.

3. Relaxin greatly increases the lengthening of ducts, and
synergizes with other mammotropic hormones to promote growth of
ducts, end-buds and lobule-alveoli.

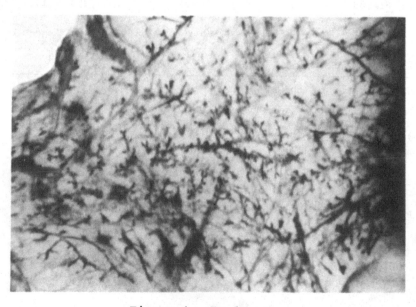

Figure 4.   Prolactin

Table 4. *EFFECT OF RELAXIN AND OTHER HORMONES IN IMMATURE HYPOPHY-SECTOMIZED FEMALE RATS ON WIDTH (cm) OF MAMMARY GLAND DUCTS.*

Group	Combined Mean $\pm$ SEMa	Group	Control Mean $\pm$ SEM	Group	Injected Mean $\pm$ SEM
5	.48 $\pm$ .02a	1	.45 $\pm$ .04a	5	.46 $\pm$ .02a
6	.49 $\pm$ .02a	6	.46 $\pm$ .02a	6	.51 $\pm$ .03ab
2	.53 $\pm$ .03ab	5	.46 $\pm$ .03a	2	.53 $\pm$ .05abc
1	.55 $\pm$ .04ab	7	.48 $\pm$ .03ab	11	.60 $\pm$ .01bcd
3	.56 $\pm$ .03ab	3	.51 $\pm$ .04abc	3	.60 $\pm$ .05bcd
7	.58 $\pm$ .03b	2	.53 $\pm$ .04abc	9	.63 $\pm$ .05bcd
9	.59 $\pm$ .03b	9	.54 $\pm$ .03abc	1	.64 $\pm$ .05bcd
11	.60 $\pm$ .06bc	8	.56 $\pm$ .04bc	10	.66 $\pm$ .05cde
10	.61 $\pm$ .03bc	10	.56 $\pm$ .04bc	7	.67 $\pm$ .05cde
8	.68 $\pm$ .04cd	4	.58 $\pm$ .05c	8	.79 $\pm$ .05ef
4	.70 $\pm$ .04d	11	.60 $\pm$ .03c	4	.81 $\pm$ .03f
LSD[b]	.09		.10		.14

[a]SEM = Standard error of the mean
[b]LSD = Least significant difference
*Column values with different subscripts are significantly different
  (α = .05)
1 = TSH
2 = TSH + EB
3 = TSH + R
4 = PRL
5 = TSH + R + EB
6 = EB + P
7 = TSH + R + EB + P
8 = PRL + EB
9 = TSH + PRL + EB + P
10 = TSH + PRL + R + EB + P
11 = TSH + PRL + R + STH + EB + P

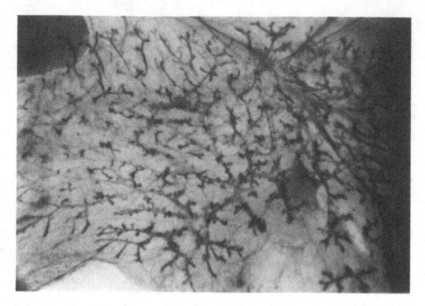

Figure 5.   Prolactin + Estrogen

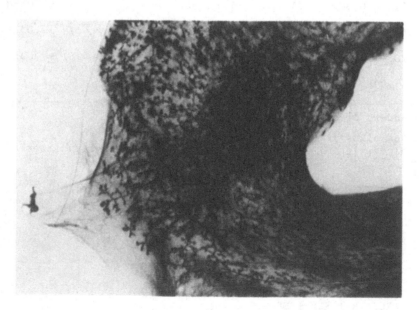

Figure 6.   TSH + Prolactin + Relaxin + Somatotropin + Estrogen + Progesterone.

4. Prolactin, and prolactin synergizing with estrogen enhances widening of ducts.

5. Growth hormone in combination with thyrotropin, relaxin, prolactin, estradiol, and progesterone enables the mammary gland to accelerate differentiation into a lobule-alveolar system.

DISCUSSION

Previous research by Harness and Anderson, (1975, 1977a,b) using DNA as a measure of mammary growth had shown that relaxin had slight mammogenic action, and augmented growth responses to the other mammogenic hormones somatotropin, prolactin, estrogen, and progesterone. Evidence as presented in this paper concludes that relaxin in absence of the primary mammogens mainly enhances the lengthening of ducts. Although other studies concering relaxin's relationship to the mammary gland suggested a synergistic role with other mammogens (Garrett and Talmage, 1952; Hamolsky and Sparrow, 1945; Smith, 1954; Trentin, 1951; Wada and Turner, 1958; Wada and Turner, 1959) none demonstrated a direct action of relaxin on the mammary gland in the absence of pituitary and ovarian hormones. New evidence in this paper supports previous research that relaxin is a potentiator of estrogen and synergizes with other mammogens to promote growth and differentiation. This is the first known evidence to establish the individual role of relaxin in growth of the mammary gland.

The mammary gland spreading factor researched by Elliott and Turner (1953, 1954) twenty-six years ago was postulated to be an enzyme similar to hyaluronidase. However, the evidence presented in this study suggests that relaxin is the long sought after mammary gland spreading factor which enables the mammogenic hormones to stimulate growth of the epithelial cells into the space previously occupied by connective tissue cells.

ACKNOWLEDGMENT

Pure porcine relaxin was generously furnished by Dr. O. D. Sherwood, Dept. of Physiology and Biophysics, University of Illinois at Urbana-Champaign.

REFERENCES

Cowie, A. T. and Folley, S. J. (1947). The role of the adrenal cortex in mammary development and its relation to the mammogenic action of the anterior pituitary. Endocrinology 40:274-285.
Elliott, J. R. and Turner, C. W. (1953). The mammary gland spreading factor. Mo. Agr. Exp. Sta. Res. Bull. 537.

Elliott, J. R. and Turner, C. W. (1954). The mammary gland spreading factor in normal pregnant animals. Endocrinology 54:284-289.

Freeman, C. S. and Topper, Y. V. (1978). Progesterone is not essential to the differentiative potential of mammary epithelium in the male mouse. Endocrinology 103:186-192.

Garrett, F. A. and Talmage, R. V. (1952). The influence of relaxin on mammary gland development in guinea pigs and rabbits. J. Endocrinol. 8:336-340.

Hall, K. (1960). Modification by relaxin of the response of the reproductive tract of mice to oestradiol and progesterone. J. Endocrinol. 20:355-364.

Hamolsky, M. and Sparrow, R. C. (1945). Influence of relaxin on mammary development in sexually immature female rats. Proc. Soc. Exp. Biol. Med. 60:8-9.

Harness, J. R. and Anderson, R. R. (1975). Effect of relaxin on mammary gland growth and lactation in the rat. Proc. Soc. Exp. Biol. Med. 148:933-936.

Harness, J. R. and Anderson, R. R. (1977). Effect of relaxin and somatotropin in combination with ovarian steroids on mammary glands in rats. Biol. Reprod. 17:599-603.

Harness, J. R. and Anderson, R. R. (1977). Effects of relaxin in combination with prolactin and ovarian steroids on mammary growth in hypophysectomized rats. Proc. Soc. Exp. Biol. Med. 156:354-358.

Hisaw, F. L. (1926). Experimental relaxation of public ligament of guinea pig. Proc. Soc. Exp. Biol. Med. 23:661-663.

Hisaw, F. L., Zarrow, M. X., Money, W. L., Talmage, R. V. N. and Abramowitz, A. A. (1944). Importance of the female reproductive tract in the formation of relaxin. Endocrinology 34:122-134.

Kahn, R. H., Baker, B. L. and Zanotti, D. B. (1965). Factors modifying the stimulatory action of norethynodrel on the mammary gland. Endocrinology 77:162-168.

Meites, J. (1965). Maintenance of the mammary lobulo-alveolar system in rats after adreno-orchidectomy by prolactin and growth hormone. Endocrinology 76:1220-1223.

Mixner, J. P., Lewis, A. A. and Turner, C. W. (1940). Evidence for the presence of a second mammogenic (lobule-alveolar) factor in the anterior pituitary. Endocrinology 27:888-892.

Smith, T. C. (1954). The action of relaxin on mammary gland growth in the rat. Endocrinology 54:59-70.

Snedecor, G. W. and Cochran, W. C. (1976). *Statisical Methods* 6th ed., Iowa State University Press, Ames, Iowa.

Steinetz, B. J., Beach, V. L., Kroc, R. L., Stasilli, N. R., Nussbaum, R. E., Nemith, P. J. and Dun, R. K. (1960). Bioassay of relaxin using a reference standard: A simple and reliable method utilizing direct measurement of interpubic ligament formation in mice. Endocrinology 67:102-115.

Trentin, J. J. (1951). Relaxin and mammary growth in the mouse. Proc. Soc. Exp. Biol. Med. 78:9-11.

Wada, H. and Turner, C. W. (1958). Role of relaxin in stimulating. mammary gland growth in mice. Proc. Soc. Exp. Biol. Med. 99:194-197.

Wada, H. and Turner, C. W. (1959). Effect of relaxin on mammary gland growth in the female rat. Proc. Soc. Exp. Biol. Med. 102:568-570.

Wada, H. and Turner, C. W. (1959). Effect of relaxin on mammary gland growth in female mice. Proc. Soc. Exp. Biol. Med. 101:707-709.

Wrenn, T. R., Bitman, J., DeLauder, W. R. and Mench, M. L. (1966). Influence of the placenta in mammary gland growth. J. Dairy Sci. 49:183-187.

DISCUSSION FOLLOWING MS. L. C. WRIGHT'S PAPER

Dr. Fred Greenwood
   (University of Hawaii): I find that absolutely fascinating, Lila, because way back when I was in breast cancer, we were looking for a duct proliferating system. Anybody who has ever dissected a mammary gland can feel sorry for a duct having to punch its way through that load of goo. We didn't get anywhere with it. We tried pro- lactin, et cetera. I think it is going to be a very useful indicator to us to where to look for receptors for relaxin, because I think we've got a hormone which is going to allow a duct to penetrate that connective tissue. I find that absolutely fascinating.

Dr. Michael Gast
   (Washington University): I would just like to say that Lila's presentation is another example of how Missouri stands in the fore- front of relaxin research and that we have witnessed that here in the latter part of this week.

Dr. Greenwood
   What's more, they're on time!

Dr. Ralph R. Anderson
   (University of Missouri): May I make one comment about relaxin?

   Twenty-five years ago, my mentor, the former Dr. Charles W. Turner, had done a series of research papers on the mammary gland spreading factor. I think perhaps relaxin will turn out to be the long-sought mammary gland spreading factor that he was searching for.

Dr. Boime
   Well, in summary, I would like to say a few things. One is that this symposium has clearly shown that the relaxin field is at a pivotal stage and there are exciting issues to be dealt with in the future. For example, the identification of relaxin in a variety of species now increases the repertoire of animal models for studying the physiology and receptor binding of relaxin.

   I think also another aspect that is involved here is the synthesis and the secretion of the hormone; what controls these two processes is something that I hope will also come out from future work.

   One point that really pervades the meeting, the need for chemically purified relaxin fractions for future experimentation. It is critical, as pointed out, for biological studies of mRNAs over the past several years, that highly purified reagents be used.

Dr. Sherwood

I am sure I speak for many of us in saying that this has been a very enjoyable and worthwhile experience. May I express thanks for all of us to the people here at the University of Missouri who have made this meeting possible.

INDEX

Printed in the United States
by Baker & Taylor Publisher Services